THE CONSUMER'S GUIDE TO

HERBAL

MEDICINE

STEVEN B. KARCH, M.D.

Copyright: © 1999 by Advanced Research Press, Inc.

All rights reserved. This book or any part thereof, may not be reproduced or recorded in any form without permission in writing from the publisher, except for brief quotations embodied in critical articles or reviews.

For information contact: Advanced Research Press, Inc.,
150 Motor Pkwy., Suite 210, Hauppauge, New York 11788.

FIRST EDITION

Library of Congress Catalog-in-Publication Data

Steven B. Karch, M.D.

The Consumer's Guide To Herbal Medicine

1. Herbs   2. Health   3. Alternative Medicine

I. Title.

ISBN 1-889462-06-3

Printed in the United States of America

Published by: **Advanced Research Press**

Publisher/President: Steve Blechman

Managing Director (Books): Roy A. Ulin

Art Director: Rob Wilner (DotCom)

Copy Editor: Carol Goldberg

Cover Design: Sam Powell

Printed by: R.R. Donnelley & Sons

HERBAL

MEDICINE

STEVEN B. KARCH, M.D.

A Professional Medical Review of the Most Popular
Medicinal and Performance Enhancing Herbs

Their Use, Benefits and Effectiveness

Safety Considerations, Drug Interactions and
German Government Commission E Recommendations
Which Every User of Herbs Should Be Aware

About The Author

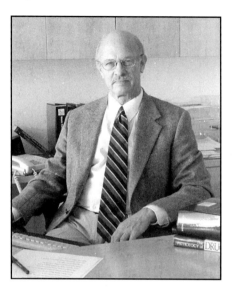

Dr. Karch received his bachelor's degree from Brown University, did graduate work in cell biology and biophysics at Stanford University, and attended Tulane University School of Medicine. He studied neuropathology at the Barnard Baron Institute at the Royal London Hospital, and cardiac pathology at Stanford University. His textbook, *The Pathology of Drug Abuse,* is generally considered to be the standard reference on that subject and is used by courts and medical examiners around the world. He is also the editor of *Drug Abuse Handbook,* a multiauthor reference book on the pharmacology and toxicology of drug abuse published in 1998, and of *A Brief History of Cocaine,* a historical and scientific analysis of the cocaine trade, from 1500 to 1945. Dr. Karch is Assistant Medical Examiner in San Francisco, a member of the American Academy of Forensic Sciences, the Society of Forensic Toxicologists, and the Royal Society of Medicine (London). He teaches and lectures regularly for those organizations, and at the Armed Forces Institute of Pathology. He and his wife, Donna, live in Berkeley, California, where they tend their herb garden and their cats.

About The Illustrations

The illustrations in this book come from two sources. Some are taken from the 4th and 5th volumes of a rare five-volume work on medical plants. The first volume was published in 1790, with new volumes appearing every few years until 1810. The work is entitled ***Medical Botany*** *containing systematic and general descriptions with plates of all the medicinal plants comprehended in the catalogues of the Materia Medica as published by the Royal Colleges of Physicians of London, Edinburgh, and Dublin.* The author was William Woodville; the publisher was a firm named John Bohn, located on Henrietta Street in London. That street is quite near Harley Street, where the most important British medical consultants, then and now, still have their offices. The beautiful illustrations were done by the famous botanist William Hooker. Hooker was appointed director of the Botanical Gardens at Kew, outside of London, in 1841. Other herb illustrations in this book were provided by Nature's Herbs of American Forks, Utah, a TWINLAB company. We are most grateful for their assistance in providing these.

Contents

Dedication

For my wife, Donna

Acknowledgments

Many thanks to Henry Urich, now retired from the Royal London Hospital, and Margaret Billingham, now retired from Stanford University, for their years of patient instruction. Thanks also to Hardwin Meade and Roger Winkle who fortunately are not retired. Without their help this book would certainly not have been possible. Thank you to Boyd Stephens for his continuing support in my research efforts; and to my wife, who had the patience and research skills to unearth the necessary documents; and to my mother-in-law, Sara Morabito, who also happens to be my favorite proofreader.

Introduction

Informed Consumers?

Serious herbalists grow their own plants and they know what to expect from the herbs they use. That description applies to very few consumers. Most of us buy our herbal remedies in stores, more often than not because they were recommended by a friend, or the clerk at the check-out counter. Whether that clerk even knows how to spell the name of the herb correctly, let alone its proper dose or what side effects to expect, seems to be irrelevant.

This book is intended for all of us who, like the author, may not be quite sure about the correct way to spell Echinacea, let alone know how it works, and who would certainly not recognize it growing in the garden. The goal is to provide enough information so consumers can decide whether they really want to take a particular herbal product. Providing details about the botany and chemistry of the herbs does little to advance that goal, and so those details have been omitted. On the other hand, details about the proper botanical names have been included, because they appear on product labels. If nothing else, the well informed consumer should at least know what it is he or she is buying.

The business of selling herbal medications has changed quite drastically since 1994, the year the U.S. Congress passed DSHEA (The Dietary Supplement Health and Education Act of 1994). Under that law manufacturers do not need to obtain any sort of license or approval from the FDA before marketing a dietary supplement; the FDA requires no proof of safety or effectiveness.

That government's legislative stance has proved a mixed blessing for consumers. On the plus side, it has made available many useful products that otherwise would never have come to market. On the minus side, the wording of the law makes it possible for a handful of unscrupulous manufacturers to imply benefits for their products that are unproven, or that simply do not exist.

There is mounting pressure in Congress to amend DSHEA. But until that happens, consumers need to be very careful about which herbal products they take and how they take them. Even if safety was not a concern, consumers need to take great care to ensure they are getting value for their money. Products containing St. John's Wort provide a good example. Some brands cost four to five times more than others. However, in a recent survey of popular brands of St. John's Wort, the least expensive brand also contained the smallest amount of active drug, making it the most expensive brand on a cost per milligram basis (see page 163 for a price comparison chart).

Fortunately, European governments have taken a much more rational approach to the regulation of herbal medicines. The German government even appointed a special committee of experts (Commission E) to review all available evidence for all herbal products sold in that country. This book builds on the recommendations of Committee E, but it also contains a good deal more recent scientific evidence published since Commission E completed its review process in 1995.

Most of this book is devoted to descriptions of individual herbs. If you are planning a trip, and a friend tells you that taking ginger can prevent nausea and vomiting from sea sickness, first look in Chapter 7 and see what Commission E has to say about the subject. If you want to know how much ginger to take, look up ginger in Chapter 6 - all of the important herbs are listed alphabetically.

An Overview

The book was written with the realistic expectation that not everyone will be interested in all the material presented. If you would like to know something about the history of the herbal drug business, how it has grown, how it is regulated, and why there are so many different products for sale at your health food store and supermarket, then take the time to read Chapter 2. It provides an overview of the herbal medicine industry and explains DSHEA, the government regulations under which the herbal medicine industry operates. The problems for consumers posed by the current regulatory climate are explained, as is the history of Commission E. The regulatory approaches of the German and American governments are contrasted.

The regulatory overview is followed by two chapters providing a brief introduction to some very important issues consumers face. Chapter 3 contains a discussion of phytoestrogens, antioxidants, and anti-inflammatory herbs, which are among the most interesting (and important) classes of herbal medicines. Antioxidants protect the heart and brain from the effects of aging; phytoestrogens aid womens' health; herbs with anti-inflammatory properties relieve the symptoms of arthritis, connective tissue disease, and autoimmune disorders. Advertising from herbal product makers is liberally spiked with such terms as flavonoids, free radical scavengers, and phytoestrogens, implying that everyone knows what these terms mean. The brief overview provided in this chapter should make some of those terms more intelligible.

Chapter 4 is about teas, tannins, pyrrolizidine alkaloids, and sesquiterpene lactones. The subjects may sound obscure, and the chemistry is complicated, but consumers need to know about these chemicals and how they can help or hurt them. A number of potentially useful herbal products have their dark sides, and side effects that need to be considered before they are used. On the other hand, many plant products that are taken for granted (such as teas and wines) may, in fact, have the power to save your life.

Any discussion about dosage forms is likely to sound a bit dry, but it is very important. Chapter 5 explains the differences between tinctures and tonics, and other dosage forms. As anyone who has ever been to a health food store knows, the same herb may be sold as a pill, elixir, tincture, or extract. It might also be sold in bulk as crushed leaves or stems. Or powdered plant material may be placed inside capsules or in a health food beverage. Not all dosage forms are the same, and some are much more likely than others to be safe and effective. This chapter contains an explanation of the basic terms. Under current federal law, none of these products are standardized. An extract from Company A might contain twice as much or half as much active ingredient as a similarly named product from Company B. If the supplement is not producing the desired effect, it may have more to do with the particular product purchased than with the pharmacologic effects of the herb!

Chapter 6 contains detailed descriptions of the most important herbal remedies. For each herb there are sections giving the name, source, history, traditional claims, Commission E recommendations, scientifically proven effects, concerns, warnings, effects on workplace drug abuse tests, dosage, summary, and recommendations for further reading. This section is followed by a summary of Commission E findings and recommendations in Chapter 7, which is divided into two parts. The first part lists all of the herbs approved by the commission and their uses. The second lists specific medical problems and the herbs that Commission E recommends for their treatment. In the absence of any other authoritative governmental source, the findings of Commission E represent the single most reliable source for such information.

The last portion of the book includes a glossary and an appendix with several useful tables. These include a listing of the herbal combinations that received Commission E approval, a listing of herbs that Commission E considered to be too toxic for general use, instructions on how to calculate your body mass index (BMI), and step-by-step instructions on how to do an Internet MEDLINE search - for free. In short, all the tools needed to make intelligent choices about which herbal products to use and when to use them.

Government Regulations of Herbal Medicines

Herbal remedies can be purchased at supermarkets, drugstores, and regular retail outlets, even Costco and Sam's Club. They are sold like any other over-the-counter (OTC) product, no differently than Tylenol™ or Sudafed™. This may explain why, in 1997, 60 million adults, nearly one-third of the U.S. population, each spent an average of $54 on herbal remedies. According to the *National Business Journal,* the total value of all herbal products sold in the United States in 1998 was expected to exceed $4 billion, more than twice what it was just two years ago.

Mostly, herbal drugs are used to treat minor medical problems like colds and allergies. They are also taken in hope of preventing illness from occurring. Increasingly, they are being taken with the goal of preventing heart attack, strengthening the immune system, promoting feelings of well-being, and preventing the effects of aging. In that sense, herbal remedies are very much like medicines prescribed by your doctor. But there are very important differences between the drugs your doctor prescribes and the herbal products sold in the grocery store. Prescriptions and OTC medicines are strictly regulated by the federal government. Herbal products are not.

When your doctor writes a prescription, you can be reasonably sure that (1) the medicine prescribed is appropriate for the condition being treated; (2) the makers of that particular drug have proven to the government's satisfaction that, in recommended doses, the drug is safe and effective; (3) except for inert binders and fillers, there is nothing else in the prescription except the prescribed drug; (4) when the prescription is refilled, it will contain exactly the same amount of the same drug as the first prescription; and (5) potentially dangerous drug interactions will be clearly stated on the package insert.

Users of herbal products lack these assurances. Recommendations posted on Internet bulletin boards do not carry the weight of large, multi-center, controlled clinical trials. Treatments recommended on the Internet, or in popular magazines, or by friends at work, may or may not be appropriate for your medical problem. Manufacturers of herbal products are not subject to the same regulations as manufacturers of prescription drugs, and if you are not buying from a large, ethical, manufacturer, you may find yourself getting both more and less than you paid for. For instance, a study conducted in 1978 found more than one-third of the commercial ginseng samples tested contained no ginseng. In 1998, a similar study of St. John's Wort-containing products, undertaken by investigative reporters at the *Los Angeles Times,* disclosed that one-third of the products tested contained less than half the amount of the product listed on the label!

The problem is not just truth-in-advertising. Compared to prescription drugs, the pathology and toxicology of herbal products have been poorly studied. Ginkgo Biloba may help treat depression and improve concentration, but it can also interfere with the way blood normally clots. The clerk at the check-out counter will almost certainly not know about this possible complication, and the label is equally unlikely to contain that bit of information.

In 1994, the United States 103rd Congress passed a law now widely referred to as DSHEA (The Dietary Supplement Health and Education Act of 1994). The law regulates herbal products as if they were foods. Regulations applying to foods are much more permissive than regulations applying to drugs. Section 6 of DSHEA has created the most problems for consumers and regulators alike; DSHEA allows product labels to contain limited discussions of known physiologic effects, but it prohibits therapeutic claims. The law allows "structure and function claims" and "statements of nutritional support," meaning that drugmakers can explain how the product they are selling affects body function and structure, but producers of medicinal herbal products are not allowed to specifically explain what medical conditions their products should be used to treat!

The wording of the law explains the wording on the packages. By now, everyone knows that St. John's Wort is a mild antidepressant, but you would never guess that from reading the label on the bottle. Instead of explaining that St. John's Wort contains chemicals that act in much the same way as antidepressants such as Prozac™, and that reports of toxicity are extremely rare, manufacturers can only claim their product contains a "nutritional factor to support general health and emotional well-being," or some other equally bland and equally uninformative statement. Product labels cannot state that valerian and hops are mild sedatives. But there is nothing to prevent the manufacturer from calling the product something like "Acme sleepy time formula." The problem is that such combinations don't always deliver what the name implies.

DSHEA does prevent manufacturers from making outrageous and unsupported claims for their products, but it also stops the flow of useful information. In fact, the Food and Drug Administration's (FDA) whole approach to herbal products has been something of a mixed blessing. The Center for Food Safety and Applied Nutrition (CFSAN), a section within the FDA, regulates "special nutritional products" including herbal products. According to the CFSAN, the decision to classify a substance as a dietary supplement or a drug is determined more by the labeling of the product than the actual contents. Products that "make claims to treat, cure, prevent, mitigate, or diagnosis (sic) a disease are regulated as drugs." If a manufacturer wants to make medical claims, the FDA requires that the manufacturer prove that the product is "safe and effective for a particular indication prior to marketing."

The CFSAN position might sound like a good idea, but it is not. The net result of CFSAN's position is that reputable supplement makers are not allowed to explain what their products actually do, while at the same time, disreputable producers are permitted to imply benefits that their product may or may not deliver. In 1995, a Presidential Commission suggested appointing an expert panel to examine data from other countries, and recommended that the FDA give serious thought to approving the sale of well studied herbal products (such as valerian) as OTC drugs. Such a measure would provide consumers with more protection and more detailed information about the products they are taking. As of this writing, the suggestion has not been acted upon. The general opinion within the industry seems to be that it never will be.

Even though the U.S. Government seems resistant to the idea of appointing an expert review panel, the German Government thought it was a good idea, and did just that. A law called the Second Medicines Act, passed in 1978, called for a complete review of the safety and effectiveness of all medicines, herbal or otherwise, sold in Germany. Commissions were established, within the German Department of Health, to review different categories of drugs. The commission tasked with reviewing herbal medicines was known as Commission E. The expert panel consisted of 24 members, drawn from all segments of the scientific community (including herbalists). They reviewed the evidence for and against hundreds of different products, and published a summary report (monograph) for each herb reviewed. These reports were subsequently published in the German equivalent of the Federal Record (*Bundesanzeiger*). The Commission stopped publishing new reports in 1995 and now acts as an advisory panel, reviewing applications from herbal product makers wanting to introduce new products.

Chapter 7 of this book contains a summary of Commission E recommendations. Some of the findings of Commission E have appeared in print before. Professor Varro E. Tyler mentions them in his book *Herbs of Choice: Use of Phytomedicinals* which was first published in 1994. A translation of all the Commission E monographs is now available (Copies of *The Complete German Commission E Monographs, Therapeutic guide to herbal medicines,* edited by Mark Blumenthal, can be obtained through the American Botanical Council - its address is given in the appendix). Readers should understand that even though Commission E was composed of very reputable scientists, very few Commission E recommendations are based on the type of clinical trials that would be required in order to bring a new blood pressure medication or antibiotic to market in the United States. On the other hand, the Commission's recommendations do take into account the hundreds of years of experience European physicians have had using these plant-derived medicines. More importantly they are, for the moment, the only game in town.

Herbs may be natural, but they do contain drugs, and there is no point in pretending otherwise. The sensible approach is to use them wisely, taking the good ones and avoiding the bad. But with regulators' heads planted firmly in the sand, consumers have been left in the dark. There have been attempts in the U.S. to improve this situation. In 1992, Congress established the Office of Alternative Medicine, a division of the National Institutes of Health (NIH). The new agency is tasked with the investigation of alternative approaches to health care, including the use of herbal products. The goal is certainly admirable, but current funding levels of $14 million dollars per year are absurdly low, and totally insufficient to fund anything like the clinical trials that are needed to evaluate these products. To put things in perspective, if an herbal product manufacturer were to seek FDA approval to sell valerian, an herbal sedative used in Europe for hundreds of years, they would probably have to spend considerably more than $14 million dollars just to complete the required clinical trials.

Antioxidants, Phytoestrogens and Anti-inflammatories

Medicinal plants contain a variety of vitamins, antibiotics, and fragrant oils. They also contain alkaloids, such as morphine and cocaine. The alkaloids and antibiotics have been intensely studied. But when judged by what is written in the popular press, and by what is being sold in health food stores, the plant components of greatest interest to the general public are those that seem capable of protecting the heart and brain, those that slow the aging process, and relieve the symptoms of menopause. That explains why so much has been written about antioxidants, phytoestrogens, and anti-inflammatory agents. The underlying biochemistry of these compounds is, in fact, very complex, and accounts in the press are hopelessly muddled. Still, some understanding of the basic biology and chemistry of the problems is required if informed decisions are to be made about whether, and what kinds of products to take.

A. Antioxidants

Antioxidant herbs are taken in hopes of counteracting the effects of free radicals. Free radicals are defined as molecules capable of independent existence, even though they contain one or more unpaired electrons. Molecules and atoms containing unpaired electrons are extremely unstable and cannot exist in a free state for very long. Because of their structure, they are inclined to react and combine with other molecules to produce a more stable unit. In the process of finding something to combine with, free radicals may cause damage. One kind of damage they produce is referred to as oxidation. Free radical reactions have been implicated in the pathology of more than 50 human diseases.

Free radicals (oxygen that is missing one electron is the most common variety of free radical, but there are many other kinds) form constantly in the human body. It would be a mistake to suppose that free radical formation is a bad thing. In fact, some cells in the body (called phagocytes) deliberately produce free radicals to help fight infections. Free radicals are also produced as a by-product of certain normal chemical reactions within the body. The only time free radicals become a problem is when there are too many of them.

Under normal circumstances, free radicals are "buffered." That is, the body produces other substances to counteract the effect of any extra free radicals introduced into the system. Free radicals can be removed by enzymes and other chemical defense systems. Usually, both enzymatic and non-enzymatic systems come into play. When too many free radicals are produced, the body's normal checks and balances fail, and a state referred to as "oxidative stress" is said to exist. The result is damage to various components of the cells. If the cell happens to be in the brain or heart, the consequence can be quite devastating.

In some disease states, natural antioxidant defenses appear to be defective. That observation has led to suggestions that oxidative damage might be reduced, and disease progression halted, by supplementing natural antioxidant defenses. To date, most attention has focused on using antioxidant therapy to treat disorders such as diabetes mellitus, reperfusion injury (a term used to describe the damage that occurs to the heart after doctors successfully open an artery that has been blocked, thereby restoring normal blood flow), inflammatory diseases, such as rheumatoid arthritis, and chronic processes, such as atherosclerosis and carcinogenesis.

The most exciting possibility, and the one for which there is the most evidence of effectiveness, is the prevention of heart attack. The number of deaths each year from heart disease has decreased substantially in the last twenty years, but coronary artery disease (CAD) still is the leading killer of men and women in the United States. In particular, it is the leading cause of death in U.S. women older than 60 years, and in men after age 40. Excessive cholesterol consumption is thought to play a role.

One type of cholesterol, low density lipoprotein (LDL), plays a key role in coronary artery disease. Laboratory studies suggest that free radicals cause oxidation of LDL cholesterol and, in the process, increase the ability of LDL to cause coronary artery disease. In theory, antioxidant vitamins, which inhibit the oxidation of LDL, could reduce the risk of CAD. The mechanism is complex, but the basic ideas have been known for some time.

If oxidized LDL becomes trapped underneath the cells that line the inside of blood vessels, it stimulates those cells to manufacture a family of related chemicals called cytokines, growth factors and several cell surface adhesion molecules. These (especially surface adhesion molecules) attract white cells that are circulating in the bloodstream (monocytes and T lymphocytes). Once attracted to the area, they stick to the inner lining of the blood vessel where they are converted into a different kind of cell called a foam cell. The latter is the earliest visible evidence of atherosclerosis - hardening of the arteries. The growth factors and cytokines stimulate the smooth muscle cells lining the blood vessel to divide and expand. As the muscle cells grow, and the foam cells multiply, there is less and less space for blood to get through the artery.

But even more is involved. Oxidized LDL can also prevent the cells lining the vessel from making two other chemicals, one called prostacyclin and the other called nitric oxide. These two chemicals cause blood vessels to dilate and allow more blood to pass through. These same substances also prevent platelets (a blood-clotting component) from sticking to the foam cells and blocking the vessel even further. Vitamin E prevents LDL oxidation, prevents the proliferation of smooth muscle cells, inhibits platelet adhesion and aggregation, and reduces production of adhesion molecules. Collectively, these biological functions of Vitamin E may account for its proven ability to protect against the development of atherosclerosis.

Two different types of antioxidants are recognized: those that occur naturally in the body, and those that are produced synthetically. The former include superoxide dismutase (SOD); alpha-tocopherol; glutathione; and its precursors; ascorbic acid; and carotenoids. The synthetic antioxidants include such substances as xanthine oxidase inhibitors; inhibitors of phagocyte function; iron ion chelators; and an anticholesterol agent called probucol.

When SOD, alpha-tocopherol, and ascorbic acid have been used to treat human disease, the results have generally been unimpressive. The evidence for xanthine oxidase inhibitors is slightly more impressive, and members of this group may yet prove to be useful in preventing human disease. Much more encouraging preliminary results have been observed with the antioxidant drug probucol in preventing atherosclerosis, and iron ion chelators in the treatment of diseases as diverse as thalassanemia, leukemia, malaria, stroke, traumatic brain injury and hemorrhagic shock. Good evidence for effectiveness has been seen in pilot studies, but the results need to be confirmed by large controlled clinical trials.

Cancer is the second leading cause of death in the United States. Dietary factors are thought to account for at least 35 percent of all human cancers, and the connection between dietary antioxidants and cancer is even better studied than the connection with heart disease. But, results in more than 100 separate population-based studies comparing dietary antioxidant intake and/or blood nutrient levels with cancer risk, have proven inconclusive. The problem, in both cases, is that antioxidants are not interchangeable. Some may be more effective than others.

The antioxidant that seems to provide the most protection is Vitamin E. The evidence might not be as overwhelming as some epidemiologists would like, but several very large studies have found that high-level Vitamin E intake, or supplementation, is associated with a significant reduction in cardiovascular disease (from 31 to 65 percent). Unfortunately, the effects are not immediately evident. They only become apparent after two years of increased intake. More time, and more studies, will be required before rational decisions can be made about other antioxidants. Many feel that there is no reason to wait. All the results may not be in, however, ask any cardiologist, and the chances are they will admit they are taking Vitamin E supplements.

B. Phytoestrogens

Plants contain molecules called flavonoids. There are many different kinds of flavonoids. The ones that have received the most attention are called the isoflavones and lignans. They are important because, in some ways, they look and act like estrogens, the female sex hormones. For that reason, they are also referred to as phytoestrogens, or plant estrogens. There is very persuasive evidence that diets rich in phytoestrogens protect against breast, bowel and prostate cancer, not to mention cardiovascular disease, menopausal symptoms, and possibly even osteoporosis.

There are two kinds of isoflavones and two kinds of lignans. Isoflavones named daidzein and genistein are found in soy beans and clover. The two lignans, called enterolactone and enterodiol are only partially produced by plants. They become active when bacteria that normally live in the colon digest plant components found in lentils, fruits, and beans. The bacteria change the structure of the lignans, converting them into their active form. The idea that plant estrogens might play a role in cancer prevention has been around for some time, but solid proof of a connection has only recently begun to emerge. Many food supplements already contain genistein, and concentrated isoflavone tablets, sold like any other food supplement, will be on the market shortly.

Interest in phytoestrogens was first prompted by the observation that vegetarians live longer, and get sick less often, than meat eaters. Soy bean consumption seemed to be the obvious explanation, because in the Far East, where soybean products are traditionally eaten instead of meat, heart disease is uncommon, rates for prostate, colon, and breast cancer are much lower than in Western meat-eating countries, and menopause is rarely associated with much in the way of disabling symptoms.

Once in the body, phytoestrogens attach at the same place in the cell nucleus where estrogens normally bind, but even though they attach to the same "receptors," they do not produce the same effects. In fact, they are classified as "anti-estrogens," because even though they attach at the right place (and thereby prevent human estrogens from attaching), phytoestrogens do not produce all the same effects produced by estrogen. Tamoxifen™ is the best known "anti-estrogen." It is used to treat breast cancer because estrogens can promote tumor growth, especially in the breast. For many women, Tamoxifen™'s anti-estrogen effects are life-saving.

Estrogens also lower cholesterol, prevent heart disease and retard bone loss (osteoporosis). The down side is that estrogens promote tumor growth, especially in the breast. What distinguishes phytoestrogens from Tamoxifen™, and what makes them so interesting, is that they produce all the desirable effects - like protecting the heart and preventing osteoporosis, without doing any of the bad things like promoting tumor growth. Soybeans are not the only source for phytoestrogens. Genisten and daidzein are also present in black beans and alfalfa. Plums and cherries contain prunetin, and dandelion contains coumesterol. Vegetable oils (linseed, cottonseed, sunflower, peanut) also have high phytoestrogen concentrations. Black cohosh root, fennel, and wild yams are also said to contain these compounds, but the claims are not well validated.

The role of estrogens in breast cancer has received the most attention. Of the many factors known to be associated with the occurrence of breast cancer in post-menopausal women, it is that the higher the estrogen levels, the greater the chance of getting breast cancer. Taking Tamoxifen™, which blocks the effects of estrogens, reduces mortality from breast cancer by more than 20 percent in the first two years. Breast cancer rates are lower for women in the Far East, but there are conflicting theories on why that should be. Diet is an obvious candidate. Not only do women in Asia consume more phytoestrogens, they also consume less fat and more fiber. Even without phytoestrogens, diets low in fat and high in fiber lower estrogen levels because they interfere with the way estrogens are metabolized in the gallbladder and intestines. Deciding which food product is providing the beneficial effects is complicated by the fact that foods rich in fiber are also rich in phytoestrogens.

Another piece of the puzzle has to do with estrogen production. The brain's pituitary gland releases chemicals (called gonadotropins) that tell the ovaries how much estrogen to make. There is very strong evidence that phytoestrogens disrupt this process. In controlled studies, gonadotropin levels are lower in women treated with soybean supplements, which means that they make less estrogen. In younger women, one consequence is that their menstrual cycle becomes longer, and longer menstrual cycles are associated with a decreased risk for breast cancer.

Altered gonadotropin production probably also explains the observation that menopausal symptoms, particularly hot flashes, are uncommon in the Far East. Contrary to popular belief, hot flashes are not the result of an absolute estrogen deficiency. Rather, they occur when there are wide swings in circulating estrogen levels. Phytoestrogens dampen those swings and reduce the symptoms. In addition, phytoestrogens act in much the same way as standard hormone supplementation; they restore the lining of the vagina to its normal premenopausal state.

Osteoporosis is another problem for aging women. All through life, bone is constantly formed and broken down ("remodeled" is the technical word), but after menopause, bone breaks down faster than it forms. When too much breaks down, the bone becomes weak and fractures, especially at the hip. It turns out that in the Far East, osteoporosis is much less of a problem than it is in the West. Tamoxifen™ prevents bone breakdown, but is far too toxic for use by otherwise healthy women. But phytoestrogens seem to be quite safe, and in animal studies, and in at least one clinical trial with post-menopausal women, adding soybeans to the diet led to increased bone formation.

There may even be some good news for men too. There is no evidence that phytoestrogens interfere with testosterone production but, as with breast cancer, prostate cancer is much less common in the Far East than in the United States. The results of population studies suggest phytoestrogen supplementation may protect against lung, stomach, and colon cancer.

All of these potential benefits do not come without some cause for concern. After all, use of the anti-estrogen Tamoxifen™, which prevents breast cancer, is limited by the fact that Tamoxifen™ promotes cancer of the lining of the uterus. In theory, any of the phytoestrogens could do the same thing. But in fact, that has never been reported, and women from countries with high intakes of soy have lower than expected rates of uterine cancer. Until more controlled trials are reported, there is no way to be certain, but currently available evidence suggests that soy supplementation may be a good idea for postmenopausal women, and possibly even for men.

C. Flavonoids and the "French Paradox"

There are other flavonoids besides the isoflavones and lignans. The term flavonoid comes from the Latin word for yellow, *flavus*, because plant extracts were used to dye linen, cotton, and silk a yellow color. Flavonoids can be divided into at least six different groups. The most important are the isoflavones (genistein) which were discussed in the section on phytoestrogens. Also included in this class are the flavones (apigenin and luteolin, found in chamomile); the flavonols (kaempferol and quercetin), found in red wine; and the catechins (found in black tea). The chemical structure of the flavonoids allows them to scavenge free radicals and function as antioxidants, and that is where most research efforts were directed during the 1990s.

Adults with the highest flavonoid intake have about three times less risk of dying from cardiovascular diseases than those with the lowest intake. Some of the flavonoids possess antioxidant and free radical-scavenging properties, and can prevent the oxidation of low density lipoprotein (LDL). No doubt that some of the benefits attributed to flavonoids are just due to their antioxidant effects. But flavonoids can also inhibit several key enzymes in cellular systems that produce free radicals, including two key enzymes systems that control the inflammatory process: cyclooxygenase and lipoxygenase.

Heavy drinking is associated with increased mortality. But a moderate intake of wine has been shown to reduce deaths from heart disease, and red wine causes more of a reduction in death rate than white. Citizens of France consume large amounts of fat and wine in their daily diets. But, paradoxically, the incidence of heart attack in France is lower than in the United States. The explanation for the paradox seems to be increased wine consumption, especially red wine.

The only consistent difference between red and white wines is the flavonoid content, which is 20 times higher in red wine. At first, it was thought the alcohol was what provided the protection, but it is now clear that it is the nonalcoholic fraction of red wine that is responsible for raising the total plasma antioxidant capacity of the blood. The good news for wine drinkers, and the bad news for tee-totalers, is that to get maximal effect, alcohol needs to be present because it facilitates the flavonoid absorption process. Drinking grape juice does not provide the protection conferred by red wine.

Compounds called procyanadins are not found in red wine. But they too are potent antioxidants, and their use may provide many of the same beneficial effects as drinking red wine. One of the best sources for the procyanadins is the seeds of the grapes used to make the wine (sold as grapeseed oil). Similar agents can be found in the green tea leaves (*Camellia sinesis),* and in the bark of the French maritime pine (*Pinus pinaster*).

There is still more to the flavonoid story. A flavonoid called apigenin, found in chamomile, binds to the same brain receptors as benzodiazepines (drugs like Valium™). Another flavonoid, called Amentoflavone, found in St. John's Wort, is thought to account for that herb's antidepressant effects. As more modern investigative techniques are applied, it is becoming increasingly obvious that many of the traditional remedies do have rational scientific explanations.

D. Linoleic Acid and the Anti-inflammatory Agents

For several decades, Americans have been urged to replace the saturated fat in their diets with polyunsaturates, such as linolenic acid. Substituting the latter for the former reduces blood cholesterol concentrations and thereby reduces the chance of developing coronary artery disease. Discussions about cholesterol lowering usually focus on dietary changes and the use of cholesterol lowering "statin" type drugs. Such a focus is too narrow. Some of the most popular herbs, including evening primrose and borage, contain substances that lower cholesterol and protect the heart.

The most common polyunsaturated fat in the American diet is linoleic acid. It is considered an "essential" fat, because it cannot be made by the human body and must be ingested. When saturated fats from meats are replaced with linolenic acid, levels of good cholesterol (HDL) stay the same, but levels of "bad" cholesterol (LDL) decrease. This is an important consideration in any cholesterol lowering program, because replacing the saturated fats with carbohydrates (as is true in most vegetarian diets), causes HDL levels to drop along with LDL. For that reason, most nutritionists now advise an increased linolenic acid intake.

What no one realized until just recently is that linolenic acid also plays a key role in regulating the inflammatory process. After injury or infection, tissues in the body release substances called cytokines. These substances, mostly interleukins-1 and -6 and tumor necrosis factor (necrosis is a medical term for the death of individual cells or tissues as a result of chemical or physical injury) are responsible for symptoms of injury such as fever, loss of appetite, and tissue wasting. But those symptoms are mostly side effects. The main thing cytokines do is coordinate the immune response and ultimately, the process of healing.

Excessive production of pro-inflammatory cytokines, or production of cytokines when they should not be produced, is seen in a range of different diseases. Cytokine abnormalities have been discovered in patients with malaria, overwhelming infection, rheumatoid arthritis, inflammatory bowel disease, cancer, and even Acquired Immune Disease Syndrome (AIDS). There are drugs that can be given to control excessive cytokine production (Advil™, Motrin™, Naprosyn™, Indocin™, etc). But cytokine production can also be modified by foods, specifically by fats. Fish oils have received the most attention. They contain substances called n-3 (or Omega 3) polyunsaturated fatty acids. These substances seem to counteract the inflammatory response, and, in the laboratory at least, show promise for treating rheumatoid arthritis, inflammatory bowel disease, psoriasis and asthma. Fish oil is not the only source for Omega 3 fatty acids. They can be found in some plant oils and even, much to the annoyance of antidrug warriors, in hemp seed oil!

Foods rich in Omega 6 fatty acids produce the opposite effects; they cause more cytokines (particularly interleukin-6 [IL6]) to be produced, and make the inflammatory response worse. IL6 production is enhanced by total unsaturated fatty acid intake. These observations are not yet fully understood, but the explanation appears to have something to do with the ability of fats to alter the composition of cell membranes. If the surface of the membrane changes in just the right way, the cytokines cannot attach to the cell, and the inflammatory response never occurs. In animals, at least, the production of tumor necrosis factor (TNF), interleukin-1 [IL1], and IL6, is a direct function of the amount of linoleic acid in the diet. The more linolenic acid in the diet, the fewer inflammatory cytokines produced. That explains why there is so much interest in supplements containing linoleic acid.

Of course, there is always a down side, and it is probably not a good idea to include too much fat in the diet. Dietary fat intake was believed by many to pose an increased risk for cancer, especially of the breast and colon. Comparisons of populations with different diets show a connection between increased saturated fat intake and cancer. However, the connection is very weak for unsaturated fats. Some people question that any relationship exists at all, and even if it did exist, the increased risk is so small compared to the increased benefits from preventing heart disease, or disorders like rheumatoid arthritis, that any sensible person would conclude that the risk is worth taking. Oils containing linolenic acid include almond (7-30 percent), peanut (13-43 percent), cottonseed (33-58 percent), evening primrose (7-14 percent), and rapeseed, also called canola (5-12 percent).

CHAPTER 4

Teas, Tannins, Pyrrozolidine Alkaloids, and Sesquiterpene Lactones

Ask a doctor whether you should take products containing tannins or saponins and the answer would almost certainly be no. Ask that same doctor about pyrrozolidine alkaloids or sesquiterpene lactones, and unless that physician has had subspecialty training in pharmacology or toxicology, the answer is likely to be "I don't know." Even though things are improving, the curricula of most medical schools is light on nutritional issues. If tannins or saponins are mentioned at all, it will probably only be to point out that taking too much of either one is likely to cause an upset stomach. The situation is even worse when it comes to more obscure compounds, such as pyrrolizidine alkaloids (very toxic compounds found in some native American plants), and sesquiterpene lactones (an important class of plant components that can block the inflammatory process and relieve pain). In a few more years, the situation will, no doubt, have improved. At the moment, however, accessible sources of information on these topics are hard to find, and even if a supplement maker does provide a chemical analysis on the product's label, most people will have no idea about what they are reading. This chapter contains a very brief introduction to some of these topics.

Teas and Tannins: Teas, meaning beverages made from the leaves of *Camellia sinesis*, as opposed to infusions, which are beverages made by soaking parts of other herbs in hot water, contain tannins. There are two kinds of teas: green and black. Green teas, such as Gunpowder tea, are made from tea leaves that are heated immediately after they are picked, then rolled and crushed. When treated in this fashion, the natural constituents of the leaves, including their color, are preserved. Black teas, such as Pekoe, are made differently. After they are picked, they are allowed to ferment before they are dried and packaged. The process of fermentation partly digests some of the leaves' components and imparts a reddish brown color. Both types of teas contain tannins, but the fermentation process greatly reduces the tannin content of black tea.

What are tannins? Traditional herbalists classify tannins as "astringents," chemicals that cause tissues to become firmer. The term is not really used in modern medicine, but the best example of what is meant by an astringent would be the styptic pencil that men use to control the bleeding that occurs when they cut themselves shaving. Tea is not the only source for tannins. Tannins can also be found in artichokes, bilberry, cranberry, guarana, hawthorn, hops, raspberry, and uva ursi. Herbalists recommend tannin-containing herbs to treat diarrhea, believing that the "firming" action of the tannins somehow helps relieve gastrointestinal symptoms. Just why making tissues firmer should be a good idea is not immediately obvious, at least not to anyone trained in modern medicine.

If the real meaning of "astringent" remains murky, the origin of the word tanin is quite clear; tannins are plant extracts used to cure leather. The soft, pliable, feel of finished leather is a result of the chemical changes that occur when rawhide is exposed to tannins. The tannins cause the protein components of leather to "denature," or lose their natural shape. Proteins that lose their normal shape acquire new properties but, as a rule, the alterations prevent them from carrying out their normal functions. To see the "denaturing" process in action, just add some vinegar to an egg white. The cloudy white material that forms is composed of "denatured" protein.

There are many different kinds of tannins, but they share some common structures. All are classified as "polyphenols," specifically as "proanthocyanidins." Large amounts of the latter are found in betel nut, and a substantial body of evidence suggests that it is the tannins in betel nut that place chronic users at an increased risk for cancer of the mouth and esophagus. Even the tannins in tea are suspect. The rate for cancer of the esophagus is much higher among Dutch tea drinkers than among the English. The difference is thought to be a function of the way tea is consumed in the two countries; British tea drinkers generally add milk to their tea, but the Dutch do not. Milk combines with tannins and makes them less toxic.

Some question whether it is the tannins that are causing the problem. There are, after all, hundreds of other molecules in tea, some more toxic than tannins. And, in fact, results of the latest laboratory studies suggest that tannins are more likely to prevent tumor growth than promote it. Tannins, it turns out, are very good antioxidants. Consuming a diet rich in tannins leads to measurable increases of antioxidant activity in the blood.

Furthermore, regular consumption of green tea, along with the regular consumption of soy protein, is thought to be the explanation for the lower rates of cancer and heart disease among the Japanese and Chinese. But the rates are only lower among Asians adhering to traditional diets. Residents of Tokyo, who eat more meat and less soy, and drink more soft drinks in preference to green tea, have cancer rates similar to those seen in Western countries. As evidence continues to mount, it is increasingly clear that tannins have "gotten a bad rap," and that they are more likely to do good than harm. Chewing betel nuts might not be such a good idea, but eating artichokes and drinking green tea is.

Saponins: Physicians hesitant about recommending tannins would be downright hostile to the idea of taking anything that contained a saponin. Certain of the saponin-containing herbs, such as *Cyclamen purpurascens*, can be very toxic if extracts are injected directly into the bloodstream. Saponins in the bloodstream destroy the membranes that surround red blood cells. But, saponins taken by mouth are quite another matter. In laboratory studies, saponins prevent tumor and bacterial growth, speed convalescence, and retard the aging process. That may sound like quite a tall order, but there is some evidence for all these claims, particularly in the case of the two best known saponins, Gingsenoside A and B.

In Latin, the word *sopa* means soap, which is where the herb soapwort derived its name. If powdered soapwort roots are added to water and shaken, the water becomes frothy and forms a lather. The reason that the lather forms is that molecules in the root extract reduce the surface tension of the water. The molecules responsible for this effect are called saponins. Saponins come in two basic forms, but both forms share a structure that very closely resemble the structure of sex hormones such as testosterone and estrogen.

Saponins can be found in many different plants. Soybeans are the best sources, but large amounts are also present in lentils, spinach and oats. Other saponin-containing herbs include asparagus, cyclamen, daisy, ginseng, horse chestnut, quillaia, violets, licorice, maize, and wild yams. Taken orally, saponins do not damage red blood cells, or anything else for that matter. However, some saponins can act as respiratory irritants, which is why traditional herbalists prescribe saponin-containing mixtures for use as expectorants.

Because of their emulsifying properties, saponins are widely used in the pharmaceutical and cosmetic industry. Until fairly recently, most commercially produced Mexican wild yams were bought up by cosmetic manufacturers. However, now that it is clear that yams, along with fenugreek (a spice used in curries) and soy, contain saponins that behave like "phytoestrogens," there has been an explosion of interest in these products (see the discussion of phytoestrogens earlier in this chapter).

Wild yams may be the most common source of saponins used by drug and cosmetic makers, but soybeans are the most important dietary source. And even in low concentrations (150 to 600 parts per million), soybean saponins can prevent the growth of human carcinoma cells. Other saponins, found in horse chestnuts, called escins, reduce the swelling seen in the legs of patients with chronic venous insufficiency. Their effectiveness has been proven in multiple European clinical trials.

Of all the saponins, ginseng is the best studied. Volumes have been written about the effects of the saponins contained in that herb, and no doubt many more will follow. Whatever the mechanism, and no one is quite sure what it is, there is convincing evidence that ginseng supplements improve mood, along with physical and mental performance, and that they do so without producing any convincing evidence of toxicity.

Sesquiterpene Lactones: This group of compounds, when they have not been ignored altogether, have also gotten a bad rap. The molecular structure of bisabolol, the active component of ginger, and the parthenolides found in feverfew, which are thought to account for that plant's ability to relieve headache pain, are just two of the members of this family. A very closely related molecule found in the essential oil of valerian (called valerianic acid), is thought to be responsible for that herb's sedative properties, and molecules with a similar structure are also found in chamomile.

Arnica has been used as an anti-inflammatory drug for many centuries, but no one knew quite why it was effective. The answer is that it contains another sesquiterpene lactone called helenalin, a potent anti-inflammatory agent. The interesting thing about this molecule is that it works by a new and totally different mechanism than that of any known anti-inflammatory drug. Prescription anti-inflammatories are effective because they inhibit an enzyme called cyclooxygenase. Helenalin does something different; it combines with a molecular complex called nuclear factor kappa beta (NFKB). Activation of NFKB is required to set off the inflammatory process in the first place. When helenalin combines with NFKB, the process never begins, and if the process never starts, inflammation cannot occur. Unfortunately, large amounts of helenalin are toxic, and arnica contains other, as yet uncharacterized, compounds that make its internal use dangerous, which is why Commission E recommends against its internal use. But that does not mean that helenalin cannot ever be used safely. It just means that we need to know more about the process.

Coltsfoot, an ancient remedy, also contains sesquiterpenes. Teas made with its leaves and flowers have been used as expectorants for more than a thousand years, and it does seem to be a reasonably effective expectorant. But it also contains a molecule called Bakkenolide G that is a natural antagonist of platelet activating factor (PAF). The presence of this molecule means that coltsfoot extracts might be used to prevent heart attacks. But, as with arnica, there is the problem of the other molecules contained in the herb. Coltsfoot has some particularly nasty molecules called pyrrolizidine alkaloids (PAs).

Pyrrolizidine Alkaloids: The backbone of the pyrrolizidine (PA) molecules is made by combining two molecules of an amino acid called ornithine. PAs are found in a great number of different plants but characteristically are found in the Boraginaceae (ie, *Heliotrope*), Leguminosae (i.e. *Crotalaria*) families. Many, but not all PAs, are extremely toxic to the liver. All species of comfrey, for example, contain PAs, but the concentrations of PAs are different in different parts of the herb. In general, the roots and rhizomes of the plants contain at least ten times the amount of pyrrolizidines as the leaves. The PA content in comfrey also varies depending on where the comfrey was grown.

The most toxic of the PAs is called echimidine. Only minute amounts are found in the leaves of comfrey that is grown in the United States, but very large amounts can be found in the leaves of Russian comfrey, and also in the leaves of the closely related prickly comfrey (*S. Aspereum*). Echimidine-containing products are banned in Canada, but they are legal in the United States. PAs are also contained in coltsfoot, and very small amounts may also be present in borage.

Pyrrolizidine alkaloids by themselves are not toxic. But once PAs get into the body, the liver converts them into compounds that may damage the lungs (primary pulmonary hypertension). Genetic material throughout the body may also be damaged, and that translates into an increased risk for cancer. Taken in sufficient doses, for a long enough time, PAs are guaranteed to cause liver damage. Specifically, they cause the linings of the veins in the liver to scar, obstructing the flow of blood through the liver, ultimately leading to liver failure and death.

The difficulty faced by American consumers is that much of the comfrey sold here is simply labeled "comfrey". The type of comfrey is often not specified, nor is mention made of which parts of the plants have been used. Reputable manufacturers will analyze their products in order to determine their PA content. Very small amounts, such as those seen in some expectorants made with coltsfoot, are almost certainly harmless. The question for consumers is whether they want to take the risk at all. Mullein, pine and wild thyme are all good expectorants, and they do not contain PAs.

CHAPTER 5

Dosage Forms

Herbal products are supplied in a confusing array of dosage forms. Consumers must decide whether to use whole herbs, teas, infusions or decoctions, not to mention capsules containing freeze dried or powdered herbs, fluidextracts, tinctures or essential oils. Many of these terms are archaic and no longer in use, at least within the established medical community. Recent medical and pharmacy school graduates have probably never heard the term decoction, let alone made one, and have only the vaguest idea of what goes into making a tincture. Worse still, most of the self-help and herbal remedy books available in bookstores repeatedly use these terms but never take the time to explain them.

The terms are of more than academic interest. Depending on which herb is involved, the product being sold may or may not produce the desired effect. Unsuspecting consumers may get too little, too much, or none at all of what they wanted. Chamomile tea is a good example. The active ingredient in chamomile (a molecule called apigenin) is contained in the herb's essential oil. That oil does not mix with water. So when teas are made from dried chamomile, the final product will be relaxing and refreshing, and it may even calm the stomach, but it only contains approximately 20 percent of the chemical responsible for those beneficial effects. To get the maximal benefit, as might be desired if the herb is being taken to promote sleep, the oil has to be used.

When it comes to tinctures and extracts great caution is required. Extracts made by one manufacturer may not contain the same concentration of active ingredients as the same product made by another manufacturer. Remember, these are food supplements, not medications regulated by the government. Remember, too, that tinctures and extracts contain the concentrated form of the herb. The greater the concentration of active ingredients, the greater the chance that undesirable side effects can occur. The other thing to remember about tinctures and extracts is that they contain alcohol, sometimes quite a bit, possibly even enough to make you test positive at a random workplace drug test, or when driving your car!

Extracts: Most of the dosage forms are extracts, a term used to describe the active portion of the plant, once it has been separated from the inert or inactive components. The resultant products may be liquids, semisolids, or powders. Extracts are classified as either decoctions, infusion, fluidextracts, tinctures, pilular (semisolid) extracts or powdered extracts. The whole group is described by the archaic term (still popular with Commission E and herbalists) "galenicals," in honor of Galen, the famous Greek physician.

Infusion: Infusions are made by soaking dried herbs in either cold or boiled water for a short period of time. The resulting concentration of active ingredients depends on which part and how much of the herb is being soaked and on how long it is allowed to steep. Because of the great variation that is possible, prescription drugs are no longer prepared in this fashion. However, many herbal products still are supplied for use in this way, often in premeasured tea bags. Depending on the manufacturer, concentrations may be quite inconsistent from batch to batch.

Decoction: Decoction is another very old term no longer used in modern medicine, but one that persists in herbal literature. Herbs with active ingredients that contain heat-stable components that are tightly connected to structures within the plant (for example, a chemical that is found only in the wood stems of the plant, as opposed to the leaves) can be boiled in water for 15 minutes, then cooled and strained into cold water. The process was used when simple infusions were not enough to get the active ingredients out of wood or fibrous plants.

Tincture: Tinctures are made from alcohol or alcohol diluted with water. Traditionally, if a very potent medicine, such as digitalis, was involved, 10 grams of plant material would be used to produce 100 milliliters of tincture. In the case of less potent drugs, i.e., most of the generally available herbal remedies, double the amount of plant material would be used. Plant material is soaked in alcohol for three to five days, after which the mixture is either strained or percolated (in much the same fashion as making coffee). Depending on which herb is involved, and which manufacturer is making it, the final potency (concentrations in milligrams per milliliter), unless it is adjusted to some standardized value, may vary by a great deal. Tincture from one maker may contain more, less, or the same amount of active ingredients as that produced by a competitor. Unless the product's label lists a specific concentration, there is no way to know how much you are taking. The nice thing about tinctures is that they are stable for a long time, and the high alcohol content prevents bacterial growth. The bad thing about tinctures is that if they are not stopped tightly, alcohol will evaporate, and the tincture remaining in the bottle will become more concentrated.

Fluidextracts: Fluidextracts are liquids prepared from herbs that contain alcohol as a solvent, or preservative, or both, made in such a way that one milliliter contains the active ingredients from one gram of the herb. In the pharmaceutical industry, when fluidextracts are made (which today is not very often), the final product is tested to make sure that some standard concentration has been achieved. That may or may not be the case with herbal remedies and food supplements. And, as with tinctures, the same caveats apply: if the final product is not standardized, then the content of active ingredients depends on which part or parts of the plant have been used, and on how the active ingredients are extracted.

Herb Profiles

Although a bewildering array of products is being offered for sale, only a dozen or so account for most of the sales. According to the 4th Annual Natural Herbal Products Sales Survey, the top ten herbs account for 54 percent of sales, with sales of the top five (echinacea, St. John's Wort, Ginkgo biloba, garlic, and saw palmetto) accounting for over a third of all herbal product sales. The top 30 sellers are shown in the table below. In Europe, where herbal products are even more widely accepted than they are in the United States, the variety of products offered (and purchased) is somewhat greater.

Top Selling Herbs in the U.S.A.

1. Echinacea	11. Cranberry	21. Feverfew
2. St. John's Wort	12. Milk Thistle	22. Kava kava
3. Ginkgo biloba	13. Cat's-claw	23. Green tea
4. Garlic	14. Grape seed extract	24. Ginger
5. Saw Palmetto	15. Bilberry	25. Pine bark extract
6. Ginseng	16. Cascara sagrada	26. Astragalus
7. Goldenseal	17. Cayenne	27. Primrose
8. Aloe	18. Dong Quai	28. Yohimbine
9. Siberian Ginseng	19. Psyllium (tie)	29. Chamomile
10. Valerian	19. Ma huang (tie)	30. Pau d'arco

Table 6:1

Individual herbs - a total of 67 different ones - are described in this section. Descriptions are divided into 12 separate sections: name, source, history, traditional claims, Commission E recommendations, proven effects, concerns, warnings, effect on drug tests, summary, dosage, and references for further readings. Some of this information might, at first, seem extraneous, but be assured it is not. You do need to know the proper botanical name of the product you are buying. American Ginseng is not the same as Siberian Ginseng and it is certainly not the same as Panax Ginseng. The amount of active ingredient you end up paying for depends on the kind of plant the manufacturer uses to make the product. Safety is an issue, and so are your chances of flunking a workplace urine drug test. Details about each of the subsections are provided below.

Name: The full botanical name is given followed by the common names used in English, French, and German. Many herbs have a number of distinct species, and it is very important to distinguish between them. For example, some types of comfrey are toxic while others are not. The comfrey that grows in the United States is *S. Officinale*. Russian comfrey, which has become increasingly popular in the United States and Europe, is called *S. X uplandicum* (formerly *S. Pergrinum*). While all species of comfrey contain toxic chemicals called pyrrolizidines (PAs), their concentration is much higher in Russian comfrey than in the comfrey grown in the U.S. If the label does not specify *S. Officinale,* you should think twice about buying it, even if it is much cheaper. Always check the botanical name on the label.

Source: This section describes where the herb comes from, and what parts of the plant are used to make the product. In most cases, you cannot just pick a plant, grind it up, and put it in capsules. Active ingredients are not distributed evenly throughout the plant. In the case of comfrey, the concentration of dangerous chemicals is much greater in the roots than in the leaves. The opposite is true for angelica (*Dong Quai*), where potentially toxic chemicals are contained in the stems and leaves, but not the roots. Even the country of origin matters. The type of calamus grown in the United States (*Acorus calamus*) is relatively nontoxic. But the kind of calamus grown in India contains beta-asarone, a known carcinogen. The container should state where the product comes from, and whether it is made from leaves, or roots, or stems, or all three.

History: Knowing how people have used the herb in the past might help an enlightened consumer decide if he wants to take it. Knowing that American Indians used calamus as a hallucinogen might persuade someone to treat an upset stomach with Tums™ instead. Knowing that valerian has been safely used as a sedative since the Middle Ages might make a person want to try valerian before requesting a prescription for Halcyon™.

Traditional Claims: Some of these herbs have been used for more than a thousand years. When a friend suggests you try herb "x" to treat problem "y," you might find it useful to check just what conditions herb "x" has been used for in the past. If the current recommendation doesn't quite agree with traditional claims, perhaps there is a reason.

Commission E Recommendations: Commission E was an expert panel commissioned by the German government to review all available research on commercially available herbal remedies, and make recommendations on the safety and effectiveness of herbal products. Commission E is the only government agency, in Europe or the United States, that has ever undertaken such a task. Their findings and recommendations are not supported by anything near the depth and quality of research that would be required to market, for example, a new antibiotic. But for the moment, Commission E recommendations are the only serious guide that we have. If Commission E says that ginger can be safely used to treat seasickness, then it probably can.

Proven Effects: The latest scientific data, both from laboratory studies and from clinical trials, is summarized in this section. Quite often results of the modern studies agree well with traditional claims, but sometimes they do not. And all too often there is very little modern information to discuss.

Concerns: Potential problems, and unanticipated effects, are discussed in this section. In general, these are important facts about herbs that consumers should know, even though such concerns are not necessarily reasons to stop using that herb. For example, the seeds and stems of angelica contain a chemical called furanocoumarin, also known as psoralen (the same molecule can also be found in limes, lemons, figs, and parsnips). Psoralen-containing drugs sensitize the skin to ultraviolet light and prolonged sun exposure can lead to severe sunburns. The possibility of photosensitivity after using angelica doesn't necessarily mean that it should not be used, just that users should avoid direct sunlight, and be aware of its effects.

Warnings: Warnings are reasons, and usually, very strong ones, not to take a particular herb. For example, compounds found in ginkgo biloba extract interfere with a natural body chemical called platelet activating factor, a key element in the blood clotting process. There have been at least three reports of brain hemorrhage in ginkgo biloba users; one individual was taking coumadin (a blood thinner) and another was taking aspirin (another blood thinner). Ginkgo biloba's anti-platelet action probably is of no consequence for any normal person, but anyone taking blood thinners (coumadin, heparin, etc.) should not be taking ginkgo biloba.

Drug Testing: Federal law requires that transportation and nuclear industry workers, along with others who have jobs that could affect the safety of others, be tested for drug abuse. Many other individuals are tested under non-regulated programs. Some herbal products can cause false positive test results; false positive tests for methamphetamine from using ephedra is a good example. In federally mandated testing programs, confirmatory testing is required, so it will eventually become clear that ephedra, and not methamphetamine, caused the positive test. Unfortunately, confirmatory testing is not required in non-federal testing programs. Employers, especially when the testing is done in the course of a preemployment examination, may elect to forgo the expense of additional testing. Even if the herb itself does not cause a false positive result, the mere presence of some herbal products (such as Goldenseal) in the urine may suggest to the drug-testing laboratory that the urine sample has been adulterated. If you work in a setting where urine drug testing is a possibility, make sure you know whether the products you are taking can cause a positive urine test.

Dosage: Dosage ranges for prescription medication are validated in clinical trials before they ever come to market. That is not the case for food supplements, and the dosage recommended on food supplement labels may or may not be appropriate for the individual consumer. The dosage lists here are taken from the recommendations of Germany's Commission E, and from the British Pharmacopeia. They are not guaranteed either to be safe or effective. They merely reflect the dosage recommended by those two organizations.

Summary: This will provide the consensus opinion on the benefits and risks of using a particular herb, and warning of any important side effects or contraindications for its use.

References: Too much of what has been written about herbal medicine is simply a rehash of what had been stated in some earlier book. Except for the sections on history, botany, and the recommendations of Commission E, all the information contained in this book is taken directly from the most recent, peer reviewed scientific literature. At the end of each section, references from the peer reviewed literature are alphabetically listed. If you want to know more about the herbs you are using, or are planning to use, you should read the articles. Even if they don't completely answer your question, they will refer you to other papers that do. Readers who have access to the Internet can find the abstracts (short versions) for all of these papers at the Website of the National Library of Medicine (NLM). In some cases, the complete paper may even be downloaded at no charge. The mechanics of doing a MEDLINE search are described in the appendix.

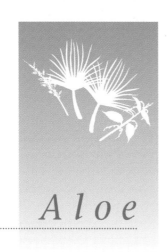

Aloe

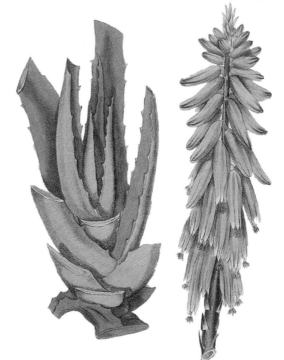

Name: *Aloe ferox,* Mil., *Aloe perryi,* Baker, called Socotrine or Zanzibar Aloe, and *Aloe barbadensis,* Mil., variously referred to as Mediterranean, Curacao, or Barbados aloe. In English, Aloe or Cape Aloe; in French, *Aloés*; in German *Aloe* and *Kap-Aloe.* All are members of the Lily family (Fam. *Liliaceae,* tribe *Aloineae*).

Source: Aloe is made by evaporating the juice of aloe leaves. Leaves are cut across the base and arranged so that their juices can be collected. The process takes roughly six hours. The juice is then heated until all the liquid is driven off, leaving large, translucent blocks of the active ingredients. The Cape Aloe comes mainly from South Africa. *Aloe barbadensis* is grown in the Caribbean. The different aloes from the Caribbean and South Africa contain essentially the same ingredients and produce the same effects. Aloe IS NOT the same thing as aloe vera gel. Aloe vera gel is made from the central part of the aloe leaf, not from the juice, and then only from the Caribbean variety, *Aloe barbadensis.*

History: According to one account, after the conquest of Persia in 333 B.C., Aristotle advised Alexander the Great to make a detour on his way home to visit the island of Socotra, in the Indian Ocean, to bring home some aloe. Whether the story is true, and scholars do have their doubts, the medicinal properties of aloe have been recognized for thousands of years. However, large scale commercial production of aloe did not begin until the late 1600s, when traders first brought Barbados aloe to London. In the 1860s, two Scottish physicians isolated aloe's active ingredient, called it Aloin (now known as babrolin), and began using it to treat constipation. Throughout much of the 18th and 19th centuries, aloe was one of the most frequently prescribed and widely used medications.

Traditional Claims: Aloe is used as a laxative and purgative.

Commission E Recommendations: Aloe is used to treat constipation.

Proven Effects: Aloe, like other members of the Lily family (including senna, cascara and rhubarb), contains molecules called anthraquinones, specifically danthrone, aloin, aloe-emodin anthrone and other anthranoids. When still in the plant, these molecules are tightly bound to sugar molecules, which makes them inactive and prevents them from being absorbed in the stomach and small intestine. When the anthraquinone-sugar complex finally gets to the large intestine, bacteria in the gut remove the sugar molecule, allowing unbound anthraquinone to react with cells on the wall of the large intestine. Anthraquinones cause cells in the intestine to transport water and salts into the intestinal tract. Increased volume stimulates the walls of the colon to contract. Bowel movements usually occur six to ten hours after aloe is taken.

Aloe also appears to have anti-bacterial and antiviral effects, and there is some evidence that using aloe can increase immunity and accelerate wound healing. In test tubes, aloes are good antioxidants, a finding that suggests they may have a role in preventing heart disease and aging. Unfortunately, these observations have not been validated in humans. Nor has anyone followed up on laboratory evidence that aloe can help speed up the rate of alcohol metabolism. If the studies could be confirmed, aloe might yet prove to be an effective hangover remedy!

Aloe vera has been used to heal radiation burns and skin irritation. Even though aloe vera is very widely used to treat an assortment of skin diseases, controlled studies testing its effectiveness in treating these conditions have produced inconclusive results. Some studies have shown that results with aloe vera are no better than with placebo. Many believe that if aloe vera does speed up wound healing, it does so by providing a protective barrier over the wound. On the other hand, there are also convincing studies showing that aloe vera does more than just provide a protective barrier, and that accelerated wound healing really does occur.

Concerns: Aloe taken as a laxative causes intense cramping, and there is something about this particular laxative that tends to make hemorrhoids worse. Hemorrhoid sufferers should consider trying another product. Small amounts of the active ingredient are absorbed from the large intestine, and may appear in mother's milk and in urine. Their presence in the urine could be a disconcerting experience since, depending on the acidity of the urine, its color may turn brown or even red. A handful of reports have described allergic skin reactions after using aloe vera, but given the large numbers of people using aloe vera on their skin, skin reactions must be quite uncommon. The greatest cause for concern is the mounting body of evidence that aloe (BUT NOT ALOE VERA), or at least some of its components, are carcinogenic. That possibility alone should be sufficient to deter the prudent consumer from using this particular laxative more than once or twice.

Warnings: Chronic use of any laxative can deplete the body of potassium, and low levels of potassium can cause dangerous irregularities in the way the heart beats. Anthraquinone-containing laxatives (not just aloe, but also senna) cause an apparently benign condition called melanosis coli. Brownish pigment accumulates in the wall of the large intestine, where it seems to do no harm. Doctors consider melanosis coli to be a marker for laxative abuse. Virtually every scientific body that has reviewed the problem recommends that none of the Lily family laxatives be used for more than 10 days. Because danthrone can cause tumors in laboratory animals, preparations made from danthrone have been withdrawn from the market. Similar tumors have not been reported after using the natural products (aloe, senna, cascara, rhubarb), but most physicians still advise against their chronic use. Aloe should not be used by nursing mothers.

Drug Testing: Aloe will not cause a false positive drug test, but chronic use may cause enough discoloration of the urine to interfere with the testing process, and that could be interpreted as an attempt to avoid being tested.

Dosage: The typical dose is 50 to 200 milligrams taken at bedtime. When aloe vera is consumed in drinks, no matter what the contents state on the label, there is really no way to know how much is being taken because it breaks down very rapidly. Neither the U.S. nor the European governments have set limits on the amount that can be added to food or beverages, and consumers should closely read the labels of all products.

Summary: Aloe and aloe vera are different products and should not be confused. Aloe-based products are effective laxatives, but there are many other laxatives that are not suspected carcinogens, that are just as effective, and that do not make urine turn brown or red. While aloe seems to have a range of interesting and potentially beneficial effects in laboratory studies, especially antioxidant effects, these alleged benefits have been hard to confirm in humans. There are no reports of significant toxicity associated with aloe vera use, and it may produce symptomatic relief for some skin conditions. More miraculous claims for aloe vera, such as accelerated wound healing, remain unproven. Unlike aloe, aloe vera is quite nontoxic and safe for use.

References:

Chung JH, Cheong JC, Lee JY, Roh HK, Cha YN. Acceleration of the alcohol oxidation rate in rats with aloin, a quinone derivative of Aloe. Biochem Pharmacol 1996;52(9):1461-8.

Haller JS, Jr. A drug for all seasons. Medical and pharmacological history of aloe. Bull N Y Acad Med 1990;66(6):647-59.

Hutter JA, Salman M, Stavinoha WB, Satsangi N, Williams RF, Streeper RT, et al. Anti-inflammatory C-glucosyl chromone from *Aloe barbadensis*. J Nat Prod 1996;59(5):541-3.

Shelton RM. Aloe vera. Its chemical and therapeutic properties. Int J Dermatol 1991;30(10):679-83.

Williams MS, Burk M, Loprinzi CL, Hill M, Schomberg PJ, Nearhood K, et al. Phase III double-blind evaluation of an aloe vera gel as a prophylactic agent for radiation-induced skin toxicity. Int J Radiat Oncol Biol Phys 1996;36(2):345-9.

Zonta F, Bogoni P, Masotti P, Micali G. High-performance liquid chromatographic profiles of aloe constituents and determination of aloin in beverages, with reference to the EEC regulation for flavoring substances. J Chromatogr A 1995;718(1):99-106.

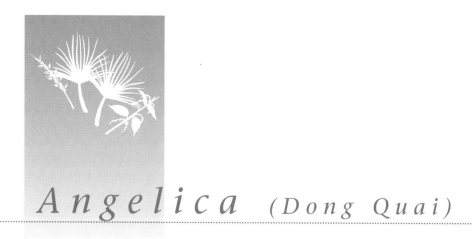

Angelica (Dong Quai)

Name: *Angelica archangelica* L. (Umbelliferae) and *Angelica atropurpurea* L., grow in Europe and North America. Related species that grow in China, *Angelica sinensis* (Oliv.) Diels, commonly called *dang-qui, dong quai, Quingui, Yangui,* and *Danggui.* In English the herb is simply known as Angelica; in French *Angéline officinale;* in German, *Angelikakraut* (herb), *Angelikawurzel* (root), *Angelikafrüchte* (seed), and *Englewurz, or Erz-Engelwurz.*

Source: Oil is extracted from the roots of European, North American, and Chinese Angelica. All of the different species seem to contain essentially the same active ingredients, including coumarin and coumarin derivatives. The seeds and stems also contain a coumarin derivative (furanocoumarin) that makes users extremely sensitive to the sun. Only products made from the roots of angelica are approved for sale by the German government.

History: In China, the herb is called dong quai, meaning "proper order." It is mentioned in medical texts dating from the year 200 AD (*Shen-nong Ben Cao Jing*). Angelica still remains one of the most frequently used herbal medicines in China, where it is prescribed for menstrual irregularities, arthritis and joint pain, anemia, and ulcers. Even in ancient times, Chinese physicians used angelica extracts to treat anemia, especially when the anemia was due to blood loss from childbirth or trauma. Today, many Chinese physicians still give patients recovering from surgery a tea or broth made with angelica. In the United States, angelica is sold as a "ginseng for women," with claims that it can reduce premenstrual discomfort and promote normal reproductive function.

Traditional Claims: Antispasmodic (stomach upset), cholagogue (gallbladder pain), and stomachic. A mixture containing angelica, called *Shi-Quan-Da-Bu-Tang* (Ten Significant Tonic Decoction), or SQT (Juzentaihoto, TJ-48) was first created by Song Dynasty administrators (Public Welfare Pharmacy Bureau) nearly 900 years ago! It is prepared by extracting a mixture of ten medicinal herbs (*Rehmannia glutinosa, Paeonia lactiflora, Liqusticum wallichii, Angelica sinensis, Glycyrrhiza uralensis, Poria cocos, Atractylodes macrocephala, Panax ginseng, Astragalus membranaceus and Cinnamomum cassia*). It was, and still is, used to treat anemia, anorexia, and extreme exhaustion.

Commission E Recommendations: Angelica is recommended for the treatment of abdominal bloating, loss of appetite, dyspepsia (upset stomach), flatulence, gastrointestinal spasm, and peptic discomfort.

Proven Effects: Laboratory studies with water-based extracts have shown that something in the herb increases coronary artery blood flow and stimulates red blood cell production. One constituent of the extract, called ferulic acid, prevents platelets from clumping, which means that its use may prevent the sort of blood clot formation that leads to heart attacks and strokes (technically, ferulic acid is a cyclooxygenase and thromboxane A2 synthetase inhibitor). Ferulic acid also plays a role in the body's defenses against some cancer causing agents, such as N-nitroso compounds. Recent studies of the old SQT formula, sponsored by the Chinese government, tend to confirm that something in the mixture does enhance immunity. But, except for one study showing positive effects in women with cervical inflammation, none of these benefits have ever been proven in a clinical trial with real patients. Moreover, benefits observed in laboratory studies were seen after animals were injected with angelica extracts. It appears that most of the active ingredients in the leaves are destroyed in the stomach, and never reach the bloodstream. Toxicity studies have been done in human volunteers. Forty stroke patients were given large doses of angelica intravenously for up to one month, and no ill effects were observed. The effects of long-term use, however, have not been studied.

Concerns: Angelica contains coumarin, the same molecule found in sweet clover and in new-mown hay. Coumarin is what gives these plants their pleasant smell. Coumarin, itself, is harmless, but under some conditions, as when sweet clover is allowed to ferment, coumarin can be converted to dicoumarol, a compound similar to the anticoagulants given to heart patients. The conversion is unlikely to occur in the case of angelica flowers, but seeds and stems do contain another coumarin derivative called furanocoumarin, also known as psoralen (the same molecule can also be found in limes, lemons, figs, and parsnips). Psoralen-containing drugs sensitize the skin to ultraviolet light, which is why they are used, under controlled conditions, to treat skin conditions such as vitiligo and psoriasis. Severe sunburns can occur if a person takes psoralen and then is exposed to the sun.

Warning: Patients taking coumadin or other blood thinners should not be taking angelica. There is laboratory evidence that the coumarin present in the herb, even though it is not an anticoagulant, will decrease the ability of the body to metabolize prescribed blood thinners, and may result in dangerous bleeding tendencies.

Drug Testing: There is no evidence that any of the components found in angelica flowers have an effect on standard workplace urine screening tests.

Dosage: The recommended dosage for dried whole root is 4.5 grams per day, equivalent to 1.5 to 3.0 grams per day of the 1:1 fluidextract, or 1.5 grams of the 1:5 tincture. If essential oil is being used, the recommended dose is 10-20 drops of oil per day. Alternatively, a tea can be made by putting one teaspoon of crushed seeds in one-half cup of boiling water.

Summary: The flowers of this herb contain a variety of promising compounds that may yet prove to be useful in treating heart diseases, anemia, and even in preventing cancer. Except for patients taking anticoagulants, use of products made from angelica flowers appears to be safe. The problem is that none of these claims have been validated in any convincing clinical trial.

References:

Baghdikian B, Lanhers MC, Fleurentin J, Ollivier E, Maillard C, Balansard G, et al. An analytical study, anti-inflammatory and analgesic effects of Harpagophytum procumbens and Harpagophytum zeyheri. Planta Med 1997;63(2):171-6.

Choy YM, Leung KN, Cho CS, Wong CK, Pang PK. Immunopharmacological studies of low molecular weight polysaccharide from *Angelica sinesis*. Am J Chin Med 1994;22(2):137-45.

Kuenzig W, Chau J, Norkus E, Holowaschenko H, Newmark H, Mergens W, et al. and ferulic acid as blockers of nitrosamine formation. Carcinogenesis 1984;5(3):309-13.

Lanhers MC, Fleurentin J, Mortier F, Vinche A, Younos C. Anti-inflammatory and analgesic effects of an aqueous extract of *Harpagophytum procumbens*. Planta Med 1992;58(2):117-23.

Mei QB, Tao JY, Cui B. Advances in the pharmacological studies of radix *Angelica sinesis* (Oliv) Diels (Chinese Danggui). Chin Med J (Engl) 1991;104(9):776-81.

Wang Y, Zhu B. [The effect of angelica polysaccharide on proliferation and differentiation of hematopoietic progenitor cell]. Chung Hua I Hsueh Tsa Chih 1996;76(5):363-6.

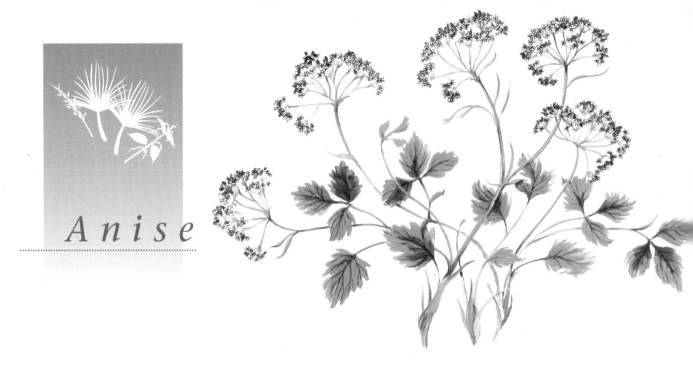

Anise

Name: *Pimpinella anisum* L. (Umbelliferae). Commonly called anise; in French, *Anis cultive,* in German, *Anis.*

Source: Anise is native to the Near East, but it is now cultivated in many countries, especially Egypt, Turkey, and Spain. Whole dried fruits are used for flavoring and medicines.

History: Anise has always been extremely popular as a food flavoring, and is especially used by bakers and candy makers. In combination with other herbs, it is widely used to treat stomach upset, particularly in Germany and France. Over the centuries, the essential oils from fennel (*Foeniculum vulgare*) and anise have been used to increase milk secretion, promote menstruation, facilitate birth and increase libido. The pattern of use also suggests that something in anise extract has estrogenic activity. In the 1930s, some interest was shown in using anise extracts for the development of synthetic estrogens, but the chemistry was never completely worked out and other alternatives were adopted.

Traditional Claims: Anise is used as a carminative, expectorant, stomachic and glactogenic.

Commission E Recommendations: Anise is used to treat dyspepsia (upset stomach), and upper respiratory catarrh (inflammation).

Proven Effects: The main constituent of the essential oils of both fennel and anise is a substance called anethole. Smaller amounts of anethole are found in other plants, including guarana. Clinical studies of anise are very few in number, but results of laboratory studies suggest that anethole is an anti-inflammatory agent and a very good antioxidant. Extracts of anise inhibit the growth of certain tumors, particularly colon cancer. An anethole derivative has been used to treat patients who do not produce enough saliva (a condition called xerostomia). There are also some laboratory studies suggesting that some ingredient in anise oil increases the movement of the cilia that line the bronchial passages. If the same thing happens in humans, that would account for the popularity of anise as an expectorant.

Concerns: Occasional allergic skin reactions have been reported, but concerns raised during the 1970s, that anise oil might be a carcinogen, have generally been rejected.

Warnings: None

Drug Testing: None of the molecules in the essential oil (>80 percent anethole), should interfere with the standard workplace urine drug screening tests.

Dosage: The recommended single oral dose for use in treating cough and upper respiratory infection is 0.1 grams, roughly the amount contained in four drops of the oil, three times a day. The average daily dose is 3 grams of drug or 0.3 grams of oil.

Summary: European physicians often combine anise oil with thyme and other fragrant oils, such as licorice, to treat upper respiratory infection and to control flatulence. Clinical trials substantiating such usage are nonexistent, but experience in Europe suggests that these remedies are effective, and that they are safe in the recommended doses.

References:

Bouthillier L, Charbonneau M, Brodeur J. Assessment of the role of glutathione conjugation in the protection afforded by anethole dithiolthione against hexachloro-1,3-butadiene- induced nephrotoxicity. Toxicol Appl Pharmacol 1996;139(1):177-85.

Ferguson MM. Pilocarpine and other cholinergic drugs in the management of salivary gland dysfunction. Oral Surg Oral Med Oral Pathol 1993;75(2):186-91.

Reddy BS. Chemoprevention of colon cancer by minor dietary constituents and their synthetic analogues. Prev Med 1996; 25(1):48-50.

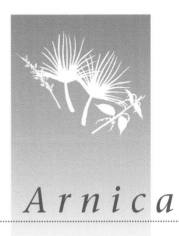

Arnica

Name: *Arnica montana* L. (Compositae). The dried flower heads are called arnica flos. The American species are named *Arnica fulgens* Pursh, *Arnica sonoria* Green, *Arnica latifolia* Bong., and *A cordifolia* Hook. Commonly called Arnica, Mountain Arnica or Mountain Tobacco; in French, *Arnica*; in German, *Arnikablüten, Arnika*, or *Berg-Wohlverleih.*

Source: The flowers are harvested from a perennial plant native to the mountainous regions of Europe. Flowers bloom from June to August. Several closely related species, members of the family Asteraceae, grow in the United States. Like angelica, the active ingredients are contained in essential oil that is extracted from the plant.

History: Medicines made from these flowers have been in use since the Middle Ages. It is unclear where the practice first began, but arnica-containing salves and ointments have been applied to sprains and bruises for hundreds of years. Modern practitioners have rediscovered arnica, and today some plastic surgeons give it to their patients in hopes of reducing postoperative pain and swelling.

Traditional Claims: Arnica is used as an anti-inflammatory.

Commission E Recommendations: Arnica-containing ointments are recommended for the treatment of bruises, contusions, dislocated bones, furunculosis (boils), hematoma, insect bites, joint pain, phlebitis, post-traumatic edema, rheumatism, and sprains. The internal use of arnica is not recommended.

Proven Effects: The essential oil contains sesquiterpene lactones. The most important component is called helenalin. It is a potent anti-inflammatory agent, and works by a new and totally different mechanism than the anti-inflammatory drugs prescribed by physicians. Prescription anti-inflammatories are effective because they inhibit an enzyme called cyclooxygenase. Helenalin does something different. Once helenalin enters a cell, it combines with a molecular complex called nuclear factor kappa beta (NFKB). Activation of NFKB is required to set off the inflammatory process (activating lymphocytes and other inflammatory cells) in the first place. When helenalin combines with NFKB, the process never begins, and therefore inflammation cannot occur. Unfortunately, helenalin does other things besides prevent inflammation. It also exerts effects on the heart (phosphodiesterase inhibitor), and on the liver (reduces the ability to metabolize certain other drugs). Helenalin also has adverse effects on blood clotting.

Concerns: As with all members of the Compositae family, allergic skin reactions are common, but the likelihood of their occurring depends on how much helenalin is in the product being applied and how the product has been manufactured. Reactions in occasional users remain unpredictable, but long-term use is very likely to cause eczema, and its use is not advised.

Warnings: Internal use of arnica is not advisable. There is only one reported arnica-related death in the medical literature, but helenalin can interact with so many of the body's enzyme systems that the risk of internal use far outweighs any possible benefits.

Drug Testing: Components of arnica-containing ointments should not be absorbed through the skin, and even if they were, there is nothing to suggest that any of those molecules would be detected by standard workplace urine drug tests.

Dosages: Commission E recommends that ointments contain no more than 15 percent arnica oil, or not more than 20-25 percent tincture.

Summary: Molecules found in Arnica have unique and potentially useful, anti-inflammatory properties. Arnica ointments may be useful for reducing the pain and swelling associated with sprains and bruises, but arnica should not be taken internally, as the risks outweigh the benefits.

References:

Haraguchi H, Ishikawa H, Sanchez Y, Ogura T, Kubo Y, Kubo I. Antioxidative constituents in *Heterotheca inuloides*. Bioorg Med Chem 1997;5(5):865-71.

Hart O, Mullee MA, Lewith G, Miller J. Double-blind, placebo-controlled, randomized clinical trial of homeopathic arnica C30 for pain and infection after total abdominal hysterectomy [see comments]. J R Soc Med 1997;90(2):73-8.

Lyss G, Schmidt TJ, Merfort I, Pahl HL. Helenalin, an anti-inflammatory sesquiterpene lactone from Arnica, selectively inhibits transcription factor NF-kappaB [see comments]. Biol Chem 1997;378(9):951-61.

Schaffner W. Granny's remedy explained at the molecular level: helenalin inhibits NF- kappaB [editorial; comment]. Biol Chem 1997;378(9):935.

Spettoli E, Silvani S, Lucente P, Guerra L, Vincenzi C. Contact dermatitis caused by sesquiterpene lactones. Am J Contact Dermat 1998;9(1):49-50.

Woerdenbag HJ, Merfort I, Passreiter CM, Schmidt TJ, Willuhn G, van Uden W, et al. Cytotoxicity of flavonoids and sesquiterpene lactones from Arnica species against the GLC4 and the COLO 320 cell lines. Planta Med 1994;60(5):434-7.

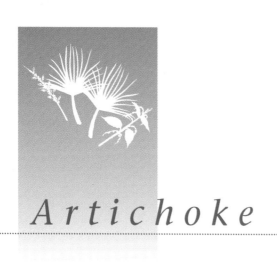

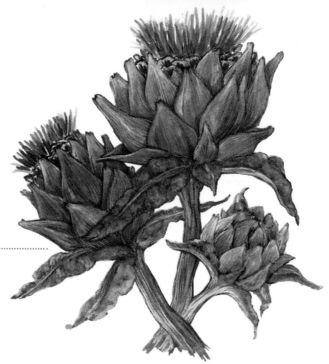

Artichoke

Name: *Cynara scolymus* L.(Compositae), commonly called the Globe Artichoke, Artichoke and Cynara; in French, *Artichaut*; in German, *Artischocke* and *Artischockenblätter*.

Source: Artichokes originally came from the Mediterranean, but are now grown in Europe and America. The artichoke is a member of the family Compositae, along with other common herbal remedies such as arnica, German chamomile, feverfew, tansy, and yarrow.

History: Dried powdered artichoke, containing fragments of the leaves, has traditionally been used to treat liver disease. Herbalists classify artichoke (along with boldo leaf and fumitory, chicory, thistle, and mugwort) as a "cholagogue," substances that can make the gallbladder contract and release bile. The human body produces hormones capable of doing just that, but it is not clear whether any of the herbal products recommended as "cholagogues" really have that ability. Extracts of the powdered plant contain large amounts of tannin and numerous enzymes. In the past, extracts of artichoke were used to curdle milk for cheese-making.

Traditional Claims: During the 17th and 18th centuries, right side abdominal discomfort, for whatever cause, was usually blamed on a defective gallbladder. Thus the interest in "cholagogues" substances to promote bile flow and normalize gallbladder function.

Commission E Recommendations: Artichoke is used to treat dyspepsia (upset stomach).

Proven Effects: Many of the traditional claims may well be true. Liver cells grown in test tubes and exposed to carbon tetrachloride (a cleaning fluid that causes liver damage in humans) quickly die, but two of the organic acids contained in artichokes, caffeic and quinic acids, prevent damage from occurring. The flavonoids and polyphenols contained in artichoke leaves are potent antioxidants, and are being investigated as water-soluble protectors against lipid peroxidation and other free radical-mediated cell injury. Claims about the ability to increase bile flow may also be true. When artichoke extract was introduced directly into the gallbladder of patients suspected of having gallbladder disease (via a tube passed through the intestines), compared to placebo, there was a very significant increase in bile flow.

Other alleged actions, including artichoke's effectiveness as a diuretic, have been harder to prove, and the therapeutic value of frequently used lipid-lowering agents, such as the essential phospholipids (EPL), pyridoxal-phosphate (PP) and cynarin are still a matter of debate. Clinical trials with EPL, PP and cynarin in patients with high cholesterol have yielded inconclusive results, but in the test tube, at least, cynarin has impressive antioxidant and hepatoprotective actions.

Concerns: Artichoke-based products seem to be very safe. The only cause for concern might be the presence of an as yet unidentified component that has adverse effects on platelets and blood clotting. When 62 volunteers took an artichoke extract for two years, the ability of their platelets to aggregate (the first phase of the clotting process), was reduced by 51 percent. It is difficult to say whether such a reduction could become clinically important, but patients who have already been diagnosed with any bleeding disorder, or those taking anticoagulants, should probably not take artichoke supplements.

Warnings: None, except for the above noted patients with blood clotting disorders.

Drug Testing: None of the chemicals found in artichoke should interfere with standard workplace urine drug screening tests.

Dosage: The typical dose for extracts and tinctures is 300 to 1,200 milligrams per day. When whole powdered artichoke is being used, the dose may range from 1.5 to 6 grams per day.

Summary: Dried artichoke powder contains potent antioxidants that may have a role in preventing cancer, heart disease, and aging. Modern laboratory studies suggest that artichokes contain compounds that can protect the liver from external toxins such as carbon tetrachloride. There is even some evidence that traditional herbalists were right that artichokes promote the flow of bile. Claims that artichokes can lower cholesterol have yet to be proven. There are no reports of serious toxicity, although patients with bleeding disorders should be concerned about possible adverse effects on clotting.

References:

Adzet T, Camarasa J, Laguna JC. Hepatoprotective activity of polyphenolic compounds from *Cynara scolymus* against CCl4 toxicity in isolated rat hepatocytes. J Nat Prod 1987;50(4):612-7.

Fraga CG, Martino VS, Ferraro GE, Coussio JD, Boveris A. Flavonoids as antioxidants evaluated by in vitro and in situ liver chemiluminescence. Biochem Pharmacol 1987;36(5):717-20.

Gebhardt R. Antioxidative and protective properties of extracts from leaves of the artichoke (*Cynara scolymus L.*) against hydroperoxide-induced oxidative stress in cultured rat hepatocytes. Toxicol Appl Pharmacol 1997;144(2):279-86.

Kirchoff R, Beckers C, G K, et al. Increase in choleresis by means of artichoke extract. Phytomedicine 1994;1:107-15.

Scheffler W, Schwartzkopff W. Frequently used lipid-lowering drugs having no guaranteed effect. Artery 1980;8(2):120-7.

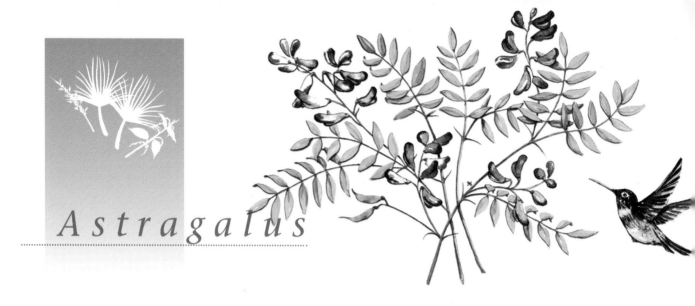

Astragalus

Name: *Astragalus membranaceus,* Fisch. (Leguminosae), commonly called Astragalus.

Source: This plant grows mainly in China. Remedies are made from the roots.

History: Roots of this plant have been used in traditional Chinese medicine for more than a thousand years. Astragalus root is the main ingredient in a medicine called "huang-qui" used to "replenish vital energy," reduce night sweats, and treat kidney disease. Astragalus is also included in another traditional formula called "Toki-shakuyaku-san" along with peony root, atractylodes lancea rhizome, alisma rhizome, hoelen, cinidium rhizome. The mixture is used to treat menstrual irregularities and vaginal infections.

Traditional Claims: Astragalus is used as a tonic and diaphoretic (something used to cause perspiration).

Commission E Recommendations: Astragalus is not on the Commission's list of approved herbs.

Proven Effects: During the 1980s there was some interest in using astragalus as a "hepatoprotective agent." In the laboratory, at least, extracts of the roots have the ability to protect liver cells from the damage that occurs after exposure to certain specific toxins. Extracts of this plant are potent lipoxygenase and cyclooxygenase (LOX and COX) inhibitors, which means they may have use as anti-inflammatory drugs. They also contain a flavonoid called astragalin (also found in many other members of the Leguminosae family), which may be a useful antioxidant. In one of the few clinical trials ever done, Chinese researchers found that treatment with "Toki-shakuyaku-san" normalized irregular menstrual cycles, healed cervical pseudo-erosions, and helped clear up vaginal discharges.

Concerns: Marketing surveys indicate that astragalus is one of the better selling herbal products in the United States, but very little has been written about the effects it produces - either good or bad. With so many individuals using this herb, and the total absence of toxicity case reports, it is reasonable to assume that astragalus is probably not very toxic.

Warning: None.

Drug Testing: It seems unlikely that any of the components of astragalus would interfere with standard workplace urine drug screening tests.

Dosage: The safe dosage range has not been determined.

Summary: Traditional healers in China and Japan have used astragalus for thousands of years, and it appears it may be useful in the treatment of some menstrual disorders. However, so little is known about this particular herb that it is difficult to make any sort of rational assessment. There are no reports of serious toxicity, but that does not necessarily mean that this particular herb can be used safely by everyone.

References:

Panter KE, James LF. Natural plant toxicants in milk: a review. J Anim Sci 1990;68(3):892-904.

Sakamoto S, Kudo H, Suzuki S, Sassa S, Yoshimura S, Nakayama T, et al. Pharmacotherapeutic effects of *toki-shakuyaku-san* on leukorrhagia in young women. Am J Chin Med 1996;24(2):165-8.

Zee-Cheng RK. *Shi-quan-da-bu-tang* (ten significant tonic decoction), SQT. A potent Chinese biological response modifier in cancer immunotherapy, potentiation and detoxification of anti-cancer drugs. Methods Find Exp Clin Pharmacol 1992;14(9):725-36.

Zhang ZL, Wen QZ, Liu CX. Hepatoprotective effects of astragalus root. J Ethnopharmacol 1990;30(2):145-9.

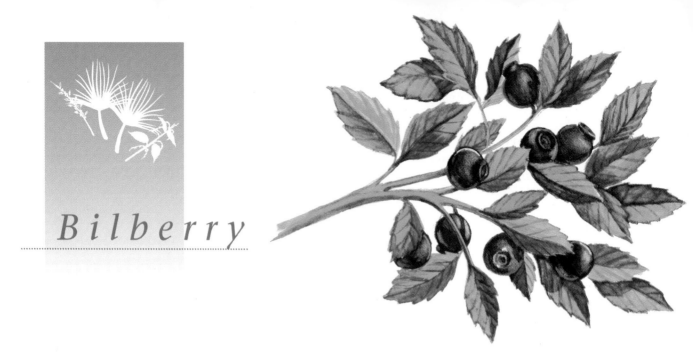

Name: *Vaccinium myrtillus* L., commonly called bilberry, huckleberry, whortleberry, and black-berry. The French for bilberry is *Myrtille;* in German, *Hiedelbeere.* Bilberry is a very close relative to cranberry and contains many of the same ingredients.

Source: *V. myrtillus,* known as bilberry, can be found in most European countries, but it is a hardier plant than its cousins, growing equally well in forests and moorlands. All contain flavonoids, phenolic acids, tannins, and glycosides in various proportions, depending on the variety, and from which part of the plant it is obtained.

Traditional Claims: Bilberry fruits have traditionally been used to treat acute cases of diarrhea. Extracts of the leaves have been used to treat diabetes, urinary tract infections, and as "metabolic stimulants."

Commission E Recommendations: Bilberry is used to treat diarrhea, oral or pharyngeal inflammation, and sore throat. Because of reports of jaundice associated with chronic use, the Commission placed the leaves on its unapproved list.

Proven Effects: Bilberry contains relatively high concentrations of flavonoids (quercetin and myrecetin) and anthocyanidins. In the test tube, these chemicals prevent the oxidation of low density cholesterol (LDL), and LDL oxidation leads to coronary artery disease. These same flavonols and anthocyanidins are found in red wines and grape juice. Many researchers believe their presence helps explain why the French, who drink much more red wine, and eat much more fat than Americans, have fewer heart attacks. In Germany, products made with bilberry fruit (but not the leaves), are used to treat diarrhea. Products made with bilberry leaf, however, are not approved for sale, because long-term use is associated with jaundice, weight loss, and possibly even seizures.

Concerns: There is not enough published information about bilberry for anyone to make an informed decision about its use. Based on the experience of European herbalists, use of the leaves could be dangerous.

Warnings: Only the fruit should be used.

Drug Testing: It seems unlikely that any of the components found in bilberry would interfere with standard workplace urine drug screening tests.

Dosage: For the treatment of diarrhea, Commission E recommends 20 to 60 grams per day of the fruit.

Summary: Bilberry seems to be an effective treatment for diarrhea (along with plantain, tormentil, and wild thyme). Whether bilberry is of value in treating elevated cholesterol is not clear. Leaves of this herb appear to contain toxic chemicals and should not be used.

References:

Cignarella A, Nastasi M, Cavalli E, Puglisi L. Novel lipid-lowering properties of Vaccinium myrtillus L. leaves, a traditional antidiabetic treatment, in several models of rat dyslipidaemia: a comparison with ciprofibrate. Thromb Res 1996;84(5):311-22.

Cristoni A, Magistretti MJ. Antiulcer and healing activity of *Vaccinium myrtillus* anthocyanosides. Farmaco [Prat] 1987;42(2):29-43.

Laplaud PM, Lelubre A, Chapman MJ. Antioxidant action of *Vaccinium myrtillus* extract on human low density lipoproteins in vitro: initial observations. Fundam Clin Pharmacol 1997;11(1):35-40.

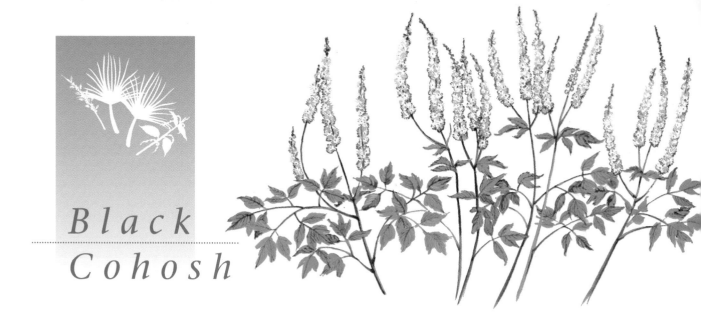

Black Cohosh

Name: *Cimicifuga racemosa* (L.), Elliot (Ranunculaceae), commonly called black cohosh. In German, it is *Cimicugawurzelstock*.

Source: A New World plant that grows mostly in the Eastern United States. Close relatives of the same *genus* grow in Europe and Asia.

History: The name *Cimicifuga* derives from the words *cimex* (a bug) and *fugo* (to drive away). Early sixteenth century physicians prescribed black cohosh to make menstrual periods regular, but also for just about every other condition they were called upon to treat.

Traditional Claims: Emmenagogue, nervine, bronchitic, snake bites, and use at birth.

Commission E Recommendations: Black cohosh is used to treat dysmenorrhea, premenstrual discomfort, PMS, and symptoms related to menopause. Black cohosh is also recommended for a variety of neurologic ailments.

Proven Effects: There have been nearly a dozen different human studies on the effectiveness of *Cimicifuga racemosa* for alleviating menopausal symptoms, especially hot flashes. Most have found that remedies made from this herb provide a safe, effective alternative to estrogen replacement therapy, but only for women who have refused estrogen replacement therapy or where estrogen replacement is contraindicated. That does not mean, however, that black cohosh contains estrogens; it does not, so any beneficial effects on menstrual or menopausal discomfort must be the consequence of some entirely unrelated action. In human volunteers, long-term treatment caused reduced levels of luteinizing hormone (LH), but levels of follice stimulating hormone (FSH) were not significantly altered.

Concerns: Black cohosh may relieve some menopausal symptoms, but since it contains no estrogen, taking this herb will do nothing to prevent osteoporosis or heart disease.

Warnings: None

Drug Testing: There are no reports of this herb interfering with any of the standard workplace urine drug screening tests.

Dosage: Commission E recommends using alcohol extracts in a dose corresponding to 40 milligrams per day. Usage should not exceed six months.

Summary: Controlled clinical trials have shown black cohosh to be an effective remedy for treating menopausal symptoms. But since it does not contain any estrogens, taking this herb will not prevent osteoporosis or heart disease. For most women, the best approach is probably to combine the use of black cohosh with standard estrogen replacement. For those who cannot take estrogen, black cohosh may offer a viable alternative. Reports of toxicity are very rare.

References:

Baillie N, Rasmussen P. Black and blue cohosh in labour [letter; comment]. N Z Med J 1997;110(1036):20-1.

Duker EM, Kopanski L, Jarry H, Wuttke W. Effects of extracts from *Cimicifuga racemosa* on gonadotropin release in menopausal women and ovariectomized rats. Planta Med 1991;57(5):420-4.

Einer-Jensen N, Zhao J, Andersen KP, Kristoffersen K. *Cimicifuga* and *Melbrosia* lack oestrogenic effects in mice and rats. Maturitas 1996;25(2):149-53.

Lieberman S. A review of the effectiveness of *Cimicifuga racemosa* (black cohosh) for the symptoms of menopause. J Womens Health 1998;7(5):525-9.

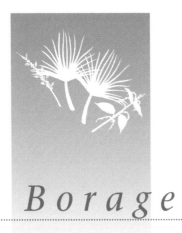

Borage

Name: *Borago officinalis L.* (Boraginceae), commonly called borage, bugloss, and burrage. In French, it is *Bourrache officinale*; in German, *Boretsch Gurkenkraut*.

Source: This family of plants came from the Mediterranean region, but borage has been cultivated in European herb gardens for many hundreds of years. Plants are said to have an odor like cucumbers, and probably for that reason, chopped leaves are sometimes added to salads. Oils extracted from borage, as well as oil extracted from evening primrose, black currant, and gooseberry (*Ribes uva crispa*) contain some of the same fatty acids found in fish oils.

History: One of the traditional uses of the herb had been to promote sweating. The name "borage" is said to derive from the arabic word *abu rach*, meaning "father of all sweat." The Greeks and Romans believed that borage could cure feelings of melancholy, but since they prepared their borage by soaking it in alcohol, it is hard to say whether it was the borage or the alcohol that improved their spirits. Traditional herbalists use borage as a diuretic. Until recently, claimed medical benefits were not taken very seriously. However, the oil extracted from the seeds, (which were never used by traditionalists) may yet turn out to be a useful food supplement.

Traditional Claims: Borage is used as a demulcent, diuretic, and stimulant.

Commission E Recommendations: Borage is not approved by Commission E, and the German government no longer permits its sale.

Proven Effects: No molecule with diuretic properties has ever been isolated from borage nor, for that matter, is there any reason to suppose borage causes sweating. But the seeds do contain large amounts (25 percent or more) of a fatty acid called gammalinolenic acid (GLA). This same product is found in fish oil and in evening primrose, the fruits of black currants, and in gooseberry. GLA plays a key role in human metabolism. Humans make GLA from another fatty acid called linoleic acid (LA), and in turn use GLA to produce components of the skin, blood cells, and a family of compounds involved in the inflammatory process (prostoglandins and leucotrienes) and in blood clotting.

Even though the body converts LA to GLA, just adding supplemental LA to the diet does not lead to increased levels of GLA in the body, and does absolutely nothing to increase levels of the important compounds made from GLA. But when GLA is added to the diet, levels of hormones made from GLA do increase. Based on these observations, GLA has been added to the diet of severely injured animals. Compared to animals that did not receive GLA, treated animals had higher levels of anti-inflammatory hormones and a higher rate of survival. Addition of GLA to the diet, but not LA, also prevented the activation of T lymphocytes, the type of white blood cells that is thought to be responsible for much of the pain and swelling in patients with rheumatoid arthritis. These effects are under active investigation at several major surgical centers.

Even more exciting are studies on using GLA to alter stress responses. It has been known for quite some time that exaggerated and inappropriate responses to stressful situations play a role in causing heart disease and high blood pressure. The traditional ways of fighting stress - exercise, relaxation and stress management training, do not always work. But, in one clinical study, men who were treated with borage oil responded better to experimental stress (their hearts did not beat as rapidly and their blood pressure did not go as high) as men treated with fish oil, olive oil, or controls (study participants who were given a placebo). The results suggest that GLA does something to counter the effects of stress hormones.

On the minus side, borage also contains very small amounts of a potentially dangerous alkaloid called pyrrolizidine. Much larger amounts of this same compound are to be found in the herb commonly known as comfrey (*Symphytum officinale*). Based on animal studies, it seems that pyrrolizidine itself is not toxic, but that once it gets into the body, the liver converts pyrrolizidine into compounds that may damage the lungs (primary pulmonary hypertension) and damage DNA. Damage to DNA translates into an increased risk for cancer.

Except for the oil extracted from the seeds, no one seriously claims any medicinal benefits for borage. But the GLA content of the oil is much higher than that of the evening primrose, and a number of conditions have been successfully treated with the latter. These include eczema, rheumatoid arthritis and premenstrual tension.

Concerns: High doses (24 grams/day) can increase the tendency of blood to clot spontaneously, but low doses normally recommended by traditional herbalists (3 grams/day) do not. The main worry is the pyrrolizidine content. Compared to other herbs, like comfrey, borage contains very little of this toxin (and apparently none in the flowers or fresh leaves), but there is some evidence that the toxin content of dried borage leaves increases with aging. The German government no longer permits the sale of borage.

Absorption is another problem. Variable amounts of GLAs are also found in black currant oil, evening primrose oil, and in the oils produced by some fungi. In animal studies comparing the effectiveness of treatment with the different GLA-containing oils, improvement could not be predicted based on GLA content alone. In experimental studies of diabetic nerve damage, improvement was seen with all the different oils, but the greatest improvement was seen after treatment with evening primrose. The different responses are explained by the fact that there are substances in all four oils that could affect GLA absorption. The message for consumers is that no matter what the label says, a high GLA content does not guarantee a greater effect or improved result. For GLA supplementation, evening primrose may be a better product than borage.

Warning: Except in certain specific disease states, there is no evidence that the body will benefit from increased GLA intake, and there is even some concern that too much GLA could dangerously increase the tendency of blood to clot. Too great an intake could also lead to increased exposure to cancer-causing toxins known to be present in the plant.

Drug Testing: Neither the plant, nor the oil extracted from the seeds, contain any compound known to interfere with workplace drug testing.

Dosage: The effective dose is not known with any certainty. Doses of 3 grams per day of oil seem to have no effect on blood clotting, but what other effect this dose might exert on the body is not known.

Summary: Fresh borage leaves and flowers might make a tasty addition to a salad, but medicinal benefits are hard to prove. The possible benefits of borage oil in the treatment of inflammatory disease are under serious investigation, but these studies are in the very early stages. Portions of the plant contain a known carcinogen, and borage products are banned in some countries.

References:

Bard JM, Luc G, Jude B, Bordet JC, Lacroix B, Bonte JP, et al. A therapeutic dosage (3 g/day) of borage oil supplementation has no effect on platelet aggregation in healthy volunteers. Fundam Clin Pharmacol 1997;11(2):143-4.

Fisher BA, Harbige LS. Effect of omega-6 lipid-rich borage oil feeding on immune function in healthy volunteers. Biochem Soc Trans 1997;25(2):343S.

Galle AM, Joseph M, Demandre C, Guerche P, Dubacq JP, Oursel A, et al. Biosynthesis of gamma-linolenic acid in developing seeds of borage (Borago officinalis L.). Biochim Biophys Acta 1993; 1158(1):52-8.

Gibson RA, Lines DR, Neumann MA. Gamma linolenic acid (GLA) content of encapsulated evening primrose oil products. Lipids 1992;27(1):82-4.

Mancuso P, Whelan J, DeMichele SJ, Snider CC, Guszcza JA, Karlstad MD. Dietary fish oil and fish and borage oil suppress intrapulmonary pro-inflammatory eicosanoid biosynthesis and attenuate pulmonary neutrophil accumulation in endotoxic rats. Crit Care Med 1997;25(7):1198-206.

Mills DE, Prkachin KM, Harvey KA, Ward RP. Dietary fatty acid supplementation alters stress reactivity and performance in man. J Hum Hypertens 1989;3(2):111-6.

Rossetti RG, Seiler CM, DeLuca P, Laposata M, Zurier RB. Oral administration of unsaturated fatty acids: effects on human peripheral blood T lymphocyte proliferation. J Leukoc Biol 1997;62(4):438-43.

Tollesson A, Frithz A. Borage oil, an effective new treatment for infantile seborrhoeic dermatitis [letter]. Br J Dermatol 1993; 129(1):95.

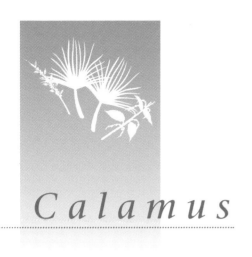

Calamus

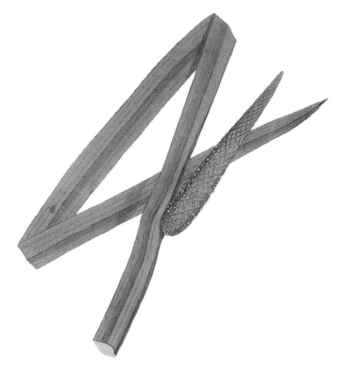

Name: *Acorus calamus* L. Var. *Americanus* Wulff or *A. calamus* L. Var. *Vulgaris* L., (Araceae) commonly called calamus, calamus root, sweet flag, rat root, sweet sedge, flag root, sweet calomel, sweet myrtle, sweet cane, sweet rush, beewort, muskrat root, and pine root. In French, it is *Acore vrai* or *Roseau aromatique*; in German, it is *Kalmus*.

Source: Calamus is a perennial herb that grows in swamps and marshes. The essential oil extracted from plants grown in Europe and Asia differs from the American variety. Roots and leaves are separated from the dried rhizomes, then ground to produce a pale, pink-tinged powder with a spicy smell and a slightly bitter taste. Calamus from Asia and India often contains so much toxic beta-asarone that it cannot (or should not) be used commercially.

History: Herbalists in India were the first to discover this plant. Ayurvedic practitioners used dried calamus to treat insomnia, melancholia, epilepsy and memory loss. Some North American Indians cultivated calamus and used it as a hallucinogen. In Europe, during the late 1800s, physicians used an alcoholic extract as a sedative and painkiller, although the main use has always been to calm upset stomachs (traditional herbalists call drugs that calm the stomach "carminatives"). For many years, American manufacturers used calamus as a flavoring in food and soft drinks. That practice was discontinued in the 1950s when it was discovered that one of the components of calamus oil caused cancer, at least in rats. Later studies showed that the offending component was not present in the variety of calamus grown in the United States, but commercial use of calamus as a food additive is still prohibited. Use of the plant by individuals, however, is legal. Today, interest has focused on the use of calamus as a hallucinogen and recreational drug.

Traditional Claims: Carminative, stomachic, stimulant and, in the Middle East, as an aphrodisiac.

Commission E Recommendations: This herb was not reviewed by Commission E.

Proven Effects: Many active constituents have been identified in the plant's oil, but the two compounds that have received the most attention are Alpha-asarone and Beta-asarone (cis-isomer). Beta-asarone is the component responsible for causing cancer in experimental animals. It is only present in calamus grown in Europe and Asia. The structure of both of the asarone molecules bears some resemblance to the structure of "ecstasy" (MDMA, 3,4-methylene-dioxymethamphetamine, an amphetamine-like drug), which probably accounts for the herb's psychoactive properties. Asarones tend to decompose overtime, and lose their psychoactive properties within a few months of harvesting.

Alpha-asarone is similar in structure to a drug called reserpine, used in the past as a sedative and as a treatment for high blood pressure. Calamus given to animals produces exactly those same effects. The structure of alpha-asarone also bears a very strong resemblance to a molecule called chlorpromazine, a very powerful medicine used to prevent vomiting, especially in surgical and chemotherapy patients. In spite of the similar structure, alpha-asarone produces exactly the opposite result - it causes vomiting. Other active ingredients are almost certainly present, but there have been so few serious pharmacologic studies that their nature remains a mystery. The main legitimate use for calamus is very much like that of chamomile - to treat stomach upset, and as a mild sedative. Large doses are said to be hallucinogenic. There is increasing interest in calamus as a legal, "recreational" drug.

Concerns: Calamus preparations, taken in sensible doses, appear to be quite safe. The problem for recreational drug users who chew whole roots in an attempt to get high, is that they have no way of knowing how much drug they are really taking. They run the risk of overdose. Taking too much calamus can lead to intractable vomiting. A few cases of skin rash (dermatitis) have also been reported. Concerns about cancer (see Federal Register 09 May 1968, 33 693) appear to be unfounded, at least for calamus grown in the United States.

Warnings: No dangerous drug interactions have been discovered.

Drug Testing: While there are no published reports, it is conceivable that calamus might cause a positive screening test for "ecstasy-like" drugs, but confirmatory testing would show that what was being detected was asarone, and not MDMA (3,4-methylenedioxymethamphetamine). Unfortunately for calamus users, if they are tested as a condition for preemployment, or under a non-federally mandated drug testing program, there is no requirement for the employer to do any confirmatory testing.

Dosage: The standard dose is 1 to 3 grams, dry or as a tea, three times a day. Liquid extracts, composed of equal parts of water and a 50 percent alcohol solution with calamus oil dissolved in it, is taken three times a day in a dose of 1-3 mL.

Summary: Calamus, in the recommended dose, may help calm an upset stomach, and perhaps calm the nerves. Large doses are said to have "ecstasy-like" (MDMA, 3,4-methylene-dioxymethamphetamine) effects, but users run the risk of intractable vomiting if they take too much. There is no evidence that calamus grown in the United States is carcinogenic, but buyers would be well advised to avoid calamus products made from plants grown in India and Asia (*A. Calamus* L. Var. *Vulgaris* L.). The possibility exists that taking large amounts of calamus may lead to a false positive urine drug test.

References:

Menon MK, Dandiya PC. The mechanism of the tranquillizing action of asarone from *Acorus calamus Linn*. J Pharm Pharmacol 1967;19(3):170-5.

Panchal GM, Venkatakrishna-Bhatt H, Doctor RB, Vajpayee S. Pharmacology of *Acorus calamus L.* Indian J Exp Biol 1989; 27(6):561-7.

Vargas CP, Wolf LR, Gamm SR, Koontz K. Getting to the root (*Acorus calamus*) of the problem [letter]. J Toxicol Clin Toxicol 1998;36(3):259-60.

Vohora SB, Shah SA, Dandiya PC. Central nervous system studies on an ethanol extract of *Acorus calamus rhizomes*. J Ethnopharmacol 1990;28(1):53-62.

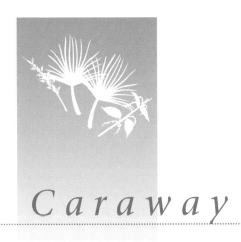

Caraway

Name: *Carum carvi*, L. (Umbelliferae), commonly called caraway seed. In French, it is *Cumin des prés* or *Carvi*; in German, *Wisenkümmel* or *Kümmel*.

Source: Caraway is a biennial that flowers from May through June. It is native to Europe and Northern Asia where it grows in the grasslands and mountainous regions. The medically active components of the plant are contained in an oil extracted from the dried seeds.

History: The name is said to come from the Arabic, *karawiya*. Caraway was cultivated in ancient Egypt, and was probably used before then. The medicinal use of caraway seeds is mentioned in the Bible. In Shakespeare's time, the roots were eaten as vegetables, and traditional herbalists recommended caraway to help improve digestion. Shakespeare even mentioned caraway in the *Merry Wives of Windsor*. Seeds were thrown at newly married couples to give them good luck. Caraway seeds have been used to make liqueurs ever since the process of alcoholic distillation was invented.

Traditional Claims: Antispasmodic, carminative, rubefacient, and to promote the appetite. Caraway was also used to treat menstrual cramps and promote the flow of breast milk.

Commission E Recommendations: Caraway is used to treat abdominal bloating, dyspepsia (upset stomach), and gastrointestinal spasm.

Proven Effects: Volatile oils from plants can be divided into two groups. Caraway oil belongs to the group containing mostly terpenoid compounds (along with camphor oil, cardamon oil, citronella, juniper, lemon, orange, pine, sandalwood, spearmint and even turpentine, among others). The two most important components of caraway oil are called carvone and limonene. Modern scientific studies are few and far between, but in a double-blind, placebo-controlled study, mixtures of caraway and peppermint (a European formulation called Enteroplant™) were more effective at relieving symptoms of indigestion than was the placebo. Anticancer effects have been demonstrated in laboratory animals, but not in humans. Nor has any clinical study ever confirmed traditional herbalist claims that caraway oil could increase the flow of breast milk or decrease menstrual cramping.

Concerns: Even minor side effects seem to be rare.

Warnings: None

Drug Testing: Caraway oil should not interfere with any of the known workplace urine drug screening tests.

Dosage: Teas can be made from crushed leaves (three teaspoons infused in one-half cup of water) or seeds (one teaspoon of finely crushed seeds allowed to steep in freshly boiled water for 15 minutes). The daily dosage of caraway seeds is 1.5-6 grams. If the oil is being used, the recommended dose is three to six drops per day.

Summary: Modern studies tend to confirm traditional claims that caraway oil, especially when it is combined with peppermint oil, can relieve stomach upset. Other claims remain unsubstantiated, but given the extremely low toxicity of caraway oil, there is no reason not to try it. Even if taking caraway does provide relief for stomach upset, persistent symptoms require medical evaluation.

References:

May B, Kuntz HD, Kieser M, Kohler S. Efficacy of a fixed peppermint oil/caraway oil combination in non-ulcer dyspepsia. Arzneimittelforschung 1996;46(12):1149-53.

Shwaireb MH. Caraway oil inhibits skin tumors in female BALB/c mice. Nutr Cancer 1993;19(3):321-5.

Zheng GQ, Kenney PM, Lam LK. Anethofuran, carvone, and limonene: potential cancer chemopreventive agents from dill weed oil and caraway oil. Planta Med 1992;58(4):338-41.

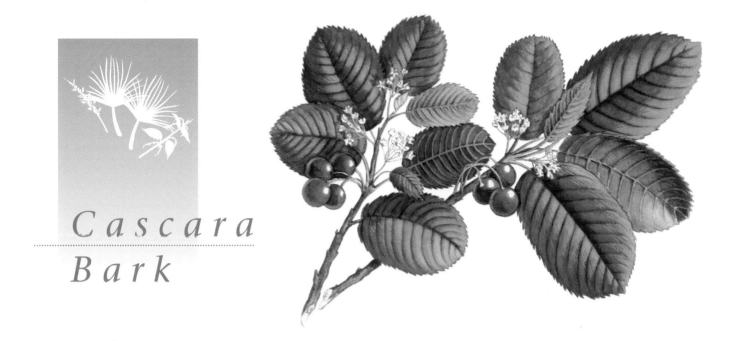

Cascara Bark

Name: *Rhamnus purshianus*, DC. (Rhamnaceae), commonly called cascara bark, or cascara. The very closely related *Rhamnus catharticus L.*, or European buckthorn is called *Neprun purgatif* in French; in German, *Kreuzdorn*.

Source: Cascara comes from the bark of a tree that is the North American relative of the Buckthorn (*Rhamnus frangula*). The latter grows throughout Europe and Asia. The active ingredients of both barks are effective laxatives. However, cascara bark must be allowed to age for at least one year before it is used. Unaged bark is much more potent than blackthorn, and if used fresh it can result in a violent gastrointestinal upset.

History: Certainly the safest of the herbal laxatives, cascara bark has been used for hundreds of years. Cascara and other anthracene-containing plants were first used for their pigments by the ancient Greeks and Romans. Their laxative properties were discovered in the Middle Ages.

Traditional Claims: Laxative and duprative (something used to purify the blood).

Commission E Recommendations: Cascara bark is used to treat constipation.

Proven Effects: Cascara bark and buckthorn belong to a group of plants that contain anthracene pigments. The name derives from the fact that they were first isolated from anthracite in 1832 (by the French chemists Dumas and Lambert). Cascara works in exactly the same way as aloe, Buckthorn, frangula bark, and senna. The active ingredients are inert in the upper gastrointestinal tract, but when they reach the large bowel they are converted to their active form (by removal of sugar molecules that are attached to the pigments). Once they have been converted, they cause water and electrolytes (vital body salts like sodium and potassium) to accumulate in the large intestine. As the volume of the large intestine increases, so does its internal pressure, and that causes the intestines to contract, resulting in a bowel movement. St. John's Wort also contains anthraquinones, but has no laxative effects because the sugar molecules are not split off in the intestines.

Concerns: As with aloe, small amounts of the anthracene pigments can be absorbed into the bloodstream. This means that the anthracene pigments may also appear in mother's milk, which is potentially dangerous for the child. As with all laxatives, chronic use may deplete the body of vital salts and electrolytes (particularly potassium), which in turn might cause the heart to beat in a dangerously irregular fashion.

Warnings: Experience has shown that cascara is an extremely safe drug, but it does contain some compounds that are known carcinogens, and used for more than a few weeks would be a very bad idea. As with aloe, prolonged use causes brownish pigment to be deposited in the wall of the intestines (melanosis coli). The pigment itself is harmless, and will go away when cascara is discontinued, but its presence is a sign of laxative abuse, and people with melanosis coli are at a much greater risk for colon cancer.

Drug Testing: Unlike aloe, cascara does not change the color of urine, and should not interfere with workplace urine drug screening tests.

Dosage: Cascara is usually taken in sugar-coated tablets, but liquid extracts and elixirs are also used. The dose is usually adjusted to contain 20-30 milligrams of the active agents (Cascarasides A, B, C, and D), the equivalent of .25 to 1 gram of the dried bark.

Summary: Cascara is a safe, effective laxative. It should not, however, be used on a long-term basis. Chronic constipation could reflect more serious underlying disease, and individuals with this problem should consult their doctor.

References:

de Witte P, Lemli L. The metabolism of anthranoid laxatives. Hepatogastroenterology 1990;37(6):601-5.

Izzo AA, Sautebin L, Rombola L, Capasso F. The role of constitutive and inducible nitric oxide synthase in senna- and cascara-induced diarrhoea in the rat. Eur J Pharmacol 1997;323(1):93-7.

Mereto E, Ghia M, Brambilla G. Evaluation of the potential carcinogenic activity of Senna and Cascara glycosides for the rat colon. Cancer Lett 1996;101(1):79-83.

Morton J. The detection of laxative abuse. Ann Clin Biochem 1987;24(Pt 1):107-8.

Petticrew M, Watt I, Sheldon T. Systematic review of the effectiveness of laxatives in the elderly. Health Technol Assess 1997;1(13):1-52.

Siegers CP, von Hertzberg-Lottin E, Otte M, Schneider B. Anthranoid laxative abuse—a risk for colorectal cancer? Gut 1993;34(8):1099-101.

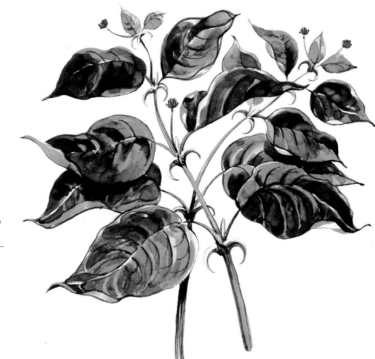

Cat's-Claw

...*mentosa* (Willdenow ex Roemer and Schultes) DC. (Rubiaceae), known in Peru ...is herb is totally unrelated to Cat's foot flower, or Cat's ear flower, *Antennaria*

...comes from the inside of the bark of a South American tree, one that is ...inchona, the source of quinine. Cat's-claw does not contain quinine, but it ...of the same compounds found in Cinchona. Cinnamon bark is another close

...ndians of Eastern Peru have traditionally used this bark to treat stomach ...is herb has recently been discovered by herbal drug manufacturers, who ...much the same way as ginseng, for its "natural immune-supporting" ...i-inflammatory, antiviral, antimutagenic and antioxidant.

...t's-claw is used to treat fevers and stomach upsets.

...nendations: Cat's-claw is not on the Commission's recommended list.

...sterol is the main sterol contained in the bark, and its presence appears ...anti-inflammatory properties. The bark also contains at least five dif-...ine, speciophylline, isopteropodine, uncarine F and isomytraphylline), ...le group alkaloids characteristically found in plants belonging to the ...hona and cinnamon). There has never been a controlled clinical trial ...-claw in humans. Results from the few toxicology studies that have ...t extracts of the bark possess little inherent toxicity.

...total and individual alkaloids, not to mention the amount of ...acids, and volatile oils vary depending on the age of the tree, where ...ot or branch bark is harvested. Producers in the United States tend ...to contain a set amount of oxindale alkaloids, but there is no ...f alkaloids (if in fact they are what confer the benefits), is present.

...al studies suggest that extracts of the bark possess little inherent ...to...clinical trials in humans are lacking, no one really knows for sure w... ...s-claw can be taken safely over an extended period.

Drug Testing: The molecular structure of some of the alkaloids found in cat's-claw is not that different from the structure of morphine, but no one has ever examined the standard workplace urine drug tests to see if they give false positive results when cat's-claw has been taken.

Dosage: Since it is not yet clear what conditions cat's-claw should be used to treat, discussing drug dosages does not make a great deal of sense. Cat's-claw is available in a number of different formulations, including dried powders, pills, and extracts. Unlike some herbs, such as chamomile, the active ingredients of cat's-claw dissolve in water. Therefore, high concentration extracts can be produced, and teas made with cat's-claw should be very effective.

Summary: Evidence suggests cat's-claw may have useful anti-inflammatory effects. Other claims are all unsubstantiated. There has never been a controlled clinical trial on this product. Animal toxicity studies suggest that there is nothing very toxic in cat's-claw bark, but long-term studies in humans are lacking.

References:

Santa Maria A, Lopez A, Diaz MM, Alban J, Galan de Mera A, Vicente Orellana JA, et al. Evaluation of the toxicity of *Uncaria tomentosa* by bioassays in vitro. J Ethnopharmacol 1997;57(3):183-7.

Senatore A, Cataldo A, Iaccarino FP, Elberti MG. [Phytochemical and biological study of *Uncaria tomentosa*]. Boll Soc Ital Biol Sper 1989;65(6):517-20.

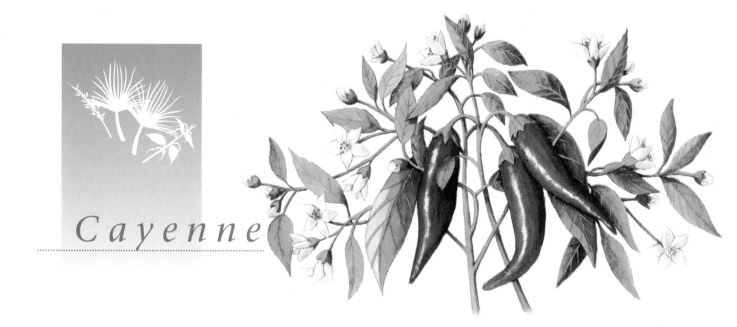

Cayenne

Name: *Capsicum frutescens* L. (Solanaceae). Also *Capsicum annuum* L., commonly called Capsicum, Chilies, Chillies, Tabasco pepper, and Paprika. In French, the herb is called *Piment* and *Paprika;* in German, *Paprika*, and *Spanischer Pfeffer.* The fleshy, bell shaped, green, red, and yellow peppers sold in supermarkets, are a related, but different, variety known as *C. annum var. Annum.*

Source: Originally native to South America, these plants are now grown in many temperate and tropical zones, especially in Africa, China and India. At least 50 different closely related cultivars are recognized. Paprika is made from the dried fruits of various *Capsicum* species. Cayenne pepper is made only from the fruits of *Capsicum frutescens*. Capsaicin is the main pungent (hot) principle of hot pepper, which is consumed in enormous quantities by people all around the world. The capsaicin content of some chili varieties ranges up to 0.53 percent. The bright red color of chilies comes from a carotenoid pigment called capsanthine.

History: The ancient Mayans used extracts of chilies as antibiotics, and modern studies confirm that, in fact, cayenne does have some antibiotic properties.

Traditional Claims: Poultices and liniments made from the dried fruits have been used to treat arthritis and muscle sprains. European herbalists recommend cayenne-containing formulations for "dyspepsia," a general term used to describe upset stomach. Within the last few years, there has been a tendency to include cayenne in formulations designed to prevent heart disease, improve memory, and enhance male sexual function.

Commission E Recommendations: Low dose capsaicin-cayenne products are used internally to treat digestive, stomach and gastrointestinal problems. External usage includes treatment for muscle spasms.

Proven Effects: In addition to containing substantial amounts of Vitamin C, chilies also contain a chemical called capsaicin (trans-8-methyl-N-vanillyl-6-nonenamide) which is what makes them taste hot. Capsaicin is currently used to treat various painful conditions such as rheumatoid arthritis and diabetic neuropathy. Initially, when capsaicin-containing creams are applied to the skin there is a burning feeling. But shortly afterwards there is pain relief. The relief is a result of interactions between the capsaicin molecule and nerves in the skin and muscles that transmit painful sensations. Capsaicin prevents these nerves from transmitting pain messages back to the brain (It does so by causing the nerves to deplete their supply of a neurotransmitter called "substance p.").

Because capsaicin is so irritating to the skin and mucous membranes, extracts are used by police as chemical crowd control agents ("pepper spray," also called oleoresin capsicum spray). When the spray comes in contact with mucous membranes, such as the insides of the eye lids, there is temporary, but very intense pain and swelling. The same sort of thing can happen if the eyes are inadvertently touched when cutting fresh chilies, or when handling capsaicin creams or herbal products. Claims that internal use of cayenne can aid digestion, or external use of cayenne can improve arthritis (as opposed to just relieving arthritis pain), have never been proven.

Capsaicin applied to the skin will cause blood vessels in the skin to dilate (which is why the skin gets red where the capsaicin has been applied), but capsaicin does not cause any changes in the blood vessels controlling blood pressure. Claims that capsaicin can be used to treat high blood pressure are spurious. Additional claims that cayenne, alone, or in combination with other herbs can improve memory and sex life, or lower cholesterol, have never been tested, let alone proven.

Concerns: Because so many people use so much cayenne, and because it appears to be such a potent agent, questions have been repeatedly raised about possible links between cancer and chili peppers. The results have been conflicting, and clear evidence, one way or the other, is lacking.

Warnings: When using these products, great care must be taken not to get them in the eyes, or in open cuts on the hands or elsewhere.

Drug Testing: Peppers are not known to contain any materials that will interfere with standard workplace drug screening tests.

Dosage: According to Commission E, liquid preparations should be standardized to contain no more than .005 to .01 percent capsaicinoids. Poultices should deliver no more than 40 grams of capsaicinoids per square centimeter and should not be used for more than two consecutive days.

Summary: Capsaicin-containing creams may well reduce some of the pain associated with arthritis and joint inflammation, as well as the pain resulting from some sprains and injuries. What good, if any, oral cayenne supplements provide is not known. Concerns about cancer in long-term users have never been substantiated and would not, in any case, apply to periodic use of a skin cream. Users should be extremely careful handling these products since they can cause severe discomfort if they get into the eyes, or any open cuts or abrasions.

References:

Cichewicz RH, Thorpe PA. The antimicrobial properties of chile peppers (Capsicum species) and their uses in Mayan medicine. J Ethnopharmacol 1996;52(2):61-70.

Govindarajan VS, Sathyanarayana MN. Capsicum—production, technology, chemistry, and quality. Part V. Impact on physiology, pharmacology, nutrition, and metabolism; structure, pungency, pain, and desensitization sequences. Crit Rev Food Sci Nutr 1991;29(6):435-74.

Surh YJ, Lee SS. Capsaicin in hot chili pepper: carcinogen, co-carcinogen or anticarcinogen? Food Chem Toxicol 1996;34(3):313-6.

Toth B, Gannett P. Carcinogenicity of lifelong administration of capsaicin of hot pepper in mice. In Vivo 1992;6(1):59-63.

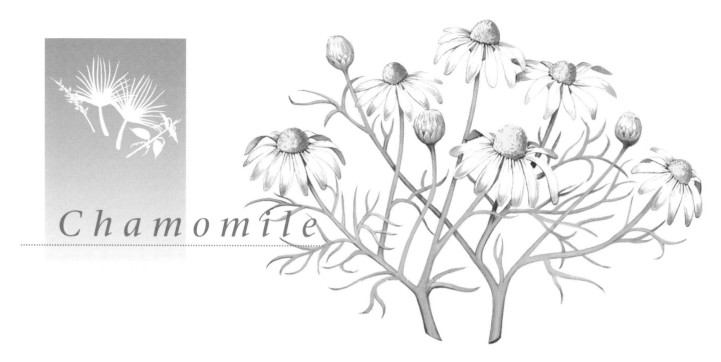

Chamomile

Name: Two different plants share the name chamomile, and a third, with a different name, contains many of the same chemicals. All three belong to the Compositae family of plants. The most widely used chamomile is known as the German or Hungarian chamomile (*Matricaria recutita* or *Chamomilla recutita,* or *Matricaria chamomilla*). The other chamomile is sometimes called Roman or English chamomile (*Chamomillae romanae flos, Chamaemelum, Anthemis, Anthemidis flos,*) and sometimes, just plain chamomile. A third, and very closely related plant is a flowering herb known as yarrow or milfoil (*Archillea millefolium*). In France the plant is variously referred to as *Chamomille, Vvraie, and Petite Chamomille*; in German, *Kamille* or *Echte Kamille.*

Source: The German chamomile is the main one grown commercially, both in Europe and the United States. It can be grown from seeds planted in any garden. Indeed, given half a chance, it will grow like a weed, which is exactly what has happened in Boulder, Colorado, where the Celestial Seasonings Company, a manufacturer of herbal teas, is located. Reportedly, seeds that have escaped from the factory have taken root all along the roadsides. Not only is German chamomile easier to grow, it also contains more of the oils that give chamomile its unique medicinal properties. Dried flowers of English chamomile have an oil content of .5 to 1.0 percent. German chamomile may contain twice that amount. Once the oil is distilled from the flowers, it takes on a characteristic blue color. Seven distinct groups of chemicals have been found in the oil, but their effects are only beginning to be understood.

History: Europeans have used chamomile, in one form or another, to treat just about every sort of affliction. *Culpeper's Complete Herbal*, published in 1827, recommends it for "drying and binding," claims "it is excellent for treating hemorrhoids," and that "it induces sleep and lessens bleeding. An ointment of the leaves cures wounds, and is good for inflammation, ulcers, fistulas, and all such runnings as about with moisture."

Traditional Claims: Chamomile is used as an antispasmodic, sedative, diuretic and demulcent.

Commission E Recommendations: Chamomile is recommended for the treatment of ano-genital irritation, bad breath, gastrointestinal tract inflammation, gastrointestinal spasm, inflamed gums, oral or pharyngeal inflammation, mucous membrane irritations, chronic respiratory infection, skin injury or irritation, spasms, and as a gargle or mouthwash.

Proven Effects: All of the active components in chamomile flowers are in the oil, which means that teas brewed from chamomile will contain only small amounts of the active components. *Culpeper's* claims are, however, at least partially true. Chamomile does have anti-inflammatory properties and it has also been shown to exert antibacterial effects. These two actions have been attributed to the molecules that give the oil its blue color, and to another molecule contained in the oil called bisabolol. The latter, along with a flavonoid molecule called apigenin, are thought to account for chamomile's ability to calm the stomach ("spasmolytic" actions). Bisabolol, because of its anti-inflammatory properties, is also said to aid in wound healing and in the treatment of chronic skin conditions such as eczema. Sugar residues contained in the oil (polysaccharides), help stimulate the immune system.

Flavonoids found in chamomile oil (apigenin) are increasingly being recognized for their important beneficial effects. Flavonoids exert multiple actions, and their presence helps explain some of the beneficial results that chamomile users have been reporting for years. For example, chamomile is widely used to treat insomnia. Now it turns out that the apigenin molecule has a shape a bit like the shape of the active ingredient in synthetic sleeping pills and tranquilizers such as Valium™ and Halcyon™. Because of the structural similarities between apigenin and Valium™, apigenin is able to attach at the same sites in the brain as Valium™ and probably exerts the same effects. Other studies suggest apigenin prevents the reuptake of neurotransmitters, which means that it acts in the same way as Prozac™-like drugs.

Chamomile's ability to reduce inflammation is also thought to be a result of its apigenin content. Like some of the anti-inflammatory drugs just now reaching the market, apigenin blocks the cytokine pathway and prevents inflammation from occurring. Other studies have shown that some components of chamomile oil prevent mast cells from releasing histamine, and since histamine is what causes many of the symptoms associated with allergic reactions, this may explain why many people claim that chamomile gives them relief from their allergies.

Chamomile is also said to be an antiseptic, but when this claim was tested in controlled trials, it turned out that iodine (povidine-iodine, known as Betadine™) was far more effective at killing bacteria than chamomile. Similar claims, that chamomile can prevent the inflammation of the mouth (stomatitis) in patients undergoing chemotherapy, also failed to stand up in control trials.

Chamomile is widely used in the cosmetics industry and can be found in shampoos, hair rinses, and even as a vegetable hair dye. Perhaps the most controversial benefit claimed for chamomile is the prevention of heart disease. A famous study published in the *Lancet* in 1993 found that high intakes of flavonoids, like the apigenin contained in chamomile, prevented heart disease. Even the vapors of chamomile oil appear to have beneficial effects. Although many of the claims made by aromatherapists remain unproven, studies in animals have shown that inhalation of chamomile oil vapor can, at least partly, block the hormonal response to stress.

Concerns: Allergic reactions to chamomile, though uncommon, are a cause for concern. During hay fever season, especially in Europe, some allergy sufferers attempt to relieve redness and itching by rinsing their eyes with chamomile tea. Unfortunately, chamomile tea also contains chamomile pollens and those pollens are very similar to pollens of other common allergens. Someone allergic to one of the related pollens could have an unpleasant, though certainly not life-threatening, reaction. Whether or not life-threatening allergic reactions ever occur is unclear. But if they do, they must be incredibly rare. A few such reports can be found in the older literature, but none has appeared for the last 15 years. Given that millions of people use chamomile on a daily basis, it is hard to imagine that this particular herb poses much of a danger.

Warnings: Individuals with serious hay fever symptoms should see their physicians before self-medicating with chamomile. Newer treatments may go a long way towards eliminating the problem, and a physician can arrange tests to see whether an individual is allergic to chamomile, and determine whether chamomile can be safely used.

Drug Testing: None of the chemicals found in chamomile oil has ever been known to cause a false positive result on any of the standard urine drug screening tests.

Dosage: Europeans have access to more dosage forms than Americans. In Germany, France, and England, chamomile is sold in rinses, gargles, ointments and alcohol extracts. Dried flowers can be added to bath water to relieve skin conditions, but it would take several pounds of flowers to produce much of a result. A standard packet of chamomile tea contains about 2 grams of the powdered flowers. In Germany, government-required labeling, which allows manufacturers to claim that their chamomile-containing products are good for bloating, flatulence, and gastrointestinal disorders, specifies that one tablespoon (2-3 grams) of flowers should be allowed to steep in hot water for 5-10 minutes before being passed through a tea strainer and drunk four times a day. External preparations are formulated to 3-10 percent herb.

Summary: Anecdotal evidence suggests that chamomile will help people sleep and may help calm their nerves and stomachs. Modern neurochemical studies seem to have provided a rational basis for these claims, but allergy suffers should be very careful about how they use these products. The jury is still out on the tranquilizing effects of the chamomile components, but some of the research looks very promising, as does the evidence that apigenin is an antioxidant that might help prevent heart disease. Serious toxicity is an extraordinarily rare event, and most people can use this herb safely.

References:

Fidler P, Loprinzi CL, O'Fallon JR, Leitch JM, Lee JK, Hayes DL, et al. Prospective evaluation of a chamomile mouthwash for prevention of 5-FU-induced oral mucositis. Cancer 1996;77(3):522-5.

Hertog MG, Feskens EJ, Hollman PC, Katan MB, Kromhout D. Dietary antioxidant flavonoids and risk of coronary heart disease: the Zutphen Elderly Study. Lancet 1993;342(8878):1007-11.

Lorenzo PS, Rubio MC, Medina JH, Adler-Graschinsky E. Involvement of monoamine oxidase and noradrenaline uptake in the positive chronotropic effects of apigenin in rat atria. Eur J Pharmacol 1996;312(2):203-7.

Read MA. Flavonoids: naturally occurring anti-inflammatory agents [comment]. Am J Pathol 1995;147(2):235-7.

Salgueiro JB, Ardenghi P, Dias M, Ferreira MB, Izquierdo I, Medina JH. Anxiolytic natural and synthetic flavonoid ligands of the central benzodiazepine receptor have no effect on memory tasks in rats. Pharmacol Biochem Behav 1997;58(4):887-91.

Subiza J, Subiza JL, Alonso M, Hinojosa M, Garcia R, Jerez M, et al. Allergic conjunctivitis to chamomile tea. Ann Allergy 1990;65(2):127-32.

Yamada K, Miura T, Mimaki Y, Sashida Y. Effect of inhalation of chamomile oil vapour on plasma ACTH level in ovariectomized-rat under restriction stress. Biol Pharm Bull 1996;19(9):1244-6.

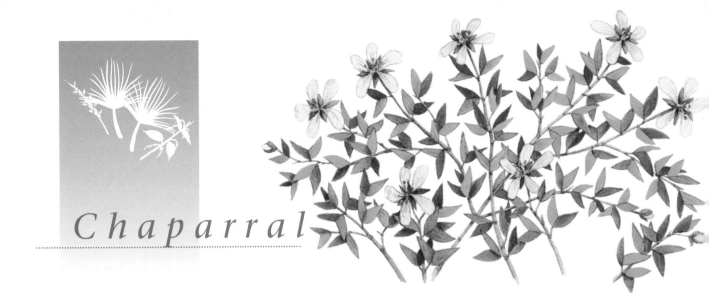

Chaparral

Name: Larrea *divaricata* Cav. and L. *mexicana* Moric., *Larrea tridentada* (De Candolle) Coville, (Zygophyllaceae) commonly called chaparral, creosote bush, or greasewood.

Source: The name chaparral refers to an assortment of shrubs that grow in the Southwest deserts of the United States and Mexico. Active ingredients are found in the leaves and twigs.

History: American Indians used a tea brewed from the leaves to treat arthritis, respiratory infections, and even cancer. Spanish explorers brewed and drank chaparral tea in hopes of curing (probably without much success) the venereal disease they brought with them to the New World. A compound found in the leaves, nordihydroguaiarectic acid (NDGA), is a potent antioxidant. Some thought it might be used to prevent cancer. NDGA was used as a food preservative in the United States until 1967 when, acting on evidence that chronic exposure can cause cancer in experimental animals, the Federal Drug Administration (FDA) removed it from the General Recognized As Safe (GRAS) list, and researchers gave up on the idea of using NDGA to prevent cancer.

Traditional Claims: Febrifuge, expectorant

Commission E Recommendations: Chaparral was not reviewed by Commission E.

Proven Effects: NDGA is classified as a cyclooxygenase and lipoxygenase inhibitor. Drugs in this category control the formation of a group of hormones known as leukotrienes which, in turn, mediate the inflammatory process. Cyclooxygenase inhibitors are used to treat arthritis, and lipoxygenase inhibitors are thought to be especially important in asthma. Zileuton™, the new asthma medication from Abbott Laboratories, is a lipoxygenase inhibitor. The down side to lipoxygenase inhibitors, naturally or synthetic, is that they may cause liver damage. In addition to using chaparral for respiratory infections and arthritis, it has also been recommended for weight loss, used as a burn salve, touted as a way to "purify" the blood and "remove toxins," and promoted as a "free radical scavenger" that can prevent aging.

Concerns: Synthetic lipoxygenase and cyclooxygenase inhibitors can cause liver damage, so it would not be very surprising if it turned out that the herbal forms of these drugs could also cause such damage. And, indeed, reports compiled by the Office of Special Nutritionals at the FDA suggest that users of chaparral products are at risk for liver damage, perhaps even liver failure. A report, published in 1997, described 13 cases of severe liver injury, but the exact mechanism in these cases remains unclear. About the only thing that is known for sure is that the liver damage was not due to NGDA. No liver damage was seen in volunteers given up to 400 mg per day of NGDA (100 times more than the amount taken per day by chaparral users who did develop liver damage). Most of the individuals with liver damage were taking powdered chaparral in capsules (400-500 mg), but investigation of the cases did not disclose any obvious connection between the total amount of chaparral taken and the severity of the reactions. Other published reports have described kidney damage and skin reactions, especially after the use of pure NDGA extracted from chaparral leaves. Such reports are, however, quite rare.

Warnings: There is no question that kidney and liver damage occurs in rats fed NDGA on a long-term basis. The same sort of reaction probably also occurs in humans. There is one case report, describing a woman who ingested very large quantities of powdered chaparral over a long period, who developed a kidney cancer with features that resembled exactly those seen in the rats fed high doses of NDGA. One case does not, of course, prove a connection, but the changes in the laboratory animals are worrisome.

Drug Testing: Chaparral should not interfere with any of the currently used workplace urine drug screening tests.

Dosage: Leaves and stems contain 7 percent NGDA, along with the other chemical constituents. When teas are brewed from the leaves, only 40 percent of the NGDA is dissolved in the water (no one knows for sure about the other constituents). The lower NGDA content may explain why the teas seem to be less toxic than products prepared from the dried leaves. The effective dosage range in humans is not known with any certainty.

Summary: Traditional claims that chaparral is an anti-inflammatory, good for treating respiratory infections and arthritis, may very well be true. Chemicals in chaparral leaf are lipoxygenase and cyclooxygenase inhibitors, no different from those now used by physicians to treat asthma and arthritis. The problem is that compounds with lipoxygenase and cyclooxygenase activity, natural or synthetic, can cause liver damage. Some evidence suggests that users are less likely to get into trouble if they confine themselves to chaparral tea, which contains a lower concentration of the active ingredients than powdered leaf. Years ago, the FDA declared NDGA unsafe for human use. If the main reason for taking NDGA is to get the antioxidant, anti-aging effects, there are many other safer options. Consumers may want to consider substituting Vitamin E. It is nontoxic, and nearly as potent an antioxidant.

References:

Alderman S, Kailas S, Goldfarb S, Singaram C, Malone DG. Cholestatic hepatitis after ingestion of chaparral leaf: confirmation by endoscopic retrograde cholangiopancreatography and liver biopsy. J Clin Gastroenterol 1994;19(3):242-7.

Batchelor WB, Heathcote J, Wanless IR. Chaparral-induced hepatic injury. Am J Gastroenterol 1995;90(5):831-3.

From the Centers for Disease Control and Prevention. Chaparral-induced toxic hepatitis—California and Texas, 1992. JAMA 1992;268(23):3295, 8.

Gordon DW, Rosenthal G, Hart J, Sirota R, Baker AL. Chaparral ingestion. The broadening spectrum of liver injury caused by herbal medications [see comments]. JAMA 1995;273(6):489-90.

Smith AY, Feddersen RM, Gardner KD, Jr., Davis CJ, Jr. Cystic renal cell carcinoma and acquired renal cystic disease associated with consumption of chaparral tea: a case report. J Urol 1994;152(6 Pt 1):2089-91.

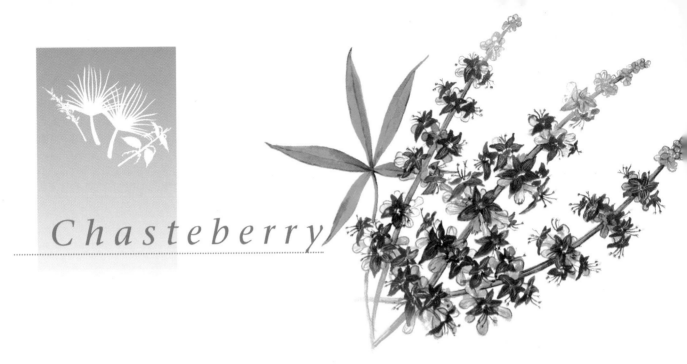

Chasteberry

Name: *Vitex agnus castus* L. (Verbenaceae), commonly called the Chaste tree, Monk's pepper tree, Abraham's balm, and wild pepper. In German it is *Keuschlammfrüchte*.

Source: Remedies are made from the fruits of wild trees, usually supplied whole. This tree came from the Mediterranean region, but now grows in the United States. The word *Vitex* is the old Latin name for the plant. *Agnus*, of course, means lamb, and *castus* is latin for chaste.

History: The name derives from the fact that, in Medieval Europe, this tree was held to be the symbol of chastity. Drinking tea made from the leaves was thought to decrease the libido, which is why the medieval monks drank it in great quantities. Chinese herbalists reached the same conclusions about this plant and used it in the same way as the Europeans. Today, this herb is widely used by Germans to treat menstrual disorders and to promote ovulation.

Traditional Claims: Galactogenic, emmenagogue, cholagogue, carminative, rheumatic, and for the treatment of impotence.

Commission E Recommendations: Chasteberry is used for the regulation of irregular menstrual cycles, premenstrual complaints, PMS, poor lactation, and sore or tender breasts.

Proven Effects: The barks of chasteberry contains at least four different flavonoids. One, called leutolin, is also found in artichokes and is thought to account for that plant's ability to lower cholesterol levels (leutolin prevents cholesterol synthesis). This same flavonoid is also a powerful anti-inflammatory agent and an antioxidant. Extracts of this plant cause the brain to produce less of a hormone called prolactin, which is why, in controlled clinical trials of women with menstrual irregularities, treatment with extracts of chaste tree fruit tends to normalize menstrual flow. Since treatment with this herb clearly reduces prolactin blood concentrations, and since the production of breast milk is partly under the control of prolactin, chaste tree may help improve milk production. That possibility, however, has never been studied in a clinical trial.

Concerns: Some individuals will experience itchy skin and possibly develop a rash if the herb is taken regularly.

Warnings: Episodes of serious toxicity have never been reported, and there are no reports of dangerous drug interactions.

Drug Testing: None of the components of chaste tree extract should interfere with any of the standard workplace urine drug screening tests.

Dosage: Commission E recommends that when this herb is used to treat menstrual irregularities, a total dose of 30 to 40 milligrams per day, of the alcohol extract should be used.

Summary: The results of controlled clinical trials indicate that chaste tree extract reduces abnormally high blood concentrations of prolactin and normalizes menstrual cycles. That action might help diminish some of the symptoms of premenstrual syndrome, although that benefit has never been proven. There is very solid laboratory evidence that the flavonoid molecules contained in this plant can lower blood cholesterol and act as free radical scavengers. Toxicity from this plant is, apparently, an extremely rare event and it should be a safe herb to use.

References:

Brown JE, Khodr H, Hider RC, Rice-Evans CA. Structural dependence of flavonoid interactions with Cu2+ ions: implications for their antioxidant properties. Biochem J 1998;330(Pt 3):1173-8.

Cahill DJ, Fox R, Wardle PG, Harlow CR. Multiple follicular development associated with herbal medicine [see comments]. Hum Reprod 1994;9(8):1469-70.

Gebhardt R. Inhibition of cholesterol biosynthesis in primary cultured rat hepatocytes by artichoke (*Cynara scolymus L.*) extracts. J Pharmacol Exp Ther 1998;286(3):1122-8.

Hirobe C, Qiao ZS, Takeya K, Itokawa H. Cytotoxic flavonoids from *Vitex agnus-castus.* Phytochemistry 1997;46(3):521-4.

Milewicz A, Gejdel E, Sworen H, Sienkiewicz K, Jedrzejak J, Teucher T, et al. [*Vitex agnus castus* extract in the treatment of luteal phase defects due to latent hyperprolactinemia. Results of a randomized placebo- controlled double-blind study]. Arzneimittelforschung 1993;43(7):752-6.

Sliutz G, Speiser P, Schultz AM, Spona J, Zeillinger R. *Agnus castus* extracts inhibit prolactin secretion of rat pituitary cells. Horm Metab Res 1993;25(5):253-5.

Ramesh M, Rao YN, Rao AV, Prabhakar MC, Rao CS, Muralidhar N, et al. Antinociceptive and anti-inflammatory activity of a flavonoid isolated from Caralluma attenuata. J Ethnopharmacol 1998;62(1):63-6.

Veal L. Complementary therapy and infertility: an Icelandic perspective. Complement Ther Nurs Midwifery 1998;4(1):3-6.

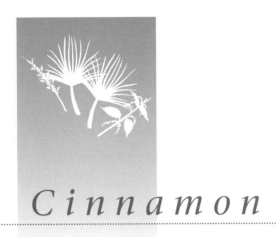

C i n n a m o n

Name: *Cinnamomum verum*, Nees (Lauraceae). Commonly called cinnamon or Ceylon cinnamon. In French it is *Cannelier de Ceylon*; in German, *Zimtbaum*. This plant is very closely related to the plant that provides camphor (*Laurus camphora or Camphora officinarum*).

Source: This widely used spice comes from the inner and outer bark of a tree that can grow to more than 40 feet high. But for commercial purposes, the plants are maintained as bushes, seven to 10 feet high, that are pruned every year. The bark and leaves contain several different fragrant spices. Cinnamaldehyde, the main component of the oil extracted from the bark, is the substance referred to when people think of cinnamon, the spice. The leaves, however, contain large amounts of eugenol, the main oil found in cloves.

History: Like pine oil, cinnamon has been used for thousand of years, but mostly as a food flavoring, and it never seemed to play a particularly important role among traditional herbalists. Eugenol has, of course, been used for years as a topical anesthetic.

Traditional Claims: Stomachic and tonic.

Commission E Recommendations: For loss of appetite, dyspepsia (upset stomach), bloating and flatulence

Proven Effects: This herb has only recently become the subject of serious research efforts, and the preliminary findings are encouraging. Studies have shown that spices such as cloves, bay leaves, tumeric, and cinnamon improve the ability of isolated cells to metabolize fats. This seems to be the result of the ability of these herbs, particularly cinnamon, to increase the effectiveness of insulin. Extracts of Brewers yeast seem to have the same effect. Although it is far too early to pass judgment, this ability might someday improve treatment outcomes for diabetics. Other studies have shown that cinnamon is a potent fungicide and suggest that it might be used to treat fungal infections of the respiratory tract, particularly some of the infections seen in patients with compromised immune systems, such as those with HIV. Controlled clinical trials have shown more rapid healing in HIV-infected patients suffering from thrush (oral candida), than in controls given only placebo. Still other laboratory tests have demonstrated antibacterial effects, but these have not been proven in humans.

Concerns: Excessive use of cinnamon (such as might be seen in gum chewers) is thought to be the cause of unexplained oral pain. Patients presenting at the dentist with unexplained oral pain and sores seem to be becoming more common. Some dentists think this increase may have to do with the increasing popularity of cinnamon as a food flavoring. The pain and sores invariably disappear when the cinnamon-containing products are discontinued.

Warnings: None. Significant episodes of toxicity have never been reported.

Drug Testing: None of the components in cinnamon, or cinnamon oil, should interact with or affect any of the normally used workplace urine drug screening tests.

Dosage: Commission E recommends 2 to 4 grams of bark per day, or the equivalent amount of essential oil (0.05 to 0.2 grams per day).

Summary: Cinnamon has been a popular flavoring for thousands of years, but has only recently attracted the attention of serious medical researchers. And what these researchers are finding is exciting, especially for diabetics. But, except for HIV patients with thrush, there is little hard evidence that there are any benefits to be derived form using cinnamon-containing products. On the other hand, the risk of use appears to be minimal, and there would certainly be no reason not to experiment with cinnamon-containing products. If unexplained mouth pain is experienced, it probably is a consequence of irritation produced by the cinnamon.

References:

Azumi S, Tanimura A, Tanamoto K. A novel inhibitor of bacterial endotoxin derived from cinnamon bark. Biochem Biophys Res Commun 1997;234(2):506-10.

Imparl-Radosevich J, Deas S, Polansky MM, Baedke DA, Ingebritsen TS, Anderson RA, et al. Regulation of PTP-1 and insulin receptor kinase by fractions from cinnamon: Implications for cinnamon regulation of insulin signalling. Horm Res 1998;50(3):177-82.

Singh HB, Srivastava M, Singh AB, Srivastava AK. Cinnamon bark oil, a potent fungitoxicant against fungi causing respiratory tract mycoses. Allergy 1995;50(12):995-9.

Smith-Palmer A, Stewart J, Fyfe L. Antimicrobial properties of plant essential oils and essences against five important food-borne pathogens. Lett Appl Microbiol 1998;26(2):118-22.

Yamasaki K, Nakano M, Kawahata T, Mori H, Otake T, Ueba N, et al. Anti-HIV-1 activity of herbs in Labiatae. Biol Pharm Bull 1998;21(8):829-33.

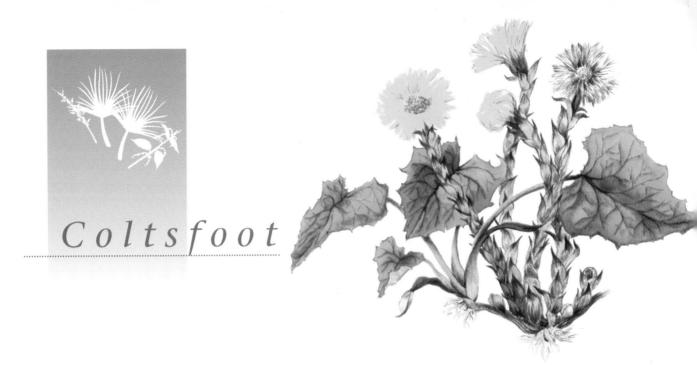

Coltsfoot

Name: *Tussilago farfara* L. (Compositae), commonly called coltsfoot. Closely related species called *Petasites* are native to the western United States. In French, it is *Tussilage*, or *Taconnet*, or *Pas-d'ane*; in German, *Huflattich*.

Source: *T. farfara* is native to Europe, but is now grown in the northeastern United States. *Petasites* species (*hybridus, formosanus*) contain many of the same ingredients, and some unique ingredients, as well.

History: Coltsfoot is an ancient remedy, mentioned both by Pliny and Dioscorides. Teas made with the leaves and flowers have been used as expectorants for more than a thousand years. Even before coltsfoot was used in Europe, traditional Chinese herbalists used Kuandong Hua (*Tussilago farfara* L.) to treat respiratory illnesses. Extracts of *Petasites hybridus* L., have been used to treat gastrointestinal pain, lung-diseases, and urinary tract pain for nearly as long as *T. Farfara*.

Traditional Claims: Coltsfoot is used as an expectorant and emollient. In Europe, a concoction called Alzoon™, containing extracts of petasites, juniper, ferns, brunellias, and dandelions, treated with oxygen and UV-light, is sold as a cure for cachexia, abdominal pain, and the anemia resulting from malignant tumors. It is still a popular, though completely unvalidated, remedy.

Commission E Recommendations: Coltsfoot is used to treat cough, hoarseness, oral or pharyngeal inflammation, respiratory catarrh, sore throat, and upper respiratory tract catarrh (inflammation).

Proven Effects: Coltsfoot seems to be a reasonably effective expectorant, although why that should be, no one knows for sure. Unfortunately, the leaves and flowers of this plant contain pyrrolizidine alkaloids (PAs). More than 150 different PAs are recognized. Taken in sufficient doses over a long period of time, PAs cause liver damage. Specifically, they cause the linings of the veins in the liver to scar, obstructing the flow of blood through the liver, and ultimately, leading to liver failure and death. They also cause cancer, at least in laboratory animals (see Chapter 4 for a more complete discussion of PAs). In addition to PAs, *Petasites* species also contain several compounds that may have important medical applications. One, called Bakkenolide G, is a natural antagonist of platelet activating factor (PAF) which means it might be used to prevent strokes and heart attacks. Another compound, contained in an alcohol-based extract of *Petasites,* blocks the production of leukotrienes - inflammatory hormones that are thought to play a role in ulcer formation.

Concerns: Liver damage may occur with high doses or long-term use of coltsfoot. There is one case report of an 18-month-old boy with liver damage, who had been fed an herbal tea mixture from the time he was three months old. The tea contained peppermint, and what the mother thought was coltsfoot. Testing showed that the tea did, indeed, contain dangerous amounts of pyrrolizidine alkaloids. But when the physicians treating the child examined the leaves the mother had picked to make the tea, they found that the mother had been mistakenly picking leaves of *Adenostyles alliariae* (alpendost), which contains even more PAs than coltsfoot. The plants are easily confused, especially after the flowering period.

Warnings: Coltsfoot is not for regular or long-term use. Users should only buy coltsfoot products which list the PA content on the label, and the content should be less than one part per million.

Drug Testings: No one has ever checked, but there is no reason to suppose that any of the chemicals present in this plant would have an effect on workplace urine tests.

Dosage: Traditional herbalists recommend using a tea made by steeping one ounce of leaves in one pint of boiling water. Commission E recommends a daily dose of 4.5-6 grams of drug per day; not to be used for more than 4-6 weeks per year.

Summary: If an expectorant is needed, there are many other herbs that are just as good as coltsfoot (mullein, wild thyme, pine oil) so that it makes little sense to risk liver damage, and possibly even cancer. Some of the components of *Petasites* species may turn out to be medically useful, but only when they can be separated and sold separately from the PAs.

References:

Debrunner B, Meier B. Petasites hybridus: a tool for interdisciplinary research in phytotherapy. Pharm Acta Helv 1998;72(6):359-62.

Lin YL, Mei CH, Huang SL, Kuo YH. Four new sesquiterpenes from Petasites formosanus. J Nat Prod 1998;61(7):887-90.

Sperl W, Stuppner H, Gassner I, Judmaier W, Dietze O, Vogel W. Reversible hepatic veno-occlusive disease in an infant after consumption of pyrrolizidine-containing herbal tea. Eur J Pediatr 1995;154(2):112-6.

Ziolo G, Samochowiec L. Study on clinical properties and mechanisms of action of Petasites in bronchial asthma and chronic obstructive bronchitis. Pharm Acta Helv 1998;72(6):378-80.

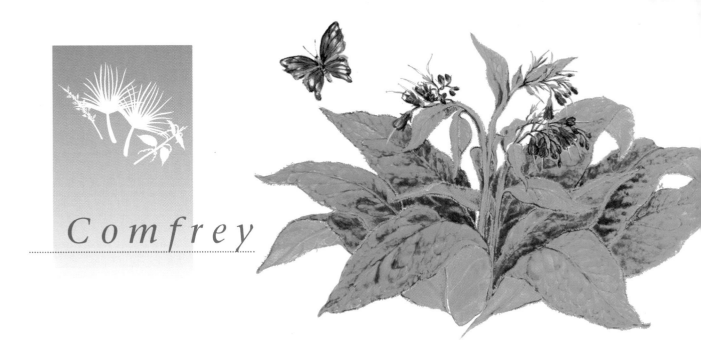

Comfrey

Name: *Symphytum officinale L.,*(Boraginaceae), commonly called Symphytum root, comfrey root, knitbone, gumplant, healing herb, slippery root, and *Consolidae radix*. Related plants, often sold as *S. Officinale* L., are *S. Aspereum,* known as prickly comfrey, and *S. X uplandicum*, commonly called Russian comfrey. In French, it is *Grande consoude*; in German, *Schwarzwurz* or *Beinwell*.

Source: Comfrey products are made from the rhizomes and roots of plants closely related to borage. Comfrey is native to Europe and Western Asia, but it can be grown in the United States. There are several distinct species, and it is very important to distinguish between them. Comfrey has the potential to produce extremely dangerous side effects, and some kinds of comfrey are much more toxic than others. The problem for consumers is finding out just which comfrey it is they are buying.

The comfrey that grows in the United States is *S. Officinale*. Russian comfrey, which has become increasingly popular in the United States and Europe, is called *S. X uplandicum* (but used to be known as *S. Pergrinum*). All species of comfrey contain chemicals called pyrrolizidine alkaloids (PAs) (see the discussion above on Coltsfoot, and Chapter 4). All pyrrolizidines are potentially toxic to the liver, but not all pyrrolizidines are equally dangerous, and the concentration of the pyrrolizidines is different in different parts of the herb. In general, the roots and rhizomes of the plants contain at least 10 times the amount of pyrrolizidines as the leaves.

The most toxic of the PAs is called echimidine. Only minute amounts are found in the leaves of *S. Officinale*, but very large amounts can be found in the leaves of Russian comfrey, and also in the leaves of prickly comfrey (*S. aspereum*). Echimidine-containing products are banned in Canada, but they are legal in the United States. The difficulty faced by American consumers is that much of the comfrey sold here is simply labeled "comfrey." The type of comfrey is often not specified, nor is mention made of which parts of the plants have been used.

History: The name derives from the Latin word *confirma,* which means "joined together. Both the Greeks and Romans believed that use of the herb would help bones to heal more quickly, which is why in the Middle Ages, comfrey came to be called "knitbone."

Traditional Claims: Comfrey is used as an emollient, sedative, astringent, demulcent, vulnerary (wound healing), and expectorant.

Commission E Recommendations: Comfrey is used externally to treat bruises, contusions, and sprains.

Proven Effects: Comfrey is mostly composed of inert mucilage, but it also has active ingredients. Allantoin was the first to be discovered, and its presence is thought to explain comfrey's ability to promote skin healing. Comfrey is not the only source for allantoin. In fact, humans convert uric acid, a breakdown product of cell metabolism, to allantoin. The conversion occurs when uric acid traps free radicals. High levels of allantoin in the body therefore equate to high levels of oxidative stress. Comfrey also contains phytosterols such as beta-sitosterol and an assortment of amino acids. Human poisoning from these compounds was first described in South Africa in the early 1900s, but cases continue to be reported in underdeveloped countries. "Bush tea" poisoning is endemic in Jamaica and Barbados, where dozens of poisoning deaths are reported each year. In Afghanistan, in the late 1970s, thousands were poisoned, and many died, when the wheat crop became contaminated with a pyrrolizidine-containing plant called *Heliotropium popovii*. The main PAs found in comfrey are 7-acetylintermedine and 7-acetyllycopsamine. The main traditional use has been to treat skin diseases and to promote bone healing. More recently, a host of other, almost entirely unsupported claims, have been advanced.

Concerns: Compared to the roots, the PA concentration in the leaves is quite low, but PAs are still present. PAs do not dissolve well in water, but tea brewed from comfrey leaves will contain small amounts of PA. Tea brewed from roots will contain even more. No one knows whether the low PA concentration found in comfrey leaf tea is sufficient to cause liver damage, but the possibility certainly exists.

Warnings: Users should only consider products made from the leaves of *S. Officinale*, and even then it would be best if the first growth leaves were discarded. The amount of echimidine contained in the leaves of *S. Officinale* is negligible. The governments of England, France, and Germany prohibit the internal use of comfrey and recommend that external application be limited to four to six weeks per year. Nursing mothers should avoid comfrey. Liver damage has been reported in infants exposed to comfrey in mother's milk.

Drug Testing: None of the compounds in comfrey should cause any interference with routine workplace urine drug screening tests.

Dosage: Tea can be made by soaking one teaspoon of leaves in one cup of boiling water. Tea should not be made from roots. Commission E monographs recommend that ointments for external use contain less than 20 percent of the dried drug, and that ointment only be applied to intact skin (cuts or abrasions will allow entrance into the bloodstream). Capsules containing 250 mg of comfrey leaf, or 250 mg of comfrey root, or mixtures of both, are sold with a recommended dose of one capsule twice a day. At that dosage, two capsules of root would supply nearly 2 mg per day of PA. In one of the few case reports where dosage can be estimated, veno-occlusive disease occurred in a woman who ingested a total of 85 mg of PA over a four-month period.

Summary: The danger of PA exposure has been very clearly demonstrated. Occasional use of a tea made from second growth leaves is unlikely to do much harm, but consumers who buy herbal remedies have no way to be certain which part of the plant they are buying. Liver failure is not a nice thing. Taking comfrey, in the hopes of achieving some ill-defined benefit, would hardly seem to be worth the risk.

References:

Betz JM, Eppley RM, Taylor WC, Andrzejewski D. Determination of pyrrolizidine alkaloids in commercial comfrey products (*Symphytum sp.*). J Pharm Sci 1994;83(5):649-53.

Garrett BJ, Cheeke PR, Miranda CL, Goeger DE, Buhler DR. Consumption of poisonous plants (*Senecio jacobaea, Symphytum officinale, Pteridium aquilinum, Hypericum perforatum*) by rats: chronic toxicity, mineral metabolism, and hepatic drug-metabolizing enzymes. Toxicol Lett 1982;10(2-3):183-8.

McDermott WV, Ridker PM. The Budd-Chiari syndrome and hepatic veno-occlusive disease. Recognition and treatment. Arch Surg 1990;125(4):525-7.

Winship KA. Toxicity of comfrey. Adverse Drug React Toxicol Rev 1991;10(1):47-59.

Yeong ML, Wakefield SJ, Ford HC. Hepatocyte membrane injury and bleb formation following low dose comfrey toxicity in rats. Int J Exp Pathol 1993;74(2):211-7.

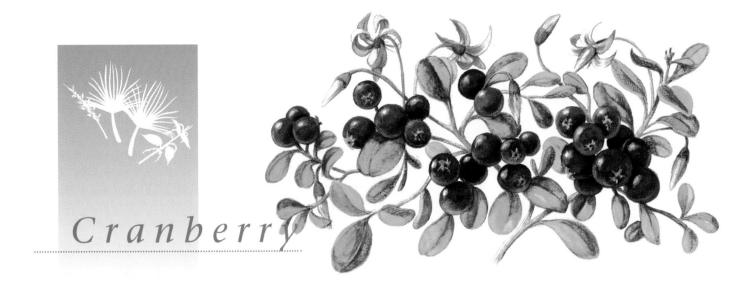

Cranberry

Name: *Vaccinium macrocarpon* Alt (Ericaceae), commonly known as cranberry, the swamp cranberry, also the trailing swamp cranberry. Its European cousins are *Vaccinium oxycoccos,* L., and *Oxycoccus quadripetalus* L. In France it is *Canneberge*; in Germany, *Moosheere*.

Source: The American cranberry grows in natural or artificial bogs on both coasts of the United States. *V. oxycoccos,* grows naturally, usually in peat-bogs, in some parts of Europe and also in Northern Asia.

History: Cranberry appears to be one of the few plants not to have generated any sort of mythology. Medical applications for the plant have only become apparent within the last decade.

Traditional Claims: The fruit of the American cranberry is used to treat and prevent urinary tract infections, particularly in older women.

Commission E Recommendations: Commission E did not review cranberry.

Proven Effects: Cranberry juice can prevent and eradicate some types of urinary tract infections. In controlled studies of postmenopausal women, drinking 300 milliliters (slightly more than one cup) per day of cranberry juice reduced the frequency of bacterial infections (bacteriuria) and the associated presence of white blood cells in the urine (pyuria) by nearly half. Young women seem to get the same benefits. Something in cranberry juice prevents bacteria from binding to the walls of the bladder, and if the bacteria cannot adhere to the surface cells, they cannot cause an infection. The tannin contained in cranberry seems to have antineoplastic effects, but it never has been tested in patients with cancer. Cranberry contains relatively high concentrations of flavonoids (quercetin and myrecetin) and anthocyanidins. In the test tube, these chemicals prevent the oxidation of low density cholesterol (LDL), and LDL oxidation leads to coronary artery disease. These same flavonols and anthocyanidins are found in red wines and grape juice. Many researchers believe their presence helps explain why the French, who drink much more red wine, and eat much more fat than Americans, have fewer heart attacks. The flavonoid content of cranberry juice is higher than that of wine or beer, but lower than that of concord grape juice.

Concerns: None

Warnings: None

Drug Testing: Cranberry juice will not interfere with standard workplace urine drug tests, but women with urinary tract infections could conceivably have a problem. When infections occur, large amounts of substances called nitrates appear in the urine. Nitrates interfere with some workplace urine tests, and some drug users try to cheat by adding nitrate to their urine samples. If large quantities of nitrates are found in the urine, some testers may consider their presence proof that the sample was adulterated. Women with urinary tract infections who are forced to submit a sample should make sure the laboratory is aware of their condition. Generally, the amount of nitrate produced by infection is much less than the amount added by cheaters, but questions could still arise.

Dosage: In clinical trials, the dose has been 300 milliliters (slightly more than a cup) per day. In the clinical trials of young women with bladder infections, the daily dose was one capsule containing 400 milligrams of dried cranberry solids.

Summary: The evidence is good that daily use of cranberry juice reduces the number of urinary tract infections in older woman, and probably in younger, sexually active women as well. Reports of serious toxicity, or even minor side effects, are nonexistent. Regular consumption of cranberry juice may help prevent coronary artery disease, but in the absence of any clinical trials, there is just no way to know. If coronary artery disease is the only concern, concord grape juice has a higher flavonoid content, and then, there is always red wine.

References:

Fleet JC. New support for a folk remedy: cranberry juice reduces bacteriuria and pyuria in elderly women. Nutr Rev 1994;52(5):168-70.

Kuzminski LN. Cranberry juice and urinary tract infections: is there a beneficial relationship? Nutr Rev 1996;54(11 Pt 2):S87-90.

Nazarko L. Infection control. The therapeutic uses of cranberry juice. Nurs Stand 1995;9(34):33-5.

Ofek I, Goldhar J, Sharon N. Anti-Escherichia coli adhesin activity of cranberry and blueberry juices. Adv Exp Med Biol 1996;408:179-83.

Walker EB, Barney DP, Mickelsen JN, Walton RJ, Mickelsen RA, Jr. Cranberry concentrate: UTI prophylaxis [letter]. J Fam Pract 1997;45(2):167-8.

Wilson T, Porcari JP, Harbin D. Cranberry extract inhibits low density lipoprotein oxidation. Life Sci 1998;62(24):L381-6.

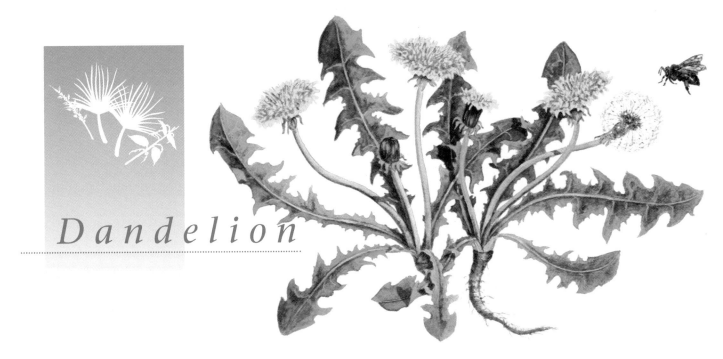

Dandelion

Name: *Taraxacum officinale* Weber (Compositae), commonly puffball, Lion's tooth, priest's crown. In French, it is *Pissenlit* or *Dent-de-lion*; in German, *Löwenzahn* or *Kuhblume.*

Source: While generally considered an annoying garden weed, dandelions are, in fact, cultivated for medicinal use. Leaves are collected before flowering, dried and crushed. Dandelion root products are composed of the roots and rhizomes, collected in the autumn, and sold in dried, broken or chopped pieces.

History: The name is derived from the French *dent de lion*, or lion's teeth, because the leaves are thought to resemble the teeth of lions. Whatever the leaves resemble, dandelion is a diuretic, which led Tudor writers to give it the name "piss-in-bed." Folklore has it that if dandelions are gathered on Midsummer's Eve, they will have the power to ward off evil spirits. Dandelion was used by ancient Greek physicians, and in the Middle Ages it was recommended by Avicenna, the famous Arab physician. A Russian variety of dandelion was cultivated during World War II because it contained a latex material that could be used to make rubber. The types of dandelions grown in the rest of Europe, and the United States, only contain inconsequential amounts of latex.

Traditional Claims: In the Middle Ages, formulations made from the leaves were used as diuretics and to promote the flow of bile. Products made with the root were used to treat constipation and indigestion, and to promote appetite. During the last century, regular use of dandelion was recommended as a way to prevent and/or cure kidney stones. Most recently, herbal product makers have promoted dandelion for "detoxifying the liver."

Commission E Recommendations: Dandelion herb is used to treat abdominal bloating, loss of appetite, biliary dyskinesia, dyspepsia (upset stomach), flatulence, and as a diuretic.

Proven Effects: On a weight-for-weight basis, dandelion extracts produce just as much fluid loss as furosemide (a very potent diuretic used to treat heart and kidney failure). Extracts of the root have been shown to increase bile flow by a factor of almost 40 percent, at least in animals. Clinical effects, in controlled trials, have been poorly studied. Encouraging results using dandelion extract to treat nonspecific colitis were reported in the early 1980s, but have not been repeated. The greatest medical potential for dandelion was not appreciated until quite recently; dandelions contain a phytoestrogen called coumesterol. The benefits of soy and dandelion phytoestrogens have never been compared head-to-head, but dandelion products are likely to be as effective as those derived from soy for treating menopausal symptoms and preventing cancer.

Concerns: Dandelion is a rich source of potassium, so the potassium depletion that often occurs with prescription diuretics may not present much of a problem. Still, long-term use of diuretics can lead to potassium depletion, and that can be dangerous. If dandelion is being used to control fluid retention, it should be done with a doctor's supervision. Like all members of the Compositae family, dandelions can cause dermatitis, especially in children who already suffer from eczema. Long-term toxicity studies are completely lacking. Long-term, unsupervised use, is not a good idea.

Warnings: It appears that something in dandelion-containing formulations can make the gallbladder contract, and that would be a bad thing if gallstones were present. Patients with gallbladder disease should only use dandelion-containing products after they have checked with their physicians.

Drug Testing: None of the components, either of the leaves or the roots, should interfere with standard workplace urine drug screening tests.

Dosage: Dried leaf, 4 to 10 grams three times a day for fluid retention. Tincture (1:5, 25 percent ethanol) 2 to 5 milliliters three times a day, or 5 to 10 milliliters of juice from fresh leaf twice daily. Dosage of the root is lower, 3 to 5 grams three times a day, either of dried root or as a tea, or as a tincture (Commission E recommends a 1:5, 25 percent formulation), 5 to 10 milliliters three times a day. Or 4 to 8 milliliters of fresh juice from the roots once a day. The British Pharmacopeia recommends a slightly higher dosage of 5 to 10 milliliters.

Summary: Dandelion is an effective diuretic and occasional use for fluid retention, as after a long airplane flight, would be a reasonable thing. There is mounting evidence that coumesterol, contained in this herb, may be an important and useful phytoestrogen, but more studies are needed. None of the other medicinal benefits suggested by laboratory studies, or by the experience of early herbalists, have been substantiated in clinical trials, although something in dandelion extract does affect the gallbladder and patients with gallstones should avoid this food supplement.

References:

Grases F, Melero G, Costa-Bauza A, Prieto R, March JG. Urolithiasis and phytotherapy. Int Urol Nephrol 1994;26(5):507-11.

Guin JD, Skidmore G. Compositae dermatitis in childhood. Arch Dermatol 1987;123(4):500-2.

Kim HM, Lee EH, Shin TY, Lee KN, Lee JS. *Taraxacum officinale* restores inhibition of nitric oxide production by cadmium in mouse peritoneal macrophages. Immunopharmacol Immunotoxicol 1998;20(2):283-97.

Racz-Kotilla E, Racz G, Solomon A. The action of *Taraxacum officinale* extracts on the body weight and diuresis of laboratory animals. Planta Med 1974;26(3):212-7.

Swanston-Flatt SK, Day C, Flatt PR, Gould BJ, Bailey CJ. Glycaemic effects of traditional European plant treatments for diabetes. Studies in normal and streptozotocin diabetic mice. Diabetes Res 1989;10(2):69-73.

Williams CA, Goldstone F, Greenham J. Flavonoids, cinnamic acids and coumarins from the different tissues and medicinal preparations of *Taraxacum officinale*. Phytochemistry 1996;42(1): 121-7.

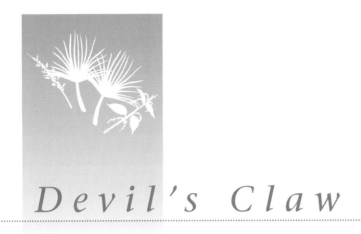

Devil's Claw

Name: *Harpagophytum procumbens DC.* (Pedaliaceae), commonly called Devil's Claw; in German, *Sudafrikanische Teufelskrallenwurzel.*

Source: Devil's claw comes from a plant native to the Kalahari and Namibian deserts. Its roots are said to resemble a claw. The active ingredients are found in the roots and tubers, with nearly twice as much active ingredient (harpagoside) in the secondary tubers as in the primary. Commercial producers buy dried slices of the tubers which are then converted to powder form or extracted.

History: Traditional herbalists have used devil's claw to treat everything from upset stomach to boils, even skin cancer. At the turn of the century, German physicians began using devil's claw to treat arthritis and joint pain.

Traditional Claims: Devil's claw is used as an anti-inflammatory, analgesic, and to stimulate appetite and digestion.

Commission E Recommendations: Devil's claw is used to treat dyspepsia (upset stomach), loss of appetite, and degenerative disorders of the locomotor system.

Proven Effects: Extracts injected into animals prevent the swelling induced by trauma. They also appear to relieve the pain induced by experimental injuries. The component thought to be responsible is called Harpagoside (members of the general class of Iridoid glycosides). The problem here is that Harpagoside both stimulates the release of, and is destroyed by, stomach acid. The highly variable rate of absorption may explain why clinical researchers have reported conflicting results. Some researchers have found that patients with arthritis get relief; others have found that use of the herb produced no measurable benefits.

Concerns: The evidence suggests that devil's claw stimulates acid secretion, and patients being treated for ulcer disease might find themselves feeling even worse. Also, there is some evidence that devil's claw works by altering the same enzyme systems that are effected by NSAIDs (nonsteroidal anti-inflammatory drugs) such as Advil™ (ibuprofen). Someone already taking an NSAID should probably not take devil's claw at the same time.

Warnings: Significant toxic side effects have never been reported, and devil's claw is not known to interact with any other medications.

Drug Testing: There are no reports of devil's claw products interfering with routine workplace urine drug screening tests.

Dosage: Commission E recommends a dose of 1.5 grams per day to stimulate appetite, and 4.5 grams per day for muscle sprains and upset stomach. Since it appears that most of the herb will be destroyed in the stomach, enteric coated formulations might be preferable. Barring that, taking the product with an antacid would also be a good idea.

Summary: Potent anti-inflammatory effects have been demonstrated in the laboratory, and devil's claw may be a good treatment for minor aches and sprains. The problem is that its effectiveness has never really been proven in a controlled clinical trial. Worse still, there is good reason to suppose that the most important components of these roots are destroyed by stomach acids. On the other hand, the potential for toxic reactions seems remote. If the product being used seems ineffective, it may just be that it is being destroyed in the stomach. Users should try taking it with an antacid, or better still, find a product that is enteric coated.

References:

Baghdikian B, Lanhers MC, Fleurentin J, Ollivier E, Maillard C, Balansard G, et al. An analytical study, anti-inflammatory and analgesic effects of *Harpagophytum procumbens* and *Harpagophytum zeyheri*. Planta Med 1997;63(2):171-6.

Lanhers MC, Fleurentin J, Mortier F, Vinche A, Younos C. Anti-inflammatory and analgesic effects of an aqueous extract of *Harpagophytum procumbens*. Planta Med 1992;58(2):117-23.

Moussard C, Alber D, Toubin MM, Thevenon N, Henry JC. A drug used in traditional medicine, *harpagophytum procumbens*: no evidence for NSAID-like effect on whole blood eicosanoid production in human. Prostaglandins Leukot Essent Fatty Acids 1992;46(4):283-6.

Soulimani R, Younos C, Mortier F, Derrieu C. The role of stomachal digestion on the pharmacological activity of plant extracts, using as an example extracts of *Harpagophytum procumbens*. Can J Physiol Pharmacol 1994;72(12):1532-6.

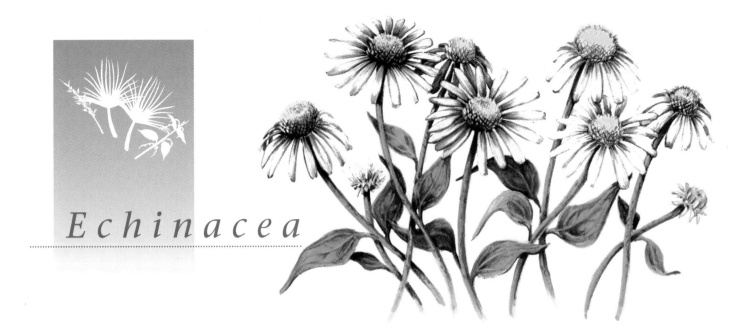

Echinacea

Name: *Echinaceae angustifolia* DC, *E. pallida* (Nutt) and *E. purpurea* (L.), Moench (Asteraceae), commonly called the American coneflower root, the narrow-leaved or purple cone flower. In French it is *Rudbeckie á feuilles étroites*; in German it is *Kegelblume.*

Source: Along with the artichoke, Echinacea is a member of the Asteraceae family. Three different kinds of echinacea are used medicinally, but many more than that grow in the United States. The active constituents of the three species differ and, until recently, there was some confusion over their naming. It now turns out that much of the *E. angustifolia* grown in Europe was (and still may be) *E. pallida*. The roots of *E. pallida* are used to stimulate the immune system, and the juice of the roots for treating skin diseases. The roots contain entirely different chemicals than are found in the flowers, and not all of the active agents have been identified.

History: Unlike many of herbal remedies, echinacea is an American discovery. A physician from Nebraska first learned about its medicinal value from American Indians. Echinacea was used to treat infections of every sort, and for a variety of other conditions including eczema and even rattle snake bites. By the early 1900s, American drug companies were selling echinacea-based products, mainly for their ability to fight infections. When sulfa, the first antibiotic, was introduced in 1930s, commercial production of echinacea essentially ceased.

Traditional Claims: Antiseptic, as a compress for infected wounds, as a gargle for dental abscess.

Commission E Recommendations: Echinacea is used to treat colds, flu, influenza, chronic respiratory infection, skin ulcers, urinary infection or inflammation, and wounds.

Proven Effects: Echinacea, taken either as fresh pressed juice or dried juice, stimulates the immune system, causing increased production of interleukin and tumor necrosis factor (a hormone that causes cell death), two members of a class of hormones called cytokines. The exact mechanism responsible for cytokine stimulation is not known, but treatment with echinacea activates white blood cells and increases their ability to fight infection, even if the white blood cells come from patients with HIV. Other components (fat soluble flavonoids like luteolin, quercetin and rutin, and water soluble components called caffeoyl derivatives) are potent free radical scavengers, capable of preventing the skin from the damage produced by intense sunlight. Results of trials done by German drugmakers (in particular the makers of a widely prescribed echinacea formulation called Resistan™) suggest that, when taken in the early stages of a cold or other mild respiratory infections, echinacea shortens the duration of symptoms by as much as one third. The results of other European studies suggest that using echinacea on a regular basis might even prevent colds in the first place.

Concerns: Buyers need to closely read labels. Root products derived from *Echinaceae anugstifolia* might not work, or at least not work as well as products made from root extract of E. *Pallida*. Except for the fact that the formulation used may not work, there is very little cause for concern. Serious episodes of toxicity related to echinacea have never been reported, and even mentions of minor complications are rare. Single oral or intravenous doses of Echinacea purpurea have proven virtually nontoxic to rats and mice, even when truly huge doses were given over a prolonged period.

Warnings: A recent report described a case of anaphylactic shock in a woman with atopic dermatitis after taking, among other dietary supplements, echinacea. Patients with atopy (very bad eczema) should be cautioned about the risk of developing life-threatening reactions.

Drug Testing: None of the constituents found in the flower or in the roots should interfere with standard workplace urine drug tests. However, echinacea is often sold in a mixture with other herbs, especially goldenseal. If you are subject to drug testing, you may want to avoid such mixtures, because goldenseal is commonly taken by drug users attempting to thwart the drug-testing process. Contrary to popular wisdom, using goldenseal will not help one pass a drug test (unless the goldenseal is taken with a gallon or so of water just before the test), but the presence of some goldenseal components in your urine sample (specifically a molecule called berberine) might suggest to the testing laboratory that you have something to hide.

Dosage: Ointments and semisolid preparations containing at least 15 percent of the juice expressed from the flowers, are used in Europe to treat superficial and poorly healing wounds. Germany's Commission E recommends that only the root extract of E. *Pallida* be used for internal consumption, and that only the juice of E. Purpurea be used for ointments and salves. The Commission also warns that E. pallida should not be used internally for more than 3 weeks or externally for more than 8 weeks.

Summary: Allopathic physicians may remain skeptical, but the evidence is quite strong that something in this herb really does give a boost to the immune process. And, unless you suffer from severe skin allergies, little or no risk is associated with taking echinacea. Whether echinacea will help patients with more serious diseases, such as HIV, is not known, but it certainly might shorten the course and minimize the symptoms of your next cold or upper respiratory infection.

References:

Burger RA, Torres AR, Warren RP, Caldwell VD, Hughes BG. Echinacea-induced cytokine production by human macrophages. Int J Immunopharmacol 1997;19(7):371-9.

Facino RM, Carini M, Aldini G, Saibene L, Pietta P, Mauri P. Echinacoside and caffeoyl conjugates protect collagen from free radical-induced degradation: a potential use of Echinacea extracts in the prevention of skin photodamage. Planta Med 1995;61(6):510-4.

Melchart D, Linde K, Worku F, Sarkady L, Holzmann M, Jurcic K, et al. Results of five randomized studies on the immunomodulatory activity of preparations of Echinacea. J Altern Complement Med 1995;1(2):145-60.

Mengs U, Clare CB, Poiley JA. Toxicity of Echinacea purpurea. Acute, subacute and genotoxicity studies. Arzneimittelforschung 1991;41(10):1076-81.

See DM, Broumand N, Sahl L, Tilles JG. In vitro effects of echinacea and ginseng on natural killer and antibody-dependent cell cytotoxicity in healthy subjects and chronic fatigue syndrome or acquired immunodeficiency syndrome patients. Immunopharmacology 1997;35(3):229-35.

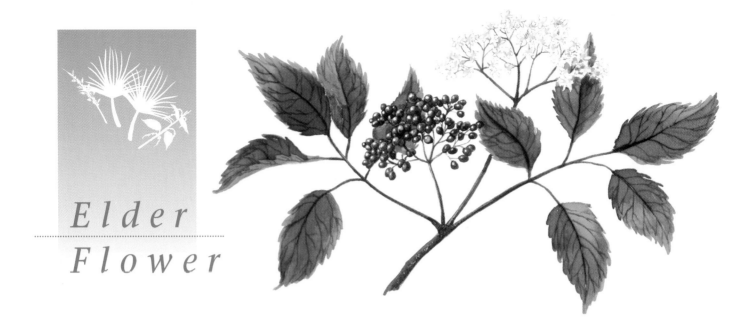

Elder Flower

Name: *Sambucus nigra* L. (Caprifoliaceae), commonly called Sambucus, European Elder Flower, Black Elder Flower, and Elder Flower. In French it is *Sureau noir;* in German, *Schwarzer Holunder* and *Holunderbluten.*

Source: Remedies are made from the dried flowers of this small tree. Elder grows in most parts of Europe, and they are sometimes planted as an ornamental.

History: Elder is one of the most ancient medicinal herbs. In medieval times, elderberries were given to women in order to bring on menstruation. In combination with peppermint, elder was used to treat colds and coughs. The tree itself, however, was thought to be the source of bad luck. Today, elder flowers are mainly used in the making of cosmetics. In Europe, it is still a popular remedy for the common cold.

Traditional Claims: Diaphoretic (something used to cause perspiration) and diuretic. Traditional healers, and even physicians until well into the 20th century, often confused cause and effect. Because profuse sweating often occurs just when a fever breaks, it only seemed natural to give something to a patient in order to make them sweat. In fact, the sweating was a result of the fever breaking (defervescence).

Commission E Recommendations: Elder is used to treat colds and flu.

Proven Effects: Elder is rich in the flavonoids (quercetin and rutin), and is, therefore, a good source of antioxidants. Unlike Hawthorn, which also contains goodly amounts of quercetin, elder does not contain substances that directly affect the heart. In addition to potential antioxidant benefits, results of more recent clinical and laboratory investigations suggest a number of other possible benefits. Quercetin is under investigation as a modulator of tumor growth, and it has shown some positive effects in clinical trials. Large doses, however, cause muscle pain and kidney damage which may limit its usefulness. Closely related synthetic molecules may yet prove to be potent anticancer medications. A placebo-controlled, double-blind study of elderberry extract as an antiviral was carried out on a group of individuals living in an agricultural community (kibbutz) during an outbreak of influenza B Panama in 1993. Volunteers treated with elderberry had fewer symptoms, recovered more quickly, and produced more antiviral antibodies than the controls (individuals given a placebo). Another potential application may be in the treatment of chronic venous insufficiency and lymphedema. When lymphatic channel obstruction occurs, whether from infection (such as elephantiasis), or even after surgery (painful arm swelling sometimes occurs after radical mastectomy), fluid accumulates, and the extremities swell. The swelling causes pain, and often breakdown of the skin. A mixture of semisynthetic flavonoids made from rutin improves the circulation and reduces the edema.

Concerns: Large doses can cause kidney and muscle damage. But the amounts required for that to happen are far in excess of those likely to be found in commercial herbal products.

Warnings: None

Drug Testing: There are no reports that any component of the elderberry flower interferes with standard workplace urine drug screening tests.

Dosage: Pour boiling water (150 milliliters) over two teaspoons of dried flowers (3-5 grams), steep for five minutes and drink as a hot tea two or three times a day; liquid extract (1:1, 25 percent ethanol, 3-5 milliliters three times a day, or tincture (1:5, 25 percent ethanol), 10-25 milliliters three times a day.

Summary: Hoping to cure a disease by inducing sweating may have seemed reasonable 100 years ago, but that is no longer the case. And, if a diuretic is needed, there are much better ones available than elderberry. But modern science has discovered some very good reasons for using this herb. There is very good evidence that elderberry may help in cases of lymphedema, and there is tantalizing evidence that it may be both antiviral and anticancer. Toxicity is possible, but the issue has been poorly studied, and if toxicity is occurring, it has not been reported in the last 15 years.

References:

Battelli MG, Citores L, Buonamici L, Ferreras JM, de Benito FM, Stirpe F, et al. Toxicity and cytotoxicity of *nigrin b*, a two-chain ribosome- inactivating protein from *Sambucus nigra*: comparison with ricin. Arch Toxicol 1997;71(6):360-4.

Casley-Smith JR. The pathophysiology of lymphedema and the action of benzo-pyrones in reducing it. Lymphology 1988;21(3):190-4.

Leads from the MMWR. Poisoning from elderberry juice. JAMA 1984;251(16):2075.

Poisoning from elderberry juice—California. MMWR Morb Mortal Wkly Rep 1984;33(13):173-4.

Wadworth AN, Faulds D. Hydroxyethylrutosides. A review of its pharmacology, and therapeutic efficacy in venous insufficiency and related disorders. Drugs 1992;44(6):1013-32.

Zakay-Rones Z, Varsano N, Zlotnik M, Manor O, Regev L, Schlesinger M, et al. Inhibition of several strains of influenza virus in vitro and reduction of symptoms by an elderberry extract (Sambucus nigra L.) during an outbreak of influenza B Panama. J Altern Complement Med 1995;1(4):361-9.

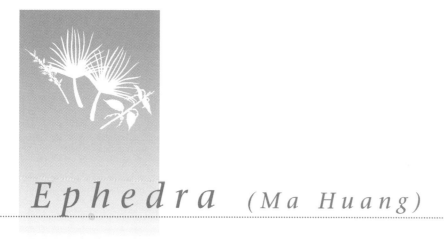

Ephedra (*Ma Huang*)

Name: *Ephedra distachya* L. (Ephedraceae), also *E. equisetina, E. sinica,* and *E. intermedia,* the name used for plants which contain the chemical ephedrine. *Ma Huang* is the name of the plant containing ephedra that grows in China and is perhaps the best known. In English it is commonly called ephedra. In French, it is *Ephédre du Valais;* in German, *Ephedrakraut* and sometimes *Walliser Meertraubchen*

Source: Ephedrine, and some of the other chemicals contained in the ephedra plant, are known as alkaloids, a term first used in the early 1800s. Until 1803, when morphine was isolated from opium, it was mistakenly believed that molecules found in plant leaves had to be acids. Morphine was an alkaloid, the first of many others (quinine and cocaine, for example) to be extracted and purified from plant materials. Ephedra contains smaller amounts of two other important alkaloids, pseudoephedrine and phenylpropanolamine. They are widely used in over-the-counter cold medications.

History: Ephedra has been used by Chinese physicians for at least 5,000 years. Chinese medical books, written at about the time Marco Polo was making his visit, recommended ephedra for the treatment of coughs and fevers. In the 16th century, Russian herbalists used ephedra to treat arthritis. During the 1800s, settlers in the U.S. Southwest brewed herbal teas from local plants that also contained small amounts of ephedrine (teamsters' tea, Mormon tea). During World War II, injections of purified ephedrine called *Philopon* (which means love of work), hundreds of times more potent than plant extract taken orally, were given to Japanese *Kamikaze* pilots.

Traditional Claims: Bronchitic, and for allergies.

Commission E. Recommendations: Ephedra is used to treat asthma, bronchospasm, colds and flu.

Proven Effects: Most of ephedrine's effects are on the heart and lungs. It causes the bronchial tubes to dilate (a good thing if one is wheezing), and the blood vessels in the nose to shrink (pseudoephedrine and phenylpropanolamine also dry up runny noses but have no effect on wheezing). Ephedrine also exerts effects on the central nervous system. In very large doses, five to 10 times the amounts found in most food supplements, ephedrine produces effects very much like methamphetamine. Recently, a compound with antibiotic activity (transtorine) has been isolated from ephedra. Its presence may help explain why ephedra products have proved so useful in treating coughs and respiratory infections. Unfortunately, large doses also mimic the effects of methamphetamine on the heart and blood vessels, leading to strokes and heart attacks.

Evidence, mostly from European studies, suggests that modest doses of ephedrine and caffeine, when combined with caloric restriction and exercise, promote weight loss. Several well-designed (technically referred to as double-blind, placebo-controlled) studies have shown that the combination of caffeine and ephedrine leads to more weight loss than can be achieved by just exercise and/or diet alone. Some believe that ephedrine causes cells to burn fat by binding to special sites on the cell surface (known as Beta 3, or even Beta 4 receptors).

Evidence for improved performance is even more convincing than the evidence for weight loss. When ephedrine is given to conditioned endurance athletes (marathon runners, bicyclists) their ability to perform at maximal levels of exertion is increased. In most cases, the increase is only modest but it is, nonetheless, quite real and well documented. This benefit may explain why ephedra-containing products are so popular among athletes.

Concerns: In 1997 the U.S. Food and Drug Administration (FDA) published a report claiming that food supplements containing ephedra could cause strokes, heart attacks, and seizures. The problem with the FDA report was that it didn't contain much in the way of evidence, and the evidence it did contain mostly had to do with the bad things that happen to people when they take too much pseudoephedrine or phenylpropanolamine, or when they take huge amounts (hundreds of times the amount contained in supplements) of ephedrine for long periods. Even though the report was unconvincing, exceeding the recommended dose range makes very little sense. Purity is also a concern, particularly with products imported from China. Cases of hepatitis and liver damage have been related to Chinese Ma Huang preparation which turned out to contain more than just ephedrine.

Warnings: Recommended doses of ephedrine do not have any significant effect on pulse rate or blood pressure, but people with heart disease should not use ephedra-containing products. That warning also applies to people with high blood pressure. Ephedrine increases blood adrenaline levels which increases blood pressure, and that makes the heart work harder. In addition to warnings about heart disease, most of the ephedra-containing food supplements carry warnings about use in prostate, liver or thyroid disease, diabetes, and seizure disorders. Obviously, anyone under the care of a physician for any of those conditions should check with his or her physician before taking any medication, not just ephedrine. Nor should ephedra-based products be used by patients taking Prozac™ and related antidepressants. The concerns are mostly theoretical. Regulators worry that, since ephedra and these drugs do share some common actions, when taken together, even in recommended dosages, toxicity may occur anyway. In theory, that is correct. Whether it is dangerous in practice, no one knows, but it does seem a risky proposition.

Drug Testing: The structure of the ephedrine molecule bears a very strong resemblance to that of all of the other amphetamines (methamphetamine and MDMA "ecstasy," to name just a few). Most urine screening tests will also detect ephedrine. If ephedra-based products have been taken, there is a very good chance of a positive test. A positive screening test should not be a problem, because confirmatory testing will disclose that it was ephedrine, and not methamphetamine, that was being used. Unfortunately, if the testing is not being done in conjunction with a federally mandated program, the employer is under no obligation to spend the extra money required to confirm the result, and many companies just don't bother. So taking an ephedra-based product and applying for a new job is not a good idea. Most traces of ephedra will be cleared from the system within 30 hours of the last dose. The International Olympic Committee (IOC), while not entirely banning ephedrine consumption, sets limits (cutoff) for the amount that may be detected. The limits is very low (500 ng/mL), a level that can easily be exceed just by taking the recommended amounts of some cold medications.

Dosage: Commission E recommends that the total daily dose of ephedrine not exceed 300 milligrams per day in adults. Most of the weight loss studies with caffeine and ephedrine mixtures have used a dose half that high, 50 milligrams three times a day, or 150 milligrams per day. Currently available food supplements contain 25 to 50 milligrams per portion, recommending up to three portions per day. In spite of Commission E recommendations, the FDA wants to limit the dose to 8 milligrams three times a day. Children should not take ephedra except under the supervision of a physician.

Summary: When used in the recommended doses, ephedra-containing products have proven themselves extremely safe, and the warning about dangerous consequences for patients with seizures, diabetes, etc. are more theoretical than real. When used sensibly, ephedra-containing supplements can promote weight loss and improve athletic performance. They should never, under any circumstances, be used by someone with heart disease or high blood pressure, and the recommended dose should not be exceeded. Ephedra products will almost certainly cause a false positive urine test for methamphetamine and related drugs. If you are being tested, make sure the company knows what products you are taking.

References:

al-Khalil S, Alkofahi A, el-Eisawi D, al-Shibib A. Transtorine, a new quinoline alkaloid from *Ephedra transitoria*. J Nat Prod 1998; 61(2):262-3.

Betz JM, Gay ML, Mossoba MM, Adams S, Portz BS. Chiral gas chromatographic determination of ephedrine-type alkaloids in dietary supplements containing Ma Huang. J AOAC Int 1997; 80(2):303-15.

Gurley BJ, Gardner SF, White LM, Wang PL. Ephedrine pharmacokinetics after the ingestion of nutritional supplements containing *Ephedra sinica* (ma huang). Ther Drug Monit 1998;20(4):439-45.

Karch S. The Pathology of Drug Abuse. Boca Raton: CRC Press; 1996.

Lefebvre, R, Surmont F, Bouckaert J, and Moerman R. Urinary excretion of ephedrine after nasal application in healthy volunteers. J Pharm Pharmacol 1992; 33:672-675

Nadir A, Agrawal S, King PD, Marshall JB. Acute hepatitis associated with the use of a Chinese herbal product, ma-huang [see comments]. Am J Gastroenterol 1996;91(7):1436-8.

White LM, Gardner SF, Gurley BJ, Marx MA, Wang PL, Estes M. Pharmacokinetics and cardiovascular effects of ma-huang (*Ephedra sinica*) in normotensive adults. J Clin Pharmacol 1997;37(2):116-22.

Young R, Glennon RA. Discriminative stimulus properties of ephedrine. Pharmacol Biochem Behav 1998; 60(3):771-5.

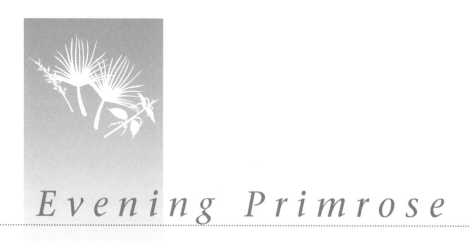

Evening Primrose

Name: *Oenothera biennis* L. (Onagraceae). In English it is called Evening Primrose, or Primrose.

Source: Evening primrose is a New World plant, but it is closely related to the European water dropwort (*Oenanthe aquatica*). The seeds of both plants contain an essential oil rich in gamma linolenic acid that is sold as a food supplement.

History: American Indians showed European settlers how to use the oil to treat stomach upsets and respiratory infections. Food supplement makers now promote evening primrose oil for conditions where sex hormones and prostoglandins are thought to be disordered such as premenstrual syndrome, benign breast disease, elevated cholesterol, atopic skin disease, and as a supplement capable of preventing abnormal blood clotting, obesity, and degenerative neurologic diseases, including multiple sclerosis and arthritis.

Traditional Claims: Expectorant and stomachic

Commission E Recommendations: Primrose is used to treat respiratory catarrh and upper respiratory tract catarrh.

Proven Effects: Evening primrose, like borage, blackcurrant, hemp oil, and oils derived from some fungi, contains a substance called gamma linolenic acid (GLA). Humans normally make GLA from linoleic acid in their diet. Patients with diabetes, however, do not convert linoleic acid to GLA very effectively. Since the protective coating that surrounds most nerves is made partly from GLA, it is believed that nerve disease in diabetics (diabetic neuropathy) is due to this GLA deficiency. In experimental animals with diabetes, adding GLA to the diet corrects the nerve damage. Gamma linolenic acid is also important because it is converted into hormones called prostoglandins. These hormones regulate multiple body functions and play a very important part in regulating the inflammatory response (such as the swelling of a joint seen in gout or rheumatoid arthritis, or even the swelling that occurs after an ankle sprain). The process of converting GLA into prostoglandins starts with a reaction called "desaturation" of linoleic acid to form GLA. Many factors can interfere with this conversion, including aging, diabetes or stress (high levels of adrenalin), to name just a few. GLA formation is also blocked when the diet contains excessive amounts of unsaturated fatty acids (the kind found in semi-solid fats such as some kinds of margarine and cooking oil) in the diet. No one knows for certain whether prostaglandin deficiencies are the cause of conditions such as premenstrual tension and breast discomfort, and clinical trials have failed to support claims that GLA supplementation would increase immunity or make platelets less sticky. However, GLA supplements clearly do improve some types of neurologic diseases, and clinical trials evaluating the other claims are ongoing.

Concerns: Not all GLA-containing natural oils are equally effective, and results cannot be predicted from just the GLA content of the product being used. In animal studies, evening primrose was substantially better at reversing diabetic neuropathy than either blackcurrant or borage. Obviously, other components of the oils have something to do with the process. The same considerations almost apply to commercial supplements. They may contain a lot of GLA, but that does not mean that all of the GLA contained in the product will be absorbed, or that some other component added to the product may not prevent the GLA from working.

Warnings: None

Drug Testing: There is no evidence that any of the components found in evening primrose oil can interfere with standard workplace urine screening tests.

Dosage: In clinical trials, patients have been given doses of 1 to 3 grams per day, but the safe and effective range, if there is one, is not known. Commission E recommends a daily dose of 2-4 grams of drug.

Summary: If you want to supplement your intake of GLAs, take evening primrose. If you are healthy, and eating a normal diet, the chances are that taking GLA supplements will not make you any healthier. But, if you do suffer from breast soreness, or PMS, or even arthritis, evening primrose oil might help, and all the available literature suggests that it can be used quite safely. There is a good possibility that this herb may help people with some neurologic diseases, but controlled trials proving effectiveness have not yet been done.

References:

Bard JM, Luc G, Jude B, Bordet JC, Lacroix B, Bonte JP, et al. A therapeutic dosage (3 g/day) of borage oil supplementation has no effect on platelet aggregation in healthy volunteers. Fundam Clin Pharmacol 1997;11(2):143-4.

Dines KC, Cotter MA, Cameron NE. Effectiveness of natural oils as sources of gamma-linolenic acid to correct peripheral nerve conduction velocity abnormalities in diabetic rats: modulation by thromboxane A2 inhibition. Prostaglandins Leukot Essent Fatty Acids 1996;55(3):159-65.

Gibson RA, Lines DR, Neumann MA. Gamma linolenic acid (GLA) content of encapsulated evening primrose oil products. Lipids 1992;27(1):82-4.

Phylactos AC, Harbige LS, Crawford MA. Essential fatty acids alter the activity of manganese-superoxide dismutase in rat heart. Lipids 1994;29(2):111-5.

Raederstorff D, Moser U. Borage or primrose oil added to standardized diets are equivalent sources for gamma-linolenic acid in rats. Lipids 1992;27(12):1018-23.

Shaw CR. The perimenopausal hot flash: epidemiology, physiology, and treatment. Nurse Pract 1997;22(3):55-6, 61-6.

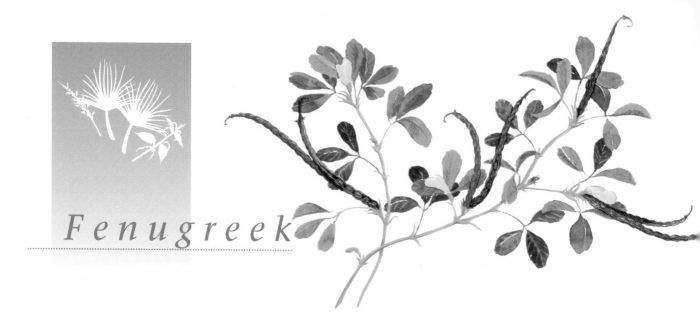

Fenugreek

Name: *Trigonella foenum-graecum* L. (Leguminosae). Commonly called Fenugreek, or Greek hay. In French, it is *Trigonelle fenugrec* or *Fenugrec*; in German, *Bockshornsamen, Bockshornklee* or *Griechisch-Heu.*

Source: Dried, ripe seeds are harvested from plants grown mainly in India and Southwest Asia. They have a mealy, unpleasant taste.

History: Fenugreek was grown by the ancient Greeks to feed animals, and Hippocrates recommended it as a treatment for respiratory infections. Fenugreek was introduced into Europe by the Benedictine monks in the 9th century. It was used by the famous Arabic physicians. At the same time, in India and Egypt, fenugreek was cultivated as a food. Europeans added it to inferior grades of hay in order to improve it's odor. Seventeenth century physicians believed that if a women who had just delivered a baby would sit over fumes of a heated fenugreek solution, they would deliver the placenta more quickly. During World War II, people began to use it as a coffee substitute.

Traditional Claims: Emollient, vulnerary, expectorant, demulcent and aphrodisiac. Pulverized seeds were used in poultices to treat boils and skin infections. The most frequent traditional use was for the treatment of upper respiratory infections, although it was sometimes also used to treat diabetes.

Commission E Recommendations: Fenugreek is used externally to treat inflammatory skin disease, and internally to stimulate the appetite.

Proven Effects: Claims about treating diabetes appear to have a basis in fact. An amino acid contained in fenugreek seeds, called 4- hydroxyisoleucine, increases glucose-induced insulin release from the pancreas. In clinical trials with diabetic patients, fenugreek supplementation lowered blood sugars and, at the same time, lowered high levels of bad cholesterol (LDL) without affecting levels of good cholesterol. The ability to lower cholesterol probably has something to do with the saponins (diosgenin and yamogenin) that make up 1-2 percent of the seeds' contents. Saponins combine with cholesterol in the intestines and prevent it from being absorbed. Remedies containing saponins are also effective expectorants. Claims that fenugreek stimulates the appetite have been validated in animal studies, but not in humans. In the absence of any hard data, it is anyone's guess whether this herb is really an aphrodisiac.

The Consumer's Guide to Herbal Medicine

Concerns: Allergic reactions, sometimes severe, have been reported. Fenugreek is a member of the Leguminosae family, and plants in this family are more likely than others to cause allergic reactions.

Warnings: Other than unpredictable allergic reactions, no serious toxicity has ever been reported. Fenugreek is a component of most curry powders, and individuals with known allergies to chickpeas (a close relative) may also have allergies to fenugreek.

Drug Testing: Saponins do not cause positive urine drug screening tests, and it is unlikely that any of the other components would either.

Dosage: For internal use, Commission E recommends 6 grams of powdered dried seeds once a day, alone or in combination with other herbs. For external use, 50 grams of powdered seeds in 250 cc of water, as a bath additive or made into an ointment.

Summary: This ancient remedy may well yet prove to be a valuable treatment for diabetes, and for elevated blood cholesterol levels. The results in clinical trials are very encouraging, but more needs to be known. Except for allergic reactions, toxicity is unheard of. Until more research is done, diabetics must rely on allopathic cures. On the other hand, eating fenugreek-containing foods on a regular basis might not be a bad idea, especially if you have a cough or cold!

References:

Bordia A, Verma SK, Srivastava KC. Effect of ginger (*Zingiber officinale* Rosc.) and fenugreek (*Trigonella foenum-graecum L.*) on blood lipids, blood sugar and platelet aggregation in patients with coronary artery disease. Prostaglandins Leukot Essent Fatty Acids 1997;56(5):379-84.

Ohnuma N, Yamaguchi E, Kawakami Y. Anaphylaxis to curry powder. Allergy 1998;53(4):452-4.

Patil SP, Niphadkar PV, Bapat MM. Allergy to fenugreek (*Trigonella foenum graecum*). Ann Allergy Asthma Immunol 1997;78(3):297-300.

Sauvaire Y, Baissac Y, Leconte O, Petit P, Ribes G. Steroid saponins from fenugreek and some of their biological properties. Adv Exp Med Biol 1996;405:37-46.

Sauvaire Y, Petit P, Broca C, Manteghetti M, Baissac Y, Fernandez-Alvarez J, et al. 4-Hydroxyisoleucine: a novel amino acid potentiator of insulin secretion. Diabetes 1998;47(2):206-10.

Sharma RD, Raghuram TC, Rao NS. Effect of fenugreek seeds on blood glucose and serum lipids in type I diabetes. Eur J Clin Nutr 1990;44(4):301-6.

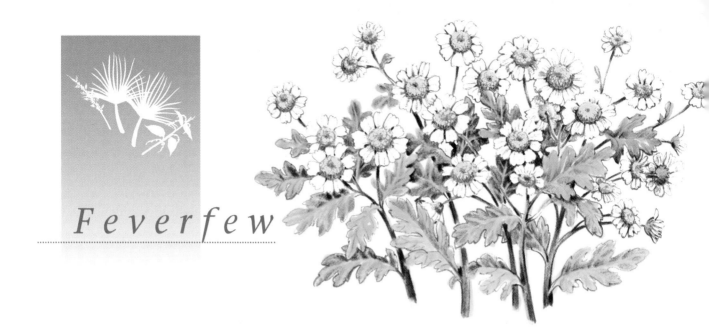

Feverfew

Name: *Tanacetum parthenium* (L) Shulz Bip., *Chrysanthemum parthenium* L. Bernh, and *Matricaria parthenium* L.(Compositae), *Pyrethrum parthenium* L Sm. Common English names include flirtwort, feverwort, and feather foil. The French call it *Grande camomille,* while the Germans refer to the same plant as *Mutterekraut.*

Source: Medicines are made from the dried upper portions of the plant, collected just when it flowers. Feverfew is native to Europe where it grows wild along roadsides and around abandoned buildings. It can also be cultivated. Depending on where the feverfew is grown, leaves contain an average of .18 to .35 percent of a substance called parthenolide, thought to be the main active ingredient. Feverfew also contains a good deal of camphor, which is the source of its powerful scent.

History: The name comes from the Latin word *febrifugia*, meaning a plant that has the ability to drive out fevers. Ancient herbalists believed that feverfew was created by Venus in order to aid womankind. Ever since, feverfew has been used by women to initiate menstruation and to help expel the placenta after childbirth. During the last decade, new uses for feverfew have emerged.

Traditional Claims: In addition to its use in obstetrics and gynecology, feverfew was also used to treat arthritis and headaches.

Commission E Recommendation: Feverfew is not mentioned in Commission E.

Proven Effects: Parthenolide is the active agent in feverfew. In Canada, where medications containing feverfew are prescribed to prevent migraine, the government requires products to be standardized to contain at least .2 percent parthenolide. Parthenolide is a sesquiterpene lactone (related to other similar lactones found in ginger and chamomile). In the laboratory it prevents platelets from releasing serotonin, a potent compound that, among other things, can cause spasm of blood vessels. Many of the older prescription drugs used to treat migraine worked by altering serotonin metabolism, and it is speculated that parthenolide acts in the same way. It is becoming increasingly obvious, however, that feverfew leaves contain other active ingredients. One of these is melatonin. Melatonin can be found in many plants (including St. John's Wort), sometimes in fairly high concentrations. For all anyone knows, it may be the melatonin, or some as yet unidentified component, that provides the beneficial effects.

Concerns: Major adverse effects have not been reported, but stomach upset and stomatitis have been reported, especially in long-term users. Fresh leaf is best eaten with some bread, as a sandwich, to protect the lining of the mouth. But in general, feverfew is so non-toxic that in two placebo control drug trials, patients taking the placebo reported more side effects than patients taking feverfew. The main concern with buying commercial products is that the parthenolide content of dried leaf deteriorates with storage. Product that has been on the shelf for any length of time may contain far less of the active ingredient than what is stated on the label.

Warnings: None

Drug Testing: There are no reports that parthenolide, or any of the other compounds contained in feverfew, interfere with standard workplace urine drug screening tests.

Dosage: Feverfew is normally prescribed in tablets or capsules, in a daily dose of 50-200 mg of dried herb per day.

Summary: Results of numerous controlled trials suggest regular use of feverfew can help prevent migraine headache, and in Canada it is sold specifically for that purpose. Other claims have not been investigated. The active ingredients of whole herb products tend to deteriorate with storage, and depending on the preparation being used, significant amounts of melatonin may also be present.

References:

Awang DV. Feverfew products. Cmaj 1997;157(5):510-1.

Brown AM, Edwards CM, Davey MR, Power JB, Lowe KC. Pharmacological activity of feverfew (*Tanacetum parthenium (L.)* Schultz- Bip.): assessment by inhibition of human polymorphonuclear leukocyte chemiluminescence in-vitro. J Pharm Pharmacol 1997;49(5):558-61.

Cottrell K. Herbal products begin to attract the attention of brand-name drug companies. Cmaj 1996;155(2):216-9.

Hausen BM. A 6-year experience with compositae mix. Am J Contact Dermat 1996;7(2):94-9.

Knight DW. Feverfew: chemistry and biological activity. Nat Prod Rep 1995;12(3):271-6.

Murch SJ, Simmons CB, Saxena PK. Melatonin in feverfew and other medicinal plants [letter]. Lancet 1997;350(9091):1598-9.

Paulsen E. Occupational dermatitis in Danish gardeners and greenhouse workers (II). Etiological factors. Contact Dermatitis 1998;38(1):14-9.

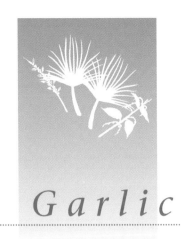

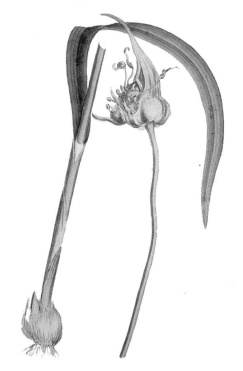

Garlic

Name: *Allium sativum* L. (Liliaceae), sometimes called allium, garlic, wild garlic, and ramsom. In French it is *Ail* (hence the term aoli used to describe garlic-flavored mayonnaise); in German, *Knoblauch.*

Source: Garlic, a member of the Lily family, is one of the oldest cultivated plants. It probably came from Central Asia, but is now grown almost everywhere. Commercial products are made from the fresh or dried bulbs. The rest of the plant is not thought to have any medicinal value. Garlic bulbs are dried immediately after harvesting and then ground to a fine powder. When prepared in this fashion, the powder contains both the water soluble and fat soluble components of the bulbs. Alternatively, garlic cloves can be soaked in corn or wheat germ oil and then put through a press. The process is called cold oil infusion, and the final product contains only the fat soluble components of the bulbs. Oil-based products generally lack the beneficial effects associated with ground whole bulbs. If the garlic is allowed to ferment, the smell disappears. Unfortunately, the medically useful components disappear as well. Another way to process garlic is by freeze drying. This process preserves the medically active components and, at the same time, prevents the reaction that leads to the formation of allicin, the compound that gives garlic its distinctive odor. Once the tablet of freeze-dried garlic has been swallowed, allicin forms, and is released into the body just as if fresh, whole garlic had been taken.

History: Garlic may have come from the Middle East, but its common name is from the Anglo-Saxon words *gar* ("lance") and *leac* ("pot herb"). Garlic bulbs worn around the neck were thought to be good protection against vampires and witches. An Egyptian medical papyrus from 1550 BC recommended 22 different garlic-containing remedies. According to Herodotus, in order to prevent workers on the Egyptian pyramids from becoming ill, they were given large rations of onions, radishes, and garlic. Benedictine monks grew garlic in their monasteries during the Middle Ages, and garlic extracts were often used to treat cases of plague (probably without much success). In addition to using garlic as an antibiotic, both European and Oriental herbalists prescribe garlic for heart disease, especially heart failure (which used to be called "dropsy").

Traditional Claims: Expectorant, nervine, and antibiotic.

Commission E Recommendations: Garlic is used to treat geriatric vascular changes, high cholesterol, hypercholestermia and hyperlipidemia.

Proven Effects: Allicin, the active ingredient, forms when an odorless compound called alliin is activated by an enzyme called allinase. The results of animal studies suggest that garlic supplementation can lower cholesterol, remove cholesterol deposits from the walls of major arteries, lower blood pressure, and protect the heart. Garlic has been recommended as a treatment for high blood pressure, as an antioxidant, and as a general "cardioprotective." It is now very widely taken by consumers hoping to lower elevated blood cholesterol levels. The idea seems to make sense because heart disease is relatively uncommon in Southern Europe, the area where the most garlic is consumed, although how allicin, or any other component found in garlic, could produce these effects is not known. Clinical trials in the early 1990s tended to confirm the folklore. When volunteers took garlic supplements, cholesterol levels dropped anywhere from 9 to 13 percent. But when more rigorously controlled studies were undertaken a few years later, no beneficial effects could be found; cholesterol levels stayed the same, and so did blood pressure.

Concerns: Toxicity from garlic, in any form, has never been reported. Too much garlic, whether taken in pill form, or in a rich butter sauce, can of course, lead to an upset stomach. If enough garlic is ingested, the smell can be quite overpowering and persistent.

Warnings: None

Drugs Testing: No interaction with standard workplace urine drug tests has been reported.

Dosage: Participants in most of the garlic-cholesterol trials took the equivalent of 800 mg per day of the dried powder. Commission E recommends a daily dose equal to 4-12 mg of alliin, 2-5 grams fresh garlic, or 2-5 grams of garlic oil.

Summary: Convincing evidence that garlic can lower cholesterol is lacking. The fact remains, however, that residents of Southern Europe eat more garlic and have less heart disease than Americans. But, they also drink more wine, consume more olive oil, and eat less meat than Americans. Obviously, more than just garlic consumption is involved. Still, it would be hard to think of a safer herbal remedy than garlic, and the only harm that could come from using too much garlic might be that people would avoid you.

References:

Berthold HK, Sudhop T, von Bergmann K. Effect of a garlic oil preparation on serum lipoproteins and cholesterol metabolism: a randomized-controlled trial. Jama 1998;279(23):1900-2.

Brown JS, Marcy SA. The use of botanicals for health purposes by members of a prepaid health plan. Res Nurs Health 1991;14(5):339-50.

Frate DA, Croom EM, Jr., Frate JB, Juergens JP, Meydrech EF. Use of plant-derived therapies in a rural, biracial population in Mississippi. J Miss State Med Assoc 1996;37(1):427-9.

Garlic oil: no impact on lipids [news]. Harv Heart Lett 1998; 9(1):6.

Isaacsohn JL, Moser M, Stein EA, Dudley K, Davey JA, Liskov E, et al. Garlic powder and plasma lipids and lipoproteins: a multicenter, randomized, placebo-controlled trial. Arch Intern Med 1998;158(11):1189-94.

Wang BH, Zuzel KA, Rahman K, Billington D. Protective effects of aged garlic extract against bromobenzene toxicity to precision cut rat liver slices. Toxicology 1998;126(3):213-221

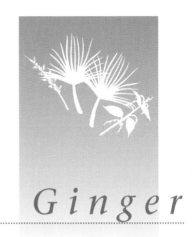

Ginger

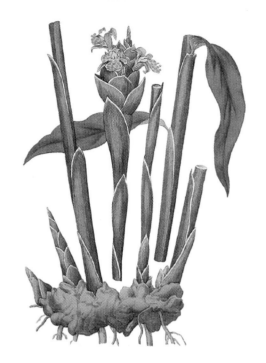

Name: *Zingiber officinale,* Roscoe (Zingiberaceae). Commonly called ginger. In French it is *Gingembre;* in German, *Ingwerwurzelstock.*

Source: Ginger comes from a perennial tropical plant that grows in many parts of the world. Ginger from Jamaica is the most prized and the most difficult to obtain. Total worldwide production is thought to exceed 100,000 tons. The plant has large flowers that look much like orchids, but the flowers produce neither fruits nor seeds - the plant reproduces through it's rhizomes. A volatile oil is distilled from ginger's rhizomes. It contains a complex mixture of molecules called terpenoids. The main terpenoid is called zingiberene, but the mix of terpenoids depends on where the plants have been grown. Gingerols, the plant components that impart the spicy taste, are not contained in the volatile oils - they are obtained by solvent extraction. The spiciest, most pungent ginger components, called shogaols, are not even found in fresh plants. They form during the drying process. Terpenoids, gingerols, and shogaols all exert effects on the body.

History: Ginger-containing medicines were used to treat nausea and indigestion by Chinese physicians more than 2000 years ago. Traditional herbalists attributed different actions to different parts of the plant. Fresh rhizomes were used to treat nausea and coughs, dried rhizomes were used to treat stomach aches and back pain. Over the years, ginger has become one of the most commonly used food additives.

Traditional Claims: Carminative and antiemetic (prevents vomiting).

Commission E Recommendations: Ginger is used to treat dyspepsia (upset stomach) and motion sickness.

Proven Effects: Ginger exerts positive effects on the digestive, cardiovascular, and central nervous systems. It may also be a powerful anti-inflammatory and antimicrobial agent. However, the only action ever to be evaluated in clinical trials is the ability of ginger to control nausea. Several different clinical trials have shown that ginger can prevent motion sickness, and that ginger (along with the use of vitamin B6 and acupressure) also helps decrease the nausea and vomiting associated with pregnancy.

Concerns: In laboratory animals, large doses can cause low blood sugar (hypoglycemia), while the gingerols and shogaols contained in ginger can induce a dangerous decrease in heart rate and blood pressure. Similar effects have not been reported in humans. It may be that they do not occur. A more likely explanation is that humans do not take doses as large as those which have been given to the experimental animals and, therefore, do not experience significant side effects.

Warnings: Gingerols, and possibly other components as well, can have a marked effect on contraction of the muscles in the bowel, and in the passages connecting the gallbladder to the intestine. There are no clinical reports of anyone with gallstones ever getting worse because they took ginger, but Commission E warns against using ginger if you have gallstones. (Commission E also warns against use by pregnant women.)

Drug Testing: No component found in ginger rhizomes, or in the volatile oil, has ever been shown to interfere with workplace urine drug screening tests.

Dosage: When used to prevent motion sickness or the morning sickness of pregnancy, the recommended dose is 1 to 2 grams of the powdered rhizome. For other purposes, the dose is .25 to 1.0 grams of powdered rhizome three times a day. According to the British Pharmacopeia, the dose of Weak Ginger Tincture (1:5, 90 percent ethanol) is 1.5 to 3 milliliters up to three times a day. For Strong Ginger Tincture (1:2, 90 percent ethanol), the dose is 0.25 to .5 milliliters up to three times a day.

Summary: Ginger seems to be an extremely safe herb, and one that can successfully prevent motion sickness and relieve the nausea and vomiting of pregnancy. Still, any pregnant woman contemplating its use should check with her physician first. Because ginger grows commercially in so many places, and because the content of the rhizomes varies depending on where the plant is grown, and because their is no industry or government standard for gingerol and shaogol content, results may vary from batch to batch, and from manufacturer to manufacturer.

References:

Aikins Murphy P. Alternative therapies for nausea and vomiting of pregnancy. Obstet Gynecol 1998;91(1):149-55.

Mascolo N, Sharma R, Jain SC, Capasso F. Ethnopharmacology of *Calotropis procera* flowers. J Ethnopharmacol 1988;22(2):211-21.

Gronstved A, Brask T, Kambskard J, Hentzer E. Ginger root against seasickness: A controlled clinical trial on the open sea. Acta Otolaryngol (Stockh) 1988;105:45-9.

Suekawa M, Ishige A, Yuasa K, Sudo K, Aburada M, Hosoya E. Pharmacological studies on ginger. I. Pharmacological actions of pungent constituents, (6)-gingerol and (6)-shogaol. J Pharmacobiodyn 1984;7(11):836-48.

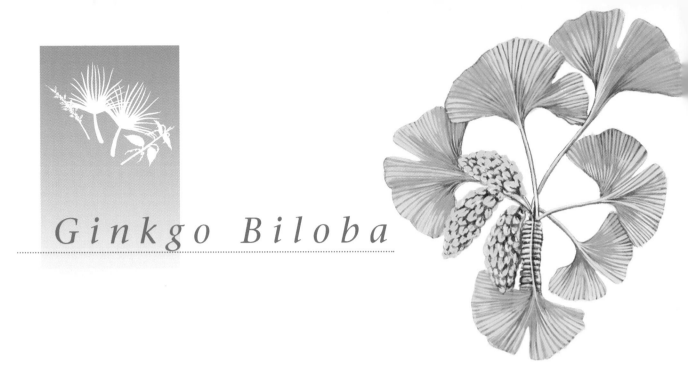

Ginkgo Biloba

Name: *Ginkgo biloba* L. (Ginkgoaceae), commonly called ginkgo or maidenhair tree. In German the leaves are *Ginkgoblätter*. It is the sole surviving species of the plant family known as Ginkgoaceae.

Source: Ginkgo was brought to Europe, from China in the 1700s as an ornamental tree, and today it can be found in parks around the world. Commercial ginkgo extracts come from the leaves. In Europe, Asia, and even the United States, trees are specifically grown for producing extract. Ginkgo leaves contain two types of molecules; flavonoids and terpenoids. Ginkgo extracts sold in Europe are standardized to contain 22-27 percent flavonoids and 5-7 percent terpenoids. At the moment, no one is quite sure which component exerts the beneficial effects.

History: Ginkgo is mentioned in Chinese texts dating back more than 3,000 years. It has been suggested that Ginkgo extract was a key component of the ancient Ayurvedic elixir called "soma." An extract of ginkgo biloba, known as EGb 761, is very widely used in Europe to treat "cerebral insufficiency." It is, in fact, the best selling herbal medication in Europe, with annual sales amounting to well over half a billion dollars a year.

Traditional Claims: For circulatory disorders and to improve memory.

Commission E. Recommendations: Ginkgo biloba leaf extract is used to treat arterial occlusive disease, circulatory disorders, depression, free radical deactivation, retinal lesions and edema, tinnitus, vertigo, and to improve memory and mental concentration.

Proven Effects: The flavonoids and the terpenoids in ginkgo are both classified as antioxidants. They combine with "free radicals," unstable molecules that are thought to play a role in aging, cancer, and Alzheimer's disease. Europeans use ginkgo extract to treat "cerebral insufficiency." Results have been mixed, partly because most of the drug trials have been poorly designed, and partly because "cerebral insufficiently" is such a vague term, referring to deficits of short-term memory and concentration, as well as lack of energy, ringing in the ears (tinnitus), headache, and even depression.

However, when the extract is used just to treat patients with dementia (Alzheimer's disease is one kind of dementia), then it does seem to help. In 1997, a highly publicized study appeared in the *Journal of the American Medical Association (JAMA)*. Standardized extract was given to hundreds of patients suffering from dementia for six months to a year, while a control group received placebo. The group taking ginkgo showed modest, but very definite signs of improvement.

The other earlier use for ginkgo, is in the treatment of circulatory disorders. Published trials claim improvement in Reynauds syndrome, in leg pain from arterial insufficiency (known as intermittent claudication) and in erectile dysfunction. The evidence for all these claims is much less substantial than for the improvements seen in the patients with dementia. Still other laboratory studies suggest that ginkgo extract may (1) be useful in preventing contact dermatitis, (2) help patients with HIV protect against recurrent pneumocystis *carinii infection,* when taken on a regular basis,(3) heal some of the blood vessel damage seen in patients with chronic venous ulcers, and, most interesting of all, (4) may prevent some of the cellular changes associated with aging when used on a regular basis. Unfortunately, the findings of these studies have never been independently confirmed in clinical trials.

Concerns: Ginkgo products made in Germany carry labels warning that the product can cause mild gastrointestinal symptoms, occasional headache, and sometimes allergic reactions. Nonetheless, years of experience have shown that ginkgo extract is an incredibly safe product. In 1991, a German drug company surveyed nearly 11,000 people with dementia who had used their ginkgo extract. Side effects were reported in fewer than 2 percent, and all of those effects were minor and transient. Given the millions and millions of prescriptions written for ginkgo in Germany, the safety record is quite extraordinary. European ginkgo extracts are standardized. Purchasers in Europe can expect to get a product containing 22-27 percent flavonoids and 5-7 percent terpenoids. That is not always the case with ginkgo supplements made in the United States. As with any other product, buyers should read the label. If the concentration is too low, the product may not work. If the concentration is too high, there may be unanticipated, adverse side effects. "Super" strength formulations of ginkgo are not necessarily a good thing!

Warnings: One of the terpenoid compounds found in ginkgo extracts interferes with a natural body chemical called platelet activating factor, and prevents it from working normally. The ability of blood to clot may be compromised. And there are, in fact, three reports of brain hemorrhage in ginkgo users; one individual was taking coumadin and another was taking aspirin (another blood thinner). Ginkgo's antiplatelet action probably is of no consequence for any normal person, but anyone taking blood thinners (coumadin, heparin, etc.) should think long and hard before taking ginkgo biloba. Another toxic compound, 4-O-Methylpyridoxine (MPN) is found only in ginkgo seeds. Seeds are not used by Western herbalists, but they are used in Japan where overdoses are not rare. Convulsions and coma can occur after large amounts of seed-containing remedies have been ingested.

Drug Testing: Ginkgo extract is not known to have any effect on any of the standard urine screening tests used for workplace testing.

Dosage: In more than 30 different European clinical trials the total dose of EGB 761 has ranged from 120-240 mg per day in divided doses.

Summary: Ginkgo biloba extract is, taken in standard dosages, very safe, and seems to produce mild improvements in patients with Alzheimer's disease. Whether it is of any value in treating other circulatory disorders, such as erectile dysfunction, is hard to say, but since it is so safe, trying the extract might be worth while. Ginkgo biloba should never be used by anyone taking coumadin or other blood thinning products. Heart patients, who take aspirin regularly, should first consult their doctors. Always read the label and only purchase products made from ginkgo leaves. The seeds are toxic and dangerous.

References:

Cohen AJ, Bartlik B. *Ginkgo biloba* for antidepressant-induced sexual dysfunction. J Sex Marital Ther 1998;24(2):139-43.

Cott J. NCDEU update. Natural product formulations available in europe for psychotropic indications. Psychopharmacol Bull 1995; 31(4):745-51.

Anon. *Ginkgo biloba*. Altern Med Rev 1998;3(1):54-7.

Kim YS, Pyo MK, Park KM, Park PH, Hahn BS, Wu SJ, et al. Antiplatelet and antithrombotic effects of a combination of ticlopidine and *Ginkgo biloba* ext (EGb 761). Thromb Res 1998;91(1):33-8.

Le Bars PL, Katz MM, Berman N, Itil TM, Freedman AM, Schatzberg AF. A placebo-controlled, double-blind, randomized trial of an extract of *Ginkgo biloba* for dementia. North American EGb Study Group [see comments]. Jama 1997;278(16):1327-32.

Lee JS, Cho YS, Park EJ, Kim J, Oh WK, Lee HS, et al. Phospholipase C-gamma1 inhibitory principles from the sarcotestas of *Ginkgo biloba*. J Nat Prod 1998;61(7):867-71.

Matthews MK, Jr. Association of *Ginkgo biloba* with intracerebral hemorrhage [letter; comment]. Neurology 1998;50(6):1933-4.

Maurer K, Ihl R, Dierks T, Frolich L. Clinical efficacy of *Ginkgo biloba* special extract EGb 761 in dementia of the Alzheimer type.J Psychiatr Res 1997;31(6):645-55.

Peters H, Kieser M, Holscher U. Demonstration of the efficacy of *Ginkgo biloba* special extract EGb 761 on intermittent claudication—a placebo-controlled, double-blind multicenter trial. Vasa 1998;27(2):106-10.

Yoneko M, Ubukata K, Sakata M, Wada K, and Haga M. The detoxification metabolism of 4-O-Methylpyridoxine (MPB), a causative substance of Ginkgo seed poisoning. Read at the Annual Meeting of the Society of Forensic Toxicologists, Albuquerque, New Mexico, October 7, 1998.

Zhu L, Gao J, Wang Y, Zhao XN, Zhang ZX. Neuron degeneration induced by verapamil and attenuated by EGb761. J Basic Clin Physiol Pharmacol 1997;8(4):301-14.

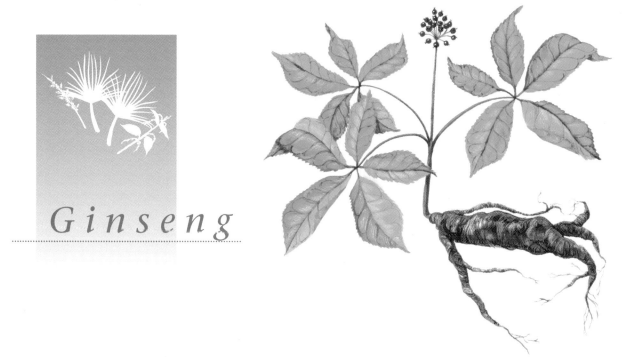

Ginseng

Name: *Panax ginseng,* Meyer (Araliaceae). Commonly called ginseng, Asian ginseng, and *Panax quinquefolius,* also known as American ginseng. Other closely related species included *Panax notoginseng* and *Panax japonicus. Eleutherococcus senticosus,* referred to as Siberian ginseng, is a close relative. In French it is called *Ginseng;* in German, it is known both as *Ginseng* and *Ginsengwurzel.*

Source: Products labeled ginseng usually contain material from the roots of *P. Ginseng* or *P. Quinquefolius.* (Asian and American ginseng). Most of the *P. Ginseng* sold in the United States and Europe is imported from Korea where it is grown commercially. Plants are harvested when they are from five to seven years old. Roots that have been allowed to air dry are the source of "white ginseng." Roots that are steamed for two to four hours yield "red ginseng." Red ginseng contains all the same active ingredients found in white ginseng, but some additional compounds are created during the steaming process. *P. quinquefolius,* which grows in the United States, is mainly exported to China. *E. senticosus* is very closely related, but contains a slightly different group of active ingredients referred to as eleutherosides. The active ingredients in *P. Ginseng* or *P. quinquefolius* are called ginsenosides. Over 20 different ginsenosides have been isolated from the roots, leaves, and flowers.

History: Traditional Chinese healers have used ginseng as a restorative "tonic" since the early Han Dynasty, more than 2,000 years ago. Europeans first learned of this plant from a Jesuit missionary, Father Petrus Jartoux (1668-1720). Jartoux was working in Northern China, and he published a book containing his observations on ginseng in 1709. Inspired by what he had read, another Jesuit, Pére Joseph Francois Lafitau (1681-1746) began looking for ginseng in America. Lafitau found that the Mohawk Indians used a plant almost identical to the one described by Jartoux. Lafitau sent a sample of American ginseng to Jartoux, and not long thereafter, North American clipper ships (including some owned by John Jacob Astor, who also realized handsome profits shipping opium to China), began carrying American-grown ginseng to China. Most American ginseng is grown in Madison County, Wisconsin. But just to make matters more confusing, Chinese farmers have planted American ginseng in China. American ginseng grown in China is referred to as "Chinese white" (no relation to China White heroin!), and is generally considered to be of poor quality. Ginseng is on the endangered species list, and ginseng harvesting is under the control of the United States government.

Traditional Claims: To maintain health and to prevent disease. It has also been used as an aid during convalescence, to improve alertness and concentration, and generally to relieve fatigue.

It was, and still is, especially recommended for the elderly, but it has also been used by the young to improve athletic performance.

Commission E Recommendations: Ginseng is used as a tonic to treat fatigue and debility and to improve mental concentration. It is also used during convalescence.

Proven Effects: Ginseng's benefits are more evident in people (or animals) who are, in some way, stressed. Many of the benefits are hard to classify, and ultimately a new word "adaptogen," was coined to described them. There is research suggesting that ginseng can improve the ability of young athletes to run, of middle-aged men to work harder, and of elderly subjects to do arithmetic. Experimental animals treated with ginseng become resistant (though not immune) to viruses, tumors, lack of oxygen, and even X-ray irradiation. The active ingredients, the ginsenosides, have two seemingly conflicting actions that could explain all of these actions: they are antioxidants, but they also stimulate production of nitric oxide. The antioxidant effects are probably what protect the heart and brain against the effects of aging. The other benefits may derive from ginseng's effects on nitric oxide production. Nitric oxide is a free radical, but not all free radicals are bad. In fact, low concentrations of free radicals are necessary for normal body function. Nitric oxide molecules are used to send messages from one nerve to another and from nerves to muscles and blood vessels. Increasing the amount of nitric oxide can cause blood vessels to dilate, and possibly increase blood flow to the brain. Increased nitric oxide production may also explain why ginseng is praised as an aphrodisiac. The nerves that control erectile function contain nitric oxide.

Concerns: Claims about ginseng toxicity are difficult to sort out. Based on animal studies of acute toxicity, the lethal dose in humans would be something on the order of two pounds! There are reports in the medical literature describing nervousness, insomnia, and gastrointestinal upset in long-term users who were taking up to 15 grams per day. No such difficulties have been reported in people taking the recommended dose of 1 to 2 grams per day. Still, ginseng does seem to activate the central nervous system, so using ginseng with too much coffee or caffeine-containing beverages might give some users more of a "buzz" than they would like. The biggest cause for concern is whether consumers will get what they are paying for. Different brands of ginseng may contain unpredictably low or high amounts of ginsenosides, which explains why it is so difficult to interpret reports in the literature - without knowing how much ginsenosides had been given, its impossible to know whether it was the ginsenosides that produced the benefits (or the undesired side effects). More recent research studies use standardized formulations containing 4 percent ginsenosides.

Warnings: There appears to be no serious health concerns, but the issue of toxicity from long-term use in humans has never really been studied. In some people, ginseng can produce moderate blood pressure elevation, which means that patients with high blood pressure need to discuss the possible use of ginseng with their doctors first. As with any other drug, ginseng use during pregnancy is not a good idea. Commission E says that ginseng use should be limited to three months, but that "a repeated course is feasible."

Drug Testing: There are no reports of any ginseng product interfering with standard workplace urine drug screening tests.

Dosage: Commission E recommends a dose of 1 to 2 grams of ginseng root per day.

Summary: So many claims have been made for ginseng for so many years that there must be something to its story. Countless laboratory studies, and some very reputable clinical trials, suggest regular use may very well increase feelings of strength and well-being, improve mental performance, particularly in the elderly and in individuals who are already pathologically stressed (from a disease or from a stressful situation). Epidemiologic studies suggesting lower cancer rates in ginseng-users are also encouraging, though in need of much more confirmation. Consumers should be sure to buy products containing standardized amounts of ginsenosides (at least 4 percent).

References:

Eliason BC, Kruger J, Mark D, Rasmann DN. Dietary supplement users: demographics, product use, and medical system interaction. J Am Board Fam Pract 1997;10(4):265-71.

Gillis CN. *Panax ginseng* pharmacology: a nitric oxide link? Biochem Pharmacol 1997;54(1):1-8.

Goldstein B. Ginseng: its history, dispersion, and folk tradition. Am J Chin Med 1975;3(3):223-34.

Lim JH, Wen TC, Matsuda S, Tanaka J, Maeda N, Peng H, et al. Protection of ischemic hippocampal neurons by ginsenoside Rb1, a main ingredient of ginseng root. Neurosci Res 1997;28(3):191-200.

Lucerno MA, McCloskey WW. Alternatives to estrogen for the treatment of hot flashes. Ann Pharmacother 1997;31(7-8):915-7.

Yun TK, Choi SY. Non-organ specific cancer prevention of ginseng: a prospective study in Korea. Int J Epidemiol 1998;27(3):359-64.

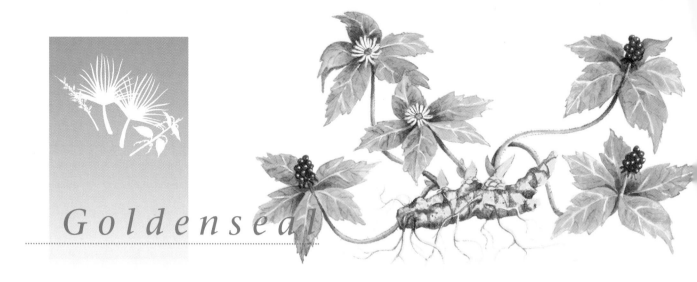

Goldenseal

Name: *Hydrastis canadensis* L., (Ranuneulaceae). Commonly called Goldenseal or hydrastis.

Source: Goldenseal comes from the dried rhizomes and roots of goldenseal, a New World plant. Modest amounts are exported to Europe.

History: Goldenseal is a native American plant, originally used by Cherokee Indians to treat skin diseases. In the early 1900s, goldenseal-containing tonics were popular for treatment of upset stomach and menstrual disorders. Teas made from goldenseal are said to relieve canker sores, and stomatitis (inflamed mouth). Use of goldenseal was negligible until the early 1990s when a false rumor began to circulate that drinking goldenseal tea would allow illicit drug users (especially marijuana smokers) to avoid detection.

Traditional Claims: Goldenseal is used for the treatment of inflamed mucous membranes, especially of the upper respiratory tract, for eye irritation, excessive menstrual bleeding, and upset stomach.

Commission E Recommendations: Goldenseal is not mentioned in Commission E.

Proven Effects: The active ingredient was thought to be a compound called hydrastine. More recently, attention has focused on another substance present in goldenseal, but in much smaller amounts, called canadine (also tetrahydroberberine or just berberine). Berberines are found in many other plants, including the opium poppy, but usually in much higher concentrations. Berberine is toxic to insects and vertebrates and prevents the growth of bacteria, fungi and viruses. Tests in the laboratory suggest that berberines have the ability to disrupt enzyme systems in bacteria and parasites. Tests on patients have shown that berberine is a very effective antimalarial and antibacterial agent. This ability to fight infections may explain why herbalists often combine goldenseal with echinacea, a herb that stimulates immunity.

Concerns: There are no reports of serious toxicity and the amount of goldenseal in an individual serving of most commercially sold products is so low that toxicity would be unlikely. But in laboratory studies, when very high doses are given to laboratory animals, irregular heartbeats have occurred. There are no relevant clinical studies. In fact, there are fewer than 20 papers in the scientific literature analyzing the actions and effects of hydrastine. Given that goldenseal is one of the best selling herbal products in the United States, the lack of serious scientific studies is distressing.

Warnings: None, except perhaps for pregnant women. Even though goldenseal has never been proven to cause uterine contractions, most European regulatory agencies recommend against its use during pregnancy.

Drug Testing: Contrary to all commercial claims and endorsements on the Internet, goldenseal-based products will not interfere with any of the commonly used workplace urine screening tests. The directions on such products almost always include drinking large quantities of water with the goldenseal, and it is the water that helps produce a negative test result, not the goldenseal. Urine drug tests are not considered positive unless a certain amount of drug (the amounts are set by the U.S. Government) is present. If marijuana metabolite is present, but at concentrations below 50 ng/mL, then the test result is called negative. If the urine contains 51 ng/mL, the result is called positive. A regular marijuana user who had smoked marijuana two days before being tested might still have 60 ng/mL of metabolite in his urine. But, if half a gallon of water was drunk just before giving the urine sample, the urine would be diluted, and the concentration might drop - just for a few hours - to below 50 ng/mL. Berberines can be detected in the urine and, in the not too distant future, some laboratories may begin testing for them.

Dosage: From .5 to 1 gram of dried rhizome and root, or 2 to 4 milliliters of 1:10 tincture two to three times a day.

Summary: Goldenseal can prevent the growth of bacteria, fungi and viruses, both in test tubes and in clinical trials. Whether the concentrations found in most herbal teas are high enough to do any good is questionable, but the combination of goldenseal and echinacea for respiratory infection does seem to make sense. Unless it is washed down with half a gallon of water, goldenseal has never helped anyone "beat" a workplace urine drug test.

References:

Facchini PJ, Penzes C, Johnson AG, Bull D. Molecular characterization of berberine bridge enzyme genes from opium poppy. Plant Physiol 1996;112(4):1669-77.

Iwasa K, Kamigauchi M, Sugiura M, Nanba H. Antimicrobial activity of some 13-alkyl substituted protoberberinium salts. Planta Med 1997;63(3):196-8.

Riccioppo Neto F, Mesquita Junior O, Olivera GB. Antiarrhythmic and electrophysiological effects of the novel KATP channel opener, rilmakalim, in rabbit cardiac cells. Gen Pharmacol 1997;29(2):201-5.

Schmeller T, Latz-Bruning B, Wink M. Biochemical activities of berberine, palmatine and sanguinarine mediating chemical defence against microorganisms and herbivores. Phytochemistry 1997;44 (2):257-66.

Sheng WD, Jiddawi MS, Hong XQ, Abdulla SM. Treatment of chloroquine-resistant malaria using pyrimethamine in combination with berberine, tetracycline or cotrimoxazole. East Afr Med J 1997;74(5):283-4.

Wu SN, Yu HS, Jan CR, Li HF, Yu CL. Inhibitory effects of berberine on voltage- and calcium-activated potassium currents in human myeloma cells. Life Sci 1998;62(25):2283-94.

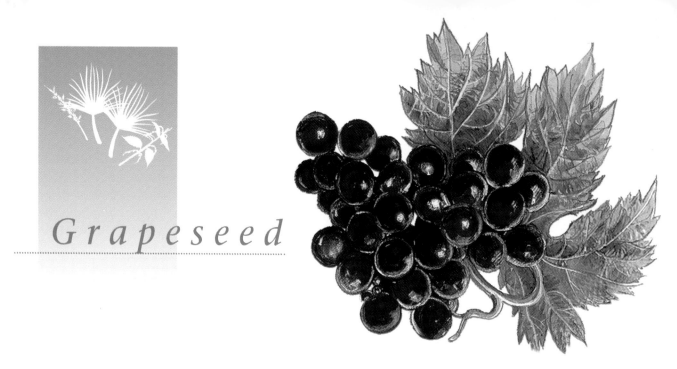

Grapeseed

Name: *Vitis vinifera* L. (Vitaceae). Commonly called grapeseed. In French, it is called *Vigne cultivé*; in German, *Weinstock*.

Source: Grape vines will grow almost everywhere, and probably were the first plant to be cultivated by man. Roughly 20 percent of the seed is comprised of a quick-drying oil with antioxidant properties.

History: The process of natural fermentation is very ancient. Beer was first brewed from fermented grain more than 3,500 years ago. The practice of making wine appears to be almost as old, and the practice of mixing medicines with wines equally ancient. The idea of using the rest of the vine for medicinal purposes is much more recent, probably dating to the Middle Ages, when sap from the vines was used to treat skin rashes and eye infections. Modern interest in grapeseed relates to its content of Vitamin E and linoleic acid.

Traditional Claims: Laxative and diuretic.

Commission E Recommendations: Grapeseed is not mentioned by Commission E.

Proven Effects: Grapeseed oil contains procyanidins, Vitamin E, and linoleic acid. The Vitamin E probably accounts for grapeseed's antioxidant effect, although the flavonoid proanthrocyanidins contained in the oil are also effective antioxidants. In two very large population studies, no benefits from Vitamin E supplementation could be found. But in other studies, double-blind at that, researchers found that supplements lowered the risk for coronary artery disease. A separate study of Finnish smokers failed to detect much of a benefit in preventing heart disease, but men taking 50 International Units (IU) a day of alpha-tocopherol had far fewer cases of prostate cancer than controls not taking the supplement. Interestingly, studies published at almost the same time reported that giving selenium also reduced the risk for prostate cancer. Since selenium is just as powerful an antioxidant as Vitamin E, it appears that the results from Finland are not a fluke. In addition to containing Vitamin E, grapeseed oil also contains linolenic acid, although not nearly as much as is found in sunflower oil and safflower oil. Conjugated linolenic acid (called, CLA, and consisting of multiple linoleic molecules bound together) prevents tumor growth. It is formed when linoleic acid in grapeseed is converted to CLA by intestinal bacteria. To the extent that linoleic acid replaces other fats in the diet, it causes good cholesterol (HDL) levels to rise and bad cholesterol levels (LDL) to fall, actions consistent with the prevention of heart disease. Antioxidant supplementation may have other benefits over and above preventing cancer and heart disease. There is an emerging consensus that "oxidative stress" plays a role in Alzheimer's disease, and that treatment with Vitamin E may help.

Concerns: There are several different types of Vitamin E. The form found naturally in our foods is gamma-tocopherol, a potent antioxidant. The Vitamin E found in supplements, such as grapeseed, is mostly alpha-tocopherol. There is laboratory evidence that when taken in very large amounts, alpha-tocopherol can block the effects of gamma-tocopherol, in effect, acting like a prooxidant!

Warning: Very high doses of Vitamin E can disrupt normal body metabolism of Vitamin K, and that can lead to bleeding tendencies. Patients taking anticoagulants such as coumadin should not be taking Vitamin E-containing products without first notifying their doctors.

Drug Testing: There is no evidence that any of the components of grapeseed oil will interfere with any of the standard workplace urine drug screening tests.

Dosage: The effective dosage has never really been determined. Most researchers feel that if Vitamin E supplements are to be taken, then at least 800 International Units a day will be required to produce any benefit. The Vitamin E content should be indicated on the label of the grapeseed product being purchased.

Summary: There is very good evidence that Vitamin E supplementation, whether from grapeseed or from some other source, helps prevent prostate cancer. There is even better evidence that linoleic acid supplementation causes good cholesterol to increase and bad cholesterol to decrease. The effects on other types of cancer, and the claimed benefits in heart disease, are still not sufficiently validated in human clinical trials. Considering the possible benefits, and the lack of evidence that grapeseed causes significant toxicity, using this supplement could provide substantial benefits with very little risk.

References:

Davey PJ, Schulz M, Gliksman M, Dobson M, Aristides M, Stephens NG. Cost-effectiveness of Vitamin E therapy in the treatment of patients with angiographically proven coronary narrowing (CHAOS trial). Cambridge Heart Antioxidant Study. Am J Cardiol 1998; 82(4):414-7.

Jain SK, Krueger KS, McVie R, Jaramillo JJ, Palmer M, Smith T. Relationship of blood thromboxane-B2 (TxB2) with lipid peroxides and effect of Vitamin E and placebo supplementation on TxB2 and lipid peroxide levels in type 1 diabetic patients. Diabetes Care 1998;21(9):1511-6.

Knopman DS. Current pharmacotherapies for Alzheimer's disease. Geriatrics 1998;53 Suppl 1:S31-4.

Nesaretnam K, Stephen R, Dils R, Darbre P. Tocotrienols inhibit the growth of human breast cancer cells irrespective of estrogen receptor status. Lipids 1998;33(5):461-9.

Peskind ER. Pharmacologic approaches to cognitive deficits in Alzheimer's disease. J Clin Psychiatry 1998;59(Suppl 9):22-7.

Teikari JM, Laatikainen L, Virtamo J, Haukka J, Rautalahti M, Liesto K, et al. Six-year supplementation with alpha-tocopherol and beta-carotene and age-related maculopathy. Acta Ophthalmol Scand 1998;76(2):224-9.

Teikari JM, Laatikainen L, Rapola JM, Virtamo J, Haukka J, Liesto K, et al. Retinal vascular changes following supplementation with alpha-tocopherol or beta-carotene. Acta Ophthalmol Scand 1998;76(1):68-73.

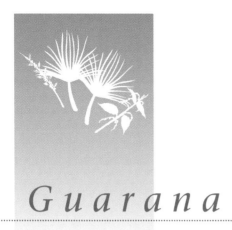

Guarana

Name: *Paullinia cupana* Mat. Var. *sorbilis,* (Sapindaceae), commonly called Guarana.

Sources: Guarana grows in the central region of the Amazon Basin. The seeds of the plant contain more caffeine, 4-5 percent, than any other plant. The leaves also contain large amounts of theobromine, a compound related to caffeine. Guarana is important because the powdered leaves and seeds are used as a source of caffeine in foods and in food supplements.

History: The Sateré-Maué Indians used guarana as a stimulant long before the first European explorers arrived in the Amazon. They used it in much the same way that ginseng is used by Chinese herbalists; to treat stress-related disorders, diarrhea and assorted aches and pains. Guarana-based products were first introduced to the United States in 1874 by Parke, Davis & Company. Parke, Davis and competing pharmaceutical companies sponsored a series of expeditions to the Amazon in an effort to discover new products. Their greatest success was, of course, cocaine, but they also discovered guarana. Until quite recently, guarana was viewed as nothing more than a source of caffeine, just as the coca plant was thought of as nothing more than a source of cocaine. Both views are clearly mistaken. There is mounting evidence that other chemicals in coca leaves, beside cocaine, helps increase endurance and protect against altitude sickness. The same is true for guarana. In addition to caffeine, guarana contains large amounts of tannins that have antioxidant activity. The essential oil from guarana has nine different components, two of which (estragole and anethole) are thought to be psychoactive. In Brazil, guarana is used to make an extremely popular carbonated soft drink.

Traditional Claims: For diarrhea and arthritic pain. Large doses of guarana oil are said to be psychoactive.

Commission E Recommendations: Guarana is not mentioned in Commission E.

Proven Effects: The caffeine found in Guarana may enhance performance. In combination with other drugs, it promotes weight loss. Caffeine is the world's most widely used stimulant drug. More than 80 percent of the U.S. population drinks or uses coffee, tea, soft drinks, or cold medications, pain relief formulas, and food supplements containing caffeine. An average cup of coffee contains 40–100 mg of caffeine. The content of cola drinks is lower, ranging from 30 to 50 mg. Caffeine supplements improve athletic performance. Elite marathon runners, given a dose of caffeine equivalent to the amount found in six or seven cups of coffee, increased the time they could run on a treadmill, and no ill effects were observed. Best of all, at least from the athletes' point of view, when their urine was tested, the caffeine content remained below the acceptable levels set by the International Olympic Committee (less than 12 µg/mL of caffeine). No one is quite sure how caffeine improves performance, but it appears caffeine promotes the use of fat as an energy source, sparing the body reserves of glycogen. Athletes who can metabolize lipid will have glycogen available for a longer period of time, and that should increase endurance. These same considerations may explain why some believe that caffeine (usually in combination with other agents, such as ephedra) helps promote weight loss.

People have been suspicious about the health effects of coffee and caffeine-containing beverages and foods ever since they were introduced in Europe more than 500 years ago. Concern focuses mainly on possible links between caffeine intake and heart attack, sudden death, fibrocystic breast disease and cancer. Alleged links to cancer have never been proven, and when controlled studies were done with heart patients, it turned out that caffeine was just as likely to make irregular ventricular beats go away as it was to cause them.

Concerns: It has been suggested that a caffeine-dependence syndrome exists, and that it meets all the generic criteria for substance dependence. Nonetheless, the evidence is really quite overwhelming that caffeine is a very safe drug, although excessive use will cause typical symptoms of sympathetic nervous system stimulation (shaky hands, racing heart).

Warnings: Caffeine may be a very safe drug, but only for adults. Children cannot handle sympathetic nervous system stimulation as well as adults, and they metabolize caffeine in such a way that toxic reactions become more likely than in adults. Excessive caffeine consumption makes children ill. Depending on the circumstances, and the size of the child, three or four bottles of caffeinated soft drink can make a child sick.

Drug Testing: The International Olympic Committee (IOC) and the National Collegiate Athletic Association have rules on the permissible amount of caffeine that may be present in an athlete's urine. Guidelines for the National Collegiate Athletic Associations are even more generous than those permitted by the IOC (15µg/mL), and at total doses of less than 9 mg/kg, no athlete is likely to be disqualified. To be sure, read the label of the product you are using and figure out how many servings you have taken, and divide by your weight in kilograms (1 kilogram = 2.25 pounds). For example, if you weigh 200 pounds and you consumed four servings of "Ripped Fuel™" containing 25 mg of caffeine per serving, your dose of caffeine would be 4 x 25 divided by your weight in kilograms, or 100 mg/88 kg = 1.4 mg/kg. Also, depending on the guarana preparation you are taking, there is a remote possibility that an initial screening test for methamphetamine might come back positive. The remote possibility exists that some components of the essential oil contained in guarana can be converted to a compound called 4-methoxyamphetamine, and that compound can cause a false positive test for methamphetamine.

Dosage: Safe and effective dose ranges for caffeine have never really been established, but millions of Americans consume three to four cups of coffee per day. Given an average caffeine content of 50 milligrams per cup, a total of 200 milligrams per day is unlikely to cause problems for anyone.

Summary: Guarana is the main source of caffeine found in food supplements, but its essential oil seems to contain other ingredients that may also be beneficial. Caffeine, itself, is a mild stimulant that improves performance and may facilitate weight loss. Questions about the safety of chronic use have been raised for years, but no solid evidence has ever been produced. Children are very sensitive to caffeine's effects, and their use of all caffeine-containing products should be limited.

References:

Bempong DK, Houghton PJ. Dissolution and absorption of caffeine from guarana. J Pharm Pharmacol 1992;44(9):769-71.

Benoni H, Dallakian P, Taraz K. Studies on the essential oil from guarana. Z Lebensm Unters Forsch 1996;203(1):95-8.

Espinola EB, Dias RF, Mattei R, Carlini EA. Pharmacological activity of Guarana (*Paullinia cupana Mart.*) in laboratory animals. J Ethnopharmacol 1997;55(3):223-9.

Galduroz JC, Carlini EdA. Acute effects of the *Paulinia cupana*, "Guarana" on the cognition of normal volunteers. Rev Paul Med 1994;112(3):607-11.

Miura T, Tatara M, Nakamura K, Suzuki I. Effect of Guarana on exercise in normal and epinephrine-induced glycogenolytic mice. Biol Pharm Bull 1998;21(6):646-8.

Morton JF. Widespread tannin intake via stimulants and masticatories, especially guarana, kola nut, betel vine, and accessories. Basic Life Sci 1992;59:739-65.

Stavric B. An update on research with coffee/caffeine (1989-1990). Food Chem Toxicol 1992;30(6):533-55.

Smith DA, Perry PJ. The efficacy of ergogenic agents in athletic competition. Part II: Other performance-enhancing agents. Ann Pharmacother 1992;26(5):653-9.

Graham TE, Spriet LL. Metabolic, catecholamine, and exercise performance responses to various doses of caffeine. J Appl Physiol 1995;78(3):867-74.

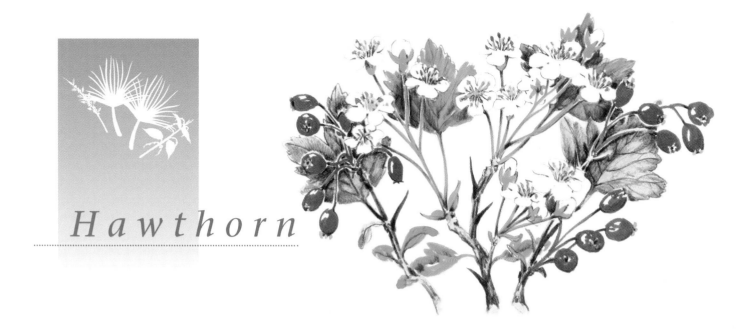

Hawthorn

Name: *Crataegus monogyna* Jacquin Emend. Lindman (Rosaceae). *Crataegus laevigata* (Poiret) DC, *Crataegus oxyacantha* L., commonly called Hawthorn, Whitethorn, May, and Haw. In French, it is *Auaépine épineuse*; in German, *Weissdorn* or *Zweigriffiger-Weissdorn*.

Source: Remedies are made from the dried ripe fruits of *C. monogyna*, a spiny tree found in woods and hedgerows across Europe. The fruits are called haws, and the tree has sharp thorns, hence hawthorn. Only fruits and leaves from the white-blooming hawthorn are thought to have medicinal value. The concentration of active ingredients in the berries is only a fraction of that found in the leaves and flowers (.1 vs 1.0 percent). The red-blooming variety of hawthorn is grown as an ornamental tree. The flowers have an unpleasant smell that serves mainly to attract flies. *C. monogyna*, which grows in the United States, appears to have the same chemical constituents as berries from the European trees.

History: Christ's crown of thorns is thought to have been made from hawthorn. In the Middle Ages, hawthorn was hung over the doorway to prevent the entry of evil spirits, although it was said to be unlucky to bring hawthorn blossoms indoors before May Day. Dioscorides, the ancient Greek physician, mentioned hawthorn, but its medically useful properties were first discovered by American physicians in the early 1800s, who used it to treat circulatory and respiratory disease. Hawthorn has only recently become popular again in the United States, but almost since the turn of the last century, European physicians, particularly those in Germany and France, have regularly used hawthorn to treat some kinds of heart disease.

Traditional Claims: A "cardiac tonic," especially useful in the treatment of irregular heartbeats, high blood pressure, hardening of the arteries and chest pain. It is also said to be antispasmodic and a sedative.

Commission E Recommendations: Hawthorn is used to treat cardiac insufficiency and geriatric vascular changes.

Proven Effects: Something in hawthorn, probably the flavonoid molecules, makes the heart beat more strongly and eliminates irregular heartbeats. These benefits occur because hawthorne (1) dilates the coronary arteries supplying the heart muscle, (2) has direct action on heart muscle causing it to contract more vigorously, and (3) relaxes the tone of the arteries that control blood pressure. There is also laboratory evidence that hawthorn can prevent the muscle damage that inevitably occurs when a coronary artery becomes occluded during a heart attack. This latter effect has not been tested clinically, but hawthorn has been given to patients with high blood pressure and mild heart failure and their conditions improved. In studies conducted by European herbalists, hawthorn seemed to work at least as well as the standard medical therapies. Other clinical benefits have been harder to demonstrate. Results from several trials suggest that using hawthorn can improve the anaerobic threshold. During maximum exercise, blood pressure and heart rate do not increase as much when patients have been treated with hawthorn. What that means, in effect, is that their hearts are working more efficiently and that hawthorn may be another "performance enhancing" drug. Unfortunately, hawthorn has never been tested in athletes. Based largely on laboratory findings, it has also been suggested that components of hawthorn extract can also lower cholesterol concentrations, but that claim has never even been studied, let alone proven, in humans.

Concerns: Test animals can tolerate massive doses (3,000 mg/kg, the equivalent of more than a half pound dose in a normal size man!) of hawthorn with very little sign of toxicity, but that does not necessarily mean the herb is harmless. The active ingredients in hawthorn, whichever they may be, take some time to exert their maximum effect. Heart failure patients treated with hawthorn do not show signs of improvement until they have been treated for more than one week. It may be that bad effects could take just as long to emerge.

Warnings: In Europe, physicians often combine hawthorn with other heart medications such as digitalis. Patients taking heart medications, or medicine for high blood pressure, MUST get a physician's approval before taking any hawthorn-containing product. If you are already taking hawthorn, make sure your doctor knows that before he prescribes any new heart medications.

Drug Testing: Hawthorn is not known to interfere with, or be detected by, any of the standard urine testing systems used to screen for drug abuse.

Dosage: Herbalists recommend making a tea by adding two tablespoons of the flowers to one cup of boiling water, and drinking two to three cups per day for one month. Commission E recommends a daily dose of 160-900 mg of hawthorn extract (standardized to contain 4-30 mg of flavonoids and 30-160 mg of oligomeric procyanidins).

Summary: Convincing laboratory and clinical trials have shown that hawthorn supplements benefit some patients with heart failure, and some patients with high blood pressure. Claims that hawthorn can lower cholesterol are unproven in clinical trials, as are claims that hawthorn is an "antispasmodic" and sedative. Performance improvement has been demonstrated in patients with heart disease, but not in healthy normal athletes. Animal studies of acute toxicity suggest hawthorn is a very safe product, but the effects of long-term use have never been studied in animals or people. If you are going to take hawthorn, it is imperative that your physician knows about it.

References:

Ammon HP, Handel M. [Crataegus, toxicology and pharmacology. Part II: Pharmacodynamics (author's transl)]. Planta Med 1981;43(3): 209-39.

Bahorun T, Trotin F, Pommery J, Vasseur J, Pinkas M. Antioxidant activities of Crataegus monogyna extracts. Planta Med 1994;60(4): 323-8.

Leuchtgens H. [Crataegus Special Extract WS 1442 in NYHA II heart failure. A placebo-controlled randomized double-blind study]. Fortschr Med 1993;111(20-21):352-4.

Popping S, Rose H, Ionescu I, Fischer Y, Kammermeier H. Effect of a hawthorn extract on contraction and energy turnover of isolated rat cardiomyocytes. Arzneimittelforschung 1995;45(11):1157-61.

Schussler M, Holzl J, Fricke U. Myocardial effects of flavonoids from *Crataegus* species. Arzneimittelforschung 1995;45(8):842-5.

Schussler M, Holzl J, Rump AF, Fricke U. Functional and antiischaemic effects of Monoacetyl-vitexinrhamnoside in different in vitro models. Gen Pharmacol 1995;26(7):1565-70.

Shanthi S, Parasakthy K, Deepalakshmi PD, Devaraj SN. Hypolipidemic activity of tincture of Crataegus in rats. Indian J Biochem Biophys 1994;31(2):143-6.

Weikl A, Assmus KD, Neukum-Schmidt A, Schmitz J, Zapfe G, Noh HS, et al. [*Crataegus* Special Extract WS 1442. Assessment of objective effectiveness in patients with heart failure (NYHA II)]. Fortschr Med 1996;114(24):291-6.

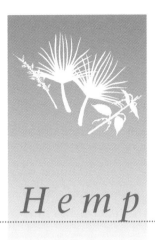

Hemp

Name: *Cannabis sativa L.* (Cannabaceae), commonly called hemp. In French, it is *Chanvre cultivé*; in German, *Hanf*.

Source: Hemp originally came from Central Asia, probably India. It will grow in almost any temperate region. Plants that are intended for producing fiber are allowed to grow quite high and are planted very close to each other. Plants intended for marijuana production tend to be short, bushy, and widely spaced. The hemp fiber is contained in the stalks. The psychoactive chemicals in marijuana are produced by the female flowers. However, all parts of the plant, including the stems, seeds and roots, contain cannabinoids, even if only in trace amounts. Hemp cannot be legally grown in the United States, however, hemp seed oil is legal, and is being promoted by some manufacturers as a health food supplement. The oil is produced by pressing hemp seeds (usually imported from China) that have been sterilized by irradiation.

History: Whether hemp was first grown for its useful fibers or its intoxicating effects is not really known, but marijuana, in one form or another, has been used for thousands of years. Hemp was an important source for commercial fiber production well into the 20th century, but now has been largely replaced by synthetic fibers.

Traditional Claims: Medical claims for the resin are limited to pain relief.

Commission E Recommendations: Commission E has not evaluated hemp.

Proven Effects: Hemp seed oil does contain sizable quantities of the same sort of beneficial oils found in borage and evening primrose, however, it also contains the active component so prized by marijuana smokers, 9-tetrahydrocannabinol (THC). In one study of 25 different hemp seed oils, THC concentrations ranged from 3 to 1,500 micrograms/g oil, often more than enough to lead to a positive urine test for marijuana. In one study, the morning urine of six volunteers who had ingested 11 or 22 g of an oil containing 1,500 micrograms of THC per gram of oil, were analyzed using a standard workplace urine drug screening test. Samples remained positive for marijuana metabolite for up to six days. In some studies, depending on the THC content of the hemp oil being taken, participants experienced psychotropic effects. In the most recent study, using low doses of a product called Cold Pressed Hemp Seed Oil, no psychotropic effects were reported, but many of the urine specimens did, nonetheless, contain substantial amounts of THC metabolites.

Concerns: Users may or may not become intoxicated, but they will almost certainly fail a workplace drug screening test.

Warnings: No matter what the intent is, under federal law, marijuana possession is illegal. Hemp seed oil contains the active ingredients in marijuana. Hemp seed oil is a legal product, but it is a bit hard to understand why, given the contents of the oil. In some jurisdictions, the mere presence of THC in the body, at any concentration, is considered proof of intoxication. If, for example, a hemp oil user was injured at work, and THC metabolites were detected in his urine, the laws of some ("zero tolerance") states would exclude him from workers' compensation insurance, even if he was totally fault-free. The presence of THC metabolites would be considered "per se" evidence of intoxication.

Drug Testing: Using hemp seed oil almost guarantees a positive urine test.

Dosage: Undetermined.

Summary: Hemp seed oil does contain some valuable nutrients, but they are not unique and they are present in other oils (borage, evening primrose and others) that are less problematic. Using hemp seed products almost guarantees a positive workplace drug test, but whether such an excuse would ever be accepted by an employer seems extremely unlikely. At the time of this writing, the government was considering what measures to take, given the real problems use of this supplement present.

References:

Alt A, Reinhardt G. Positive cannabis results in urine and blood samples after consumption of hemp food products [letter; comment]. J Anal Toxicol 1998;22(1):80-1.

Costantino A, Schwartz RH, Kaplan P. Hemp oil ingestion causes positive urine tests for delta 9- tetrahydrocannabinol carboxylic acid. J Anal Toxicol 1997;21(6):482-5.

Callaway JC, Weeks RA, Raymon LP, Walls HC, Hearn WL. A positive THC urinalysis from hemp (Cannabis) seed oil [letter]. J Anal Toxicol 1997;21(4):319-20.

Struempler RE, Nelson G, Urry FM. A positive cannabinoids workplace drug test following the ingestion of commercially available hemp seed oil [see comments]. J Anal Toxicol 1997;21(4):283-5.

Vasaliades J, Glass L, Urry M. Cannabinoid Urine Positive after Ingestion of Hemp Seed Oil. 1998. Presented at the Annual Meeting of the Society of Forensic Toxicologists, Albuquerque, New Mexico, October 6, 1998.

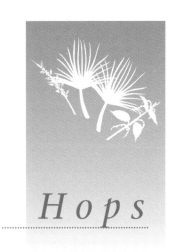

Hops

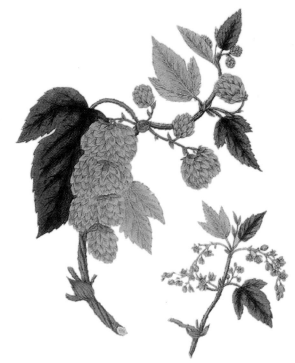

Name: *Humulus lupulus* L., Cannabinaceae, and *Lupul strobulus,* commonly known as hops, humulus, lupulus, hop bine, and willow wolf in English. In French, it is *Houblon grimpant;* in German, *Hopfenzapfen* or just *Hopen.*

Source: This herb is a perennial with green flowers that bloom in late summer. Herbal remedies are made from a part of the plant called the strobile, essentially a cone-like fruit. Inside the fruit, surrounding the seed, is a yellow granular powder called lupulin; it contains the active ingredients. Hops are, of course, cultivated worldwide for beer production. Hops are members of the Cannabis family and are, indeed, closely related to marijuana.

History: The common name, hops, is thought to be from the Old English *hopen,* meaning "to climb." In the wild, leaves of this herb tend to be found growing around willow trees (hence the name "willow wolf"). Since Medieval times, hops have been grown for beer-making, and pillows stuffed with hops were used during the Middle Ages to treat insomnia. Oils from hops are also used in perfume manufacturing.

Traditional Claims: For anxiety and sleep disturbances, as an antispasmodic, and as a digestive aid.

Commission E Recommendations: Hops is used for anxiety, insomnia, mood disturbance, restlessness and sleep disturbances.

Proven Effects: The main ingredients in hops are resins and compounds known as alpha and beta acids. The alpha acids consist of humulone, cohumulone, and adhumulone. The beta acids are lupuplone, colupulone, and adlupulone. Both types of acids tend to break down and disappear with storage. The ability of hops to induce sleep is thought to be due to the presence of a chemical called 2-methyl-3-butne-2-ol. Once the alpha acids enter the body, some of them are converted to 2-methyl-3-butne-2-ol. In clinical, double-blind controlled clinical trials using health volunteers, hops induced sleep just as efficiently as flunitrazepam (Rohypnol™ is sold on the street as "roofies"). Equally important, volunteers treated with hops had less of a hangover the next morning. Hops also contain substances called phytoestrogens - molecules that in some way look and act like estrogens. Many believe that phytoestrogen can prevent coronary artery disease, osteoporosis, and other age-related diseases.

Concerns: Hops also contain quercetin, the same flavonol found in cranberries, and substances called terpenes. Terpenes are also found in other plants known to cause contact dermatitis (citrus fruit peels and pines to name just two), which probably explains why allergy to hops can occur. But given the number of people who work in the industry, it is an uncommon occurrence, even among brewery workers. Life-threatening reactions have never been reported.

Warnings: None

Drug Testing: Hops belongs to the only other genus of family Cannabinaceae. But that does not mean that hops contains THC (the active ingredient in marijuana), or any molecules closely related to THC. Therefore, taking a hops-containing product is no excuse for a positive marijuana test. Since hops is a sedative, and can cause impairment, it should not be used with alcohol. Don't drink and drive.

Dosage: Hops may be used two to three times a day and, again, at bedtime. The standard dose is one cup of tea made with .5 to 1 gram of dried strobiles. The same amount could be taken in capsule form, though it may take longer to exert its effect.

Summary: Results of European trials strongly suggest that hops, like valerian, can be used as an effective, and very safe, sleeping aid. Users go to sleep more quickly when they have taken hops, and they awake with clearer heads than when using prescription sleeping pills. There are no reports of serious toxicity. The phytoestrogens contained in hops may provide additional benefits in terms of preventing heart disease and relieving menopausal symptoms.

References:

Gerhard U, Linnenbrink N, Georghiadou C, Hobi V. [Vigilance-decreasing effects of 2 plant-derived sedatives]. Schweiz Rundsch Med Prax 1996;85(15):473-81.

Kammerer E. [Phytogenic sedatives-hypnotics—does a combination of valerian and hops have a value in the modern drug repertoire?]. Z Arztl Fortbild (Jena) 1993;87(5):401-6.

Newmark FM. Hops allergy and terpene sensitivity: an occupational disease. Ann Allergy 1978;41(5):311-2.

Siniscalco Gigliano G, Caputo P, Cozzolino S. Ribosomal DNA analysis as a tool for the identification of *Cannabis sativa L.* specimens of forensic interest. Sci Justice 1997;37(3):171-4.

Williams CS, Eastoe BV, Slaiding IR, Walker MD. Analysis of pesticide residues in hops and their extraction by liquid CO_2 during the production of hop extracts. Food Addit Contam 1994; 11(5):615-9.

Zava DT, Dollbaum CM, Blen M. Estrogen and progestin bioactivity of foods, herbs, and spices. Proc Soc Exp Biol Med 1998;217(3): 369-78.

Zuskin E, Mustajbegovic J, Sitar-Srebocan V. [Pharmacologic study of the effects of the components of beer in vitro]. Lijec Vjesn 1997;119(3-4):103-5.

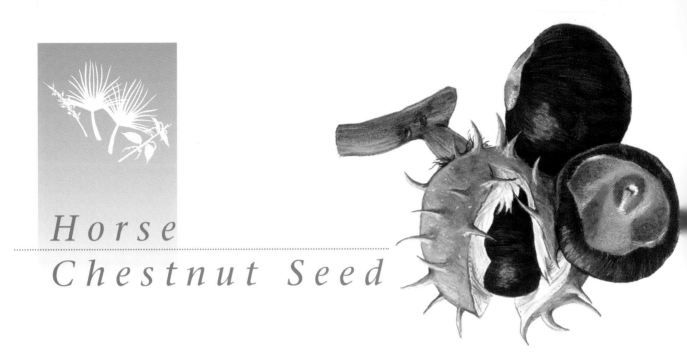

Horse Chestnut Seed

Name: *Aesculus hippocastanum,* L. (Hippocastanaceae), commonly called the Horse Chestnut or Conker tree seed in English. In French, it is *Marronier d'inde;* in German, *Rosskastiensamen* or *Rosskastanie.*

Source: Remedies are made from the horse chestnut seed, supplied whole or in powdered form. Horse chestnut probably came from India originally, but it is now grown in most temperate climates. Large amounts are produced in Eastern Europe.

History: The naming of this plant is a bit confusing, because *Aesculus* is the word the Greeks used to describe oak trees. The name horse chestnut probably derives from the fact that during the Middle Ages, fruits of this tree were used to feed cattle and horses. One of the components of the plant, cyclamin, is particularly toxic to fish. In India, fishermen used to put horse chestnut extracts into the water in order to paralyze the fish and make them easier to catch. During the 1500s, horse chestnut made its way from India to Europe where herbalists used the fruits to treat hemorrhoids.

Traditional Claims: In addition to treating hemorrhoids, tea from the fruit was used for arthritis. Fluidextracts of horse chestnut were used to protect the skin from prolonged sun exposure - the first sun block. Before quinine became widely available, horse chestnut extracts were used to treat fevers. Today, it is mostly recommended as a treatment for venous insufficiency and for treating prostate disease. In Germany, it is the agent most widely used to treat swelling of the legs from venous disease.

Commission E Recommendations: Horse chestnut is used for itching, leg cramps, post-operative or post-traumatic swelling and varicose veins.

Proven Effects: Horse Chestnut's beneficial effects are thought to derive from a group of chemical compounds called saponins - a name given to a group of molecules that resemble steroids, except that they have a sugar molecule attached. Saponins have soap-like effects; when mixed with water, they produce a lather. The saponins contained in horse chestnut are collectively called escins (Ia, Ib, IIa, and IIb). It is not clear whether all the escins, or just one of the subtypes, is medically effective, but horse chestnut extract clearly reduces the swelling seen in the legs of patients with chronic venous insufficiency. The effectiveness of this remedy has been proven in multiple European clinical trials.

Concerns: Saponins can be irritating to the stomach. When taken in full therapeutic doses, gastrointestinal upset is likely to result, and some people report itching when large doses are taken. Some recent animal studies suggest that taking too much extract could cause blood sugar concentrations to drop, but such an occurrence has never been reported in humans.

Warnings: The first-line treatment for leg swelling is compression - wearing surgical stockings to prevent fluid from accumulating, and to force accumulated fluid back into the circulatory system. If horse chestnut is to be used for leg swelling, it should only be used in conjunction with surgical stockings.

Drug Testing: Nothing in horse chestnut extract should interfere with standard workplace urine drug screening tests.

Dosage: Commission E recommends use of powdered extract standardized to contain 16-20 percent of dried escin to deliver a dose of 250-313 milligrams twice a day.

Summary: Physicians in the Middle Ages knew that horse chestnut extract reduced the swelling of hemorrhoids, and modern medical research has shown that this extract will also reduce the swelling associated with disease of the leg veins. Except for the possibility of stomach upset associated with large doses, there is no evidence that horse chestnut is capable of causing any sort of serious toxicity.

References:

Diehm C, Trampisch HJ, Lange S, Schmidt C. Comparison of leg compression stocking and oral horse-chestnut seed extract therapy in patients with chronic venous insufficiency [see comments]. Lancet 1996;347(8997):292-4.

Dworschak E, Antal M, Biro L, Regoly-Merei A, Nagy K, Szepvolgyi J, et al. Medical activities of *Aesculus hippocastaneum* (horse-chestnut) saponins. Adv Exp Med Biol 1996;404:471-4.

Greeske K, Pohlmann BK. [Horse chestnut seed extract—an effective therapy principle in general practice. Drug therapy of chronic venous insufficiency]. Fortschr Med 1996;114(15):196-200.

Matsuda H, Li Y, Murakami T, Ninomiya K, Yamahara J, Yoshikawa M. Effects of escins Ia, Ib, IIa, and IIb from horse chestnut, the seeds of *Aesculus hippocastanum L.*, on acute inflammation in animals. Biol Pharm Bull 1997;20(10):1092-5.

Rehn D, Unkauf M, Klein P, Jost V, Lucker PW. Comparative clinical efficacy and tolerability of oxerutins and horse chestnut extract in patients with chronic venous insufficiency. Arzneimittelforschung 1996;46(5):483-7.

Yoshikawa M, Murakami T, Matsuda H, Yamahara J, Murakami N, Kitagawa I. Bioactive saponins and glycosides. III. Horse chestnut. (1): The structures, inhibitory effects on ethanol absorption, and hypoglycemic activity of escins Ia, Ib, IIa, IIb, and IIIa from the seeds of *Aesculus hippocastanum L.* Chem Pharm Bull (Tokyo) 1996;44(8):1454-64.

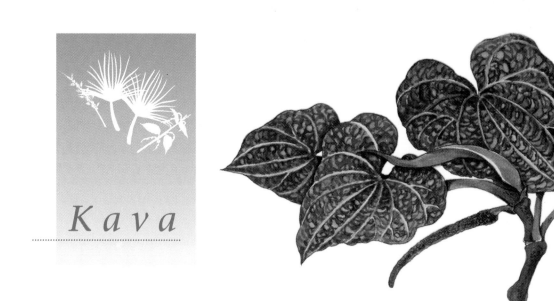

Kava

Name: *Piper methysticum,* G. Forst. (Family Piperaceae), commonly known as kava kava, 'ava, or kawa. Fijians call it *yaqona*, and sometimes "grog." In German it is *Kava-kava-Wurzelstock.*

Source: Kava belongs to the pepper family (Piperaceae) and grows in Polynesia, Melanesia, and Micronesia. Kava kava is made from the dried rhizomes of *Piper methysticum* G. Forster. There are dozens of different but related strains and they all contain the same psychoactive principles.

History: Pacific Islanders use kava as a depressant drug. The first published account in European literature was written by the Dutch explorers, Jacob LeMaire and William Schouten in 1616, when they visited the Horne Islands (now part of the French Wallis and Futuna) and watched a kava ceremony. The Dutchmen were a bit put off by the way the kava was prepared - roots were chewed and the pulpy material expectorated into one bowl that everyone drank from. Schouten wrote, "They presented also their desirable drink to our people, as a thing rare and delicate, but the sight of their brewing had quenched our thirst."

The Dutch reports did not create much of a sensation, but Captain James Cook's account, written in 1770, found a wider audience. A botanist sailing with Cook on his second expedition drew detailed descriptions of the plant and named it *Piper methysticum* ("intoxicating pepper"). In some areas, especially Tonga, Fiji, and in the islands of Micronesia, kava is still used ritually, although it can be, and is, used as an intoxicant. The first modern studies of kava were done in the early 1900s, when parts of Samoa belonged to Germany. Representatives of the German pharmaceutical industry began to experiment with kava extracts. For a time, kava-based products were used as diuretics, and as a not very successful treatment for gonorrhea. After World War II, Riker Laboratories, an American pharmaceutical maker, tested one of the kava pyrones (dihydromethysticin) in volunteers. They found that large doses (500 mg a day) produced effects much like those produced by any other minor tranquilizer, but that it also caused skin disease (a scaly rash and yellow discoloration) in so many of the participants that the study had to be discontinued.

During the early 1980s, excessive kava consumption became a problem among Australian Aborigines in an area known as the Arnhem Land, in the Northern Territory. There, ritual kava consumption has been replaced by heavy daily usage. Medical surveys done by Australian researchers uncovered a number of undesirable health consequences. A decade later, kava abuse is still a problem for the Aborigines, and the situation does not appear to be improving.

Kava-containing preparations are now very widely available in the United States and in Europe. Kava is used as a minor tranquilizer and as a treatment for anxiety. Kava is sold under the brand name Laitan™ or Kavasporal™ in Germany, as Potter's Antigian Tablets™ in the United Kingdom, and as Viocava™ in Switzerland. In the last few years, more American manufacturers have been adding kava products to their product lines and kava is available under a variety of different names.

Traditional Claims: Sedative

Commission E Recommendations: Kava is used to treat anxiety, muscle pain, restlessness and stress.

Proven Effects: The chemically active components of kava are called pyrones. The two main pyrones are dihydromethysticin and kawain. In addition to being depressants, producing effects very much like those of any benzodiazepine (such as Valium™ or Librium™), these drugs have anticonvulsant activity, analgesic effects, and muscle relaxing properties. In 1990, the Federal Board of Health in Germany approved kava products for treating the symptoms of anxiety. At the molecular level, kava pyrones behave very much like the antiepileptic drug Dilantin™. Kava also has an unexplained effect on the smooth muscles that control pupil size, an action that can sometimes lead to trouble focusing. In addition, some of the pyrones can prevent the reuptake of neurotransmitters. Preventing reuptake means that the effects of the neurotransmitters are exaggerated and prolonged. Prozac™, for example, is thought to improve the symptoms of depression because it prevents the reuptake of serotonin. Cocaine causes euphoria by preventing the reuptake of another neurotransmitter called dopamine.

Concerns: Heavy users develop a reversible, scaly skin rash known as kava dermopathy. This disorder was first described by the botanist who sailed with Captain Cook. It is thought to be the result of a kava-related abnormality in cholesterol metabolism. In addition to the distinctive skin rash, Australian researchers studying aboriginal kava abusers have found evidence of weight loss and liver damage (elevated levels of certain enzymes in the blood which are markers for liver disease). Long-term follow-up is not available, so it is not known whether the liver damage is reversible. Results from the same set of Australian studies also suggested that kidney damage might be detected in long-term users, but the evidence was less convincing. Users should know that kava can cause dry mouth, dilated pupils, and trouble focusing (collectively these are known as anticholinergic symptoms). Another consequence of long-term kava use is discoloration of the hair and nails.

Warnings: Kava is not known to interact with any medications, but it is not a good idea to combine depressants. Also, kava should not be used with alcohol. Anyone who takes kava for a long enough period is guaranteed to get the distinctive skin rash, discolored hair and nails, but it will go away if the drug is discontinued. There are recent reports in the literature suggesting that use of kava-based commercial products can cause movement disorders (called choreoathetosis), much like those seen in patients taking medication for schizophrenia (drugs like Haldol™). This disorder is self-limiting and quite rare, but should it occur it is imperative you tell your physician which herbal products you are taking.

Drug Testing: Kava pyrones are not known to interfere with, or be detected by, any of the standard screening tests used for workplace drug testing.

Dosage: Dosage is problematic. Kava for export is usually sold as a dry powder to be mixed with cold water. Total dose will depend on the type of powder, the amount of water added, and how long it is allowed to sit. This makes the dosage extremely unpredictable. When Riker Laboratories gave volunteers 500 mg per day they became ill. But in another study, no problems were encountered with the 100 mg per day dose. Commission E recommends a daily dose of 60-120mg Kava Pyrones.

Summary: In moderate doses, kava produces the same effects as any mild tranquilizer. Large doses may have additional effects, not all of which are desirable. There is no evidence that occasional use produces any serious or long lasting side effects, but there is evidence that using large amounts for prolonged periods has adverse health consequences. Some of the active components of the extract hold promise for the treatment of epilepsy and stroke.

References:

Gleitz J, Beile A, Wilkens P, Ameri A, Peters T. Antithrombotic action of the kava pyrone (+)-kavain prepared from *Piper methysticum* on human platelets. Planta Med 1997;63(1):27-30.

Backhauss C, Krieglstein J. Extract of kava (*Piper methysticum*) and its methysticin constituents protect brain tissue against ischemic damage in rodents. Eur J Pharmacol 1992;215(2-3):265-9.

Mathews JD, Riley MD, Fejo L, Munoz E, Milns NR, Gardner ID, et al. Effects of the heavy usage of kava on physical health: summary of a pilot survey in an aboriginal community. Med J Aust 1988; 148(11):548-55.

Magura EI, Kopanitsa MV, Gleitz J, Peters T, Krishtal OA. Kava extract ingredients, (+)-methysticin and (+/-)-kavain inhibit voltage-operated Na(+)-channels in rat CA1 hippocampal neurons. Neuroscience 1997;81(2):345-51.

Norton SA, Ruze P. Kava dermopathy. J Am Acad Dermatol 1994;31(1):89-97.

Schelosky L, Raffauf C, Jendroska K, Poewe W. Kava and dopamine antagonism [letter]. J Neurol Neurosurg Psychiatry 1995;58(5):639-40.

Seitz U, Ameri A, Pelzer H, Gleitz J, Peters T. Relaxation of evoked contractile activity of isolated guinea-pig ileum by (+/-)-kavain. Planta Med 1997;63(4):303-6.

Singh YN. Kava: an overview. J Ethnopharmacol 1992;37(1):13-45.

Spillane PK, Fisher DA, Currie BJ. Neurological manifestations of kava intoxication [letter] [see comments]. Med J Aust 1997;167(3):172-3.

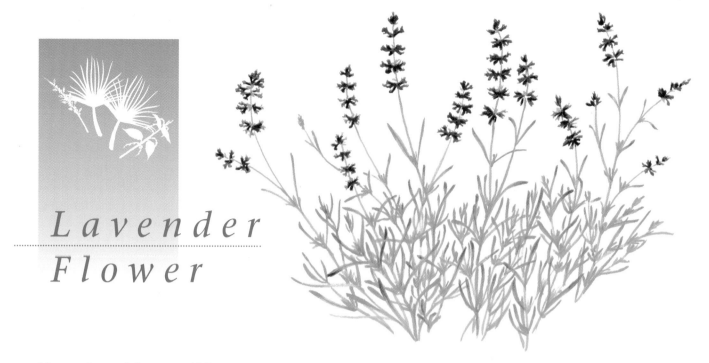

Lavender Flower

Name: *Lavandula angustifolia* L. (Labiatae), commonly called lavender flower; in French, it is *Lavande officinale*; in German, *Lavendel*

Source: The plant originally came from the Mediterranean region and Southern Europe, but is now cultivated in almost any area with a sunny, dry climate.

History: The name of the plant almost surely derives from the Latin *lavare*, meaning to wash. The ancient Romans added the flowers and the essential oil to their baths, and stored sachets of the flowers with their clothes. The Greeks used the oil to treat skin diseases, and in the Middle Ages lavender was used to kill lice and bedbugs.

Traditional Claims: Stimulant, antispasmodic and tonic. Also carminative and diuretic. More recently aromatherapists have recommended it as a "harmonizing" agent, good for the treatment of headache and sleeplessness.

Commission E Recommendations: Lavender is used to treat circulatory and gastrointestinal disorders, flatulence, insomnia, mood disturbances, nervous stomach and restlessness.

Proven Effects: There has been pathetically little modern research on this herb. Laboratory studies suggest that it is both antimicrobial and antifungal. Very limited clinical trials with inhalation suggest some improvement in chronic bronchitis. For many centuries, the essential oil has been recommended as an antiseptic, but clinical trials have never been undertaken. The two main ingredients of the oil, linalyl acdetate (25-45 percent), and linalool (25-38 percent) are not known to possess any useful medicinal properties, though they do have a lovely aroma.

Concerns: Plants belonging to the Labiatae family seem to show cross-sensitivity on the basis of clinical history. So someone allergic to marjoram might very well be allergic to lavender and other related Labiatae family members.

Warnings: None

Drug Testing: The tests have never been done, but it is unlikely that either linalyl acdetate or linalool would have an effect on standard workplace urine drug screening tests.

Dosage: One to two teaspoon of dried herb soaked in one cup of boiling water for 15 minutes may be consumed as a tea three times a day.

Summary: Substantial medical benefits for lavender have never been demonstrated. On the other hand, there is no evidence of serious toxicity either, and the smell is very pleasing.

References:

Benito M, Jorro G, Morales C, Pelaez A, Fernandez A. Labiatae allergy: systemic reactions due to ingestion of oregano and thyme. Ann Allergy Asthma Immunol 1996;76(5):416-8.

Larrondo JV, Agut M, Calvo-Torras MA. Antimicrobial activity of essences from labiates. Microbios 1995;82(332):171-2.

Shubina LP, Siurin SA, Savchenko VM. [Inhalations of essential oils in the combined treatment of patients with chronic bronchitis]. Vrach Delo 1990(5):66-7.

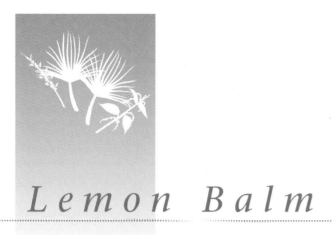

Lemon Balm

Name: *Melissa officinalis* L., (Labiatae), commonly called as Lemon Balm, or balm, garden balm, bee balm, Milissae folium, melissa, or Scholar's herb. In French, it is Mélisse officina*le,* and in German, *Melisse* or *Zitronekraut or Melissenblätter.*

Source: Remedies are made from the dried leaves and flowering tops of lemon balm. *Melissae* originally was grown in Southern Europe and the Mediterranean. The leaves have the smell of lemons because like lemons, they contain citronella.

History: Lemon balm was used by the ancient Greeks (Hippocrates) and Romans (Dioscorides) and is mentioned in the Bible. The pleasant smelling essential oil was highly prized and used in various liniments and balms. In the 17th century, lemon balm was a key ingredient in *Eau des Carmes,* a remedy produced by the Carmelite nuns for inducing sleep (the other ingredients were lemon rind, cinnamon, cloves, nutmeg, and coriander in a white wine).

Traditional Claims: Lemon balm is used as a sedative, antispasmodic, diaphoretic, carminative and stomachic (an antiquated term used by herbalists to describe agents that "stimulate" the stomach).

Commission E Recommendations: Lemon balm is used to treat dyspepsia (upset stomach), insomnia and functional gastrointestinal complaints.

Proven Effects: Extracts of *Melissa* have demonstrated antiviral, antibacterial, and antitumor activity, at least in animals. Other experimental studies have shown that extracts of the whole plant, as opposed to just the oil, are reasonably potent sedatives, with an effect comparable to that of phenobarbital. Rosmarinic acid, which has been isolated from *Melissa officinalis* L. extracts, inhibits complement-dependent inflammatory processes (the systems involved in disorders such as lupus erythematosus and rheumatoid arthritis). Unfortunately, none of these actions has ever been validated in a real placebo-controlled clinical trial.

Concerns: None. There are no reports of toxic reactions or side effects.

Warnings: None known.

Drug Testing: No component of *Melissae officinalis* L. is known to interfere with any of the standard workplace urine screening tests.

Dosage: Lemon balm is made into a tea by steeping 1.5 to 4.5 grams of dried leaves in a cup of hot water. It can be consumed several times per day, as needed.

Summary: Lemon balm teas have been used as mild sedatives for hundreds of years. The Carmelite nuns thought the herb was effective and laboratory studies tend to confirm the sedative properties of this herb. Clinical studies are lacking, but so are any reports of toxicity or side effects.

References:

Galasinski W, Chlabicz J, Paszkiewicz-Gadek A, Marcinkiewicz C, Gindzienski A. The substances of plant origin that inhibit protein biosynthesis. Acta Pol Pharm 1996;53(5):311-8.

Dimitrova Z, Dimov B, Manolova N, Pancheva S, Ilieva D, Shishkov S. Antiherpes effect of *Melissa officinalis L.* extracts. Acta Microbiol Bulg 1993;29:65-72.

Larrondo JV, Agut M, Calvo-Torras MA. Antimicrobial activity of essences from labiates. Microbios 1995;82(332):171-2.

Soulimani R, Fleurentin J, Mortier F, Misslin R, Derrieu G, Pelt JM. Neurotropic action of the hydroalcoholic extract of *Melissa officinalis* in the mouse. Planta Med 1991;57(2):105-9.

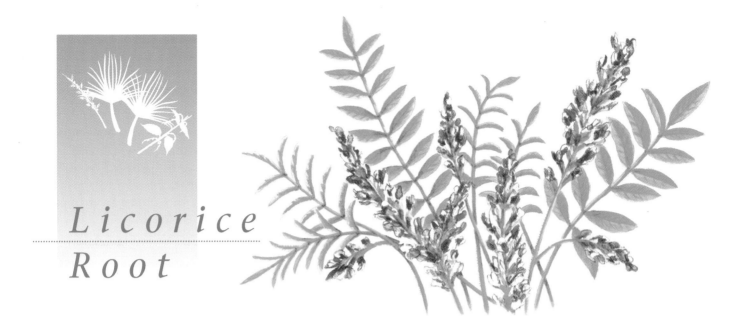

Licorice Root

Name: *Glycyrrhiza glabra*, L. (Leguminosae), Liquiritiae radix., commonly called licorice and licorice root.

Source: More than 20 different species of *Glycyrrhiza* are recognized. Licorice is a member of the pea family and contains some of the same phytoestrogens found in soy beans. Extracts of licorice are made from dried roots and stolons by steam distillation. In the United States, most "licorice" candies are, in fact, made from anise.

History: Wild licorice was used by German healers during the Dark Ages, but it was first cultivated in Spain during the 13th century. In 1302, King Edward I of England began taxing licorice imports in order to help pay for repairs on the London Bridge. Traditional Chinese herbalists included licorice in formulations prescribed to promote women's health. Modern herbalists recommend licorice as a cough remedy, but the main use for licorice today, in the United States, at least, is in the making of cigarettes and smokeless tobacco. Licorice is added to both products in order to impart a pleasant taste and smell.

Traditional Claims: Teas made from the dried and peeled roots were recommended for cough and upper respiratory symptoms, also purgative and stomachic (stomach stimulant).

Commission E Recommendations: Licorice root is used to treat gastrointestinal ulcers, respiratory catarrh, and upper respiratory tract catarrh (inflammation).

Proven Effects: The sweet taste of licorice comes from a substance called glycyrrhizic acid. In the body, glycyrrhizic acid is converted to a substance called glycyrrhetic acid. A derivative of glycyrrhizic acid, called carbenoxolone, has been used to treat peptic ulcers, but it is not approved for use in the United States. Carbenoxolone makes the stomach lining more resistant to stomach acid. Intake of too much carbenoxolone, or too much glycyrrhizic acid, causes sodium and fluid retention while, at the same time, promoting potassium loss, a combination that predictably leads to high blood pressure, muscle damage, and potassium levels so low that dangerous irregularities in heartbeat can occur. Traditional Chinese herbalists have, for thousands of years, treated menopausal symptoms with a combination of licorice and jujube. The success of such treatments may have to do with the fact that licorice, like other members of the Leuminosae family, contains phytoestrogens. The type of phytoestrogens found in licorice have not received the attention afforded soy products, but they certainly are present, and probably active. Licorice extract contains compounds that can kill parasites, such as malaria, and they may have antibiotic effects as well, though these laboratory findings have not been validated in humans.

Concerns: The biggest concern is deciding how much can be safely taken. Medical text books say that an intake of 100 mg glycyrrhizic acid per day (equivalent to 50 grams licorice sweets or candies containing 0.2 percent glycyrrhizic acid) is enough to cause problems. However, results of studies with human volunteers indicate that when the glycyrrhizic acid came from licorice extract, rather than from pure glycyrrhizic acid that had been added to candies as a food flavoring, much less was absorbed into the body, and that as much as 200 mg per day of glycyrrhizic acid could be taken safely (provided it came from licorice extract).

Warnings: In studies with volunteers, women in general, and those taking birth control pills in particular, were much more likely to experience side effects than men. Pregnant rats fed licorice delivered low birth weight offspring, and they often had high blood pressure and heart damage. Pregnant women should not be using licorice. Nor should breast feeding mothers, at least until someone takes the time to measure the glycyrrhetic acid content of breast milk.

Drug Testing: There are no published studies suggesting that glycyrrhizic acid, or anything contained in the extract, can interfere with standard workplace urine drug screening tests.

Dosage: In human volunteers, dried extracts of licorice, containing up to 217 mg per day of glycyrrhizic acid, produced no side effects. But doses higher than that did, if the extract was used daily for more than two weeks. Average daily dose is 5-15 grams of root, equal to 200-600 mg of glycyrrhizin.

Summary: Licorice derivatives seems to be effective anti-ulcer medications, but they do not appear to be any more effective than drugs like Tagamet™ and Zantac™ (H2 blockers), and the risk of developing side effects with licorice is greater. The same could be said about using licorice as a cough suppressant. It may be effective, but so are allopathic cough syrups, and they are much safer. Use of licorice extract is much less likely to cause problems than purified glycyrrhizic acid, and studies with volunteers have shown that side effects are quite unlikely, even with doses as high as 400 milligrams, provided the 400 milligrams come from extract.

References:

Bernardi M, D'Intino PE, Trevisani F, Cantelli-Forti G, Raggi MA, Turchetto E, et al. Effects of prolonged ingestion of graded doses of licorice by healthy volunteers. Life Sci 1994;55(11):863-72.

Cantelli-Forti G, Maffei F, Hrelia P, Bugamelli F, Bernardi M, D'Intino P, et al. Interaction of licorice on glycyrrhizin pharmacokinetics. Environ Health Perspect 1994;102 Suppl 9:65-8.

Chen M, Christensen SB, Blom J, Lemmich E, Nadelmann L, Fich K, et al. Licochalcone A, a novel antiparasitic agent with potent activity against human pathogenic protozoan species of Leishmania. Antimicrob Agents Chemother 1993;37(12):2550-6.

Langley-Evans SC. Maternal carbenoxolone treatment lowers birthweight and induces hypertension in the offspring of rats fed a protein-replete diet. Clin Sci (Colch) 1997;93(5):423-9.

Zava DT, Dollbaum CM, Blen M. Estrogen and progestin bioactivity of foods, herbs, and spices. Proc Soc Exp Biol Med 1998;217(3): 369-78.

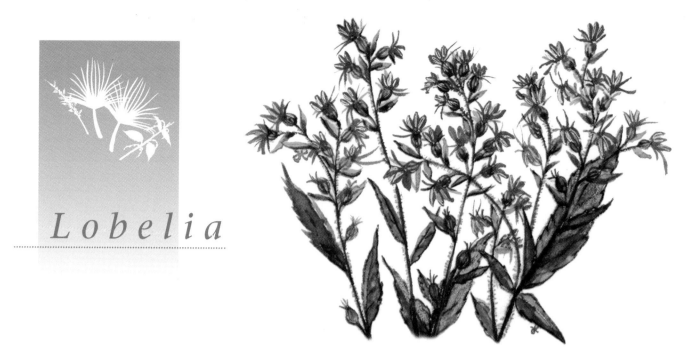

Lobelia

Name: *Lobelia inflata* L. (Campanulaceae), commonly called Indian Tobacco, gag root, and puke weed in English. A closely related variety, *Lobelia dortmanna* L., which grows in Europe, contains the same active ingredients. In France, it is called *Lobélie de Dortman*. In German, it is *Wasser Spleisse or Wasser-Lobelie*.

Source: Lobelia is grown commercially in North America, and in the Netherlands. Remedies are made from the crushed dried flowers of the plant.

History: During the late 1700s, and the first part of the nineteenth century, American physicians used lobelia to induce vomiting and remove "toxins." Some physicians recommended smoking it to relieve the wheezing of asthma. For the last several decades, one of the components, called lobeline, has been used to help people stop smoking.

Traditional Claims: Lobelia is used as a diaphoretic (something that causes sweating), expectorant, sedative and purgative (laxative).

Commission E Recommendations: The Commission makes no mention of this herb.

Proven Effects: The leaves, stems and flowers of lobelia contain nearly two dozen different alkaloids, most of which are closely related to nicotine (piperidine alkaloids). Some of these alkaloids have the ability to prevent inflammation, or at least reduce it and work in much the same way as commercial products, such as Advil™. Lobeline, a slightly different sort of alkaloid, is used in smoking cessation. How, and even whether, it helps a person to stop smoking is not clear, but at the molecular level, this alkaloid shares common mechanisms with cocaine and methamphetamine, and even antidepressants, like Prozac™, i.e., it prevents the reuptake of dopamine. Reuptake is the way the body turns off neurotransmitters. If reuptake is prevented, then the effects of the hormone are exaggerated. Lobeline has a molecular structure very similar to that of nicotine and it produces many of the same effects. In large doses, both lobeline and nicotine cause nausea and vomiting. Even the dose prescribed in smoking cessation programs, 2-4 milligrams several times a day, may leave some users nauseated. Claims that extract of lobelia, or smoked lobelia, are effective treatments for asthma or stomach cramps have never been validated in a clinical trial.

Concerns: Lobelia is generally considered a fairly toxic plant. Like nicotine, the lobeline contained in lobelia stimulates sympathetic nerve ganglia. Large doses, in addition to causing nausea and vomiting, can also cause profound sweating, rapid heart rate and low blood pressure. It should only be used under a doctor's supervision.

Warnings: Remedies made from lobelia should not be used by pregnant women. Taking very large doses can lead to convulsions and even death in both men and women.

Drug Testing: Insurance companies test urine to see if applicants are cigarette smokers. The chemical they test for is a nicotine metabolite called conitine. Lobeline is very closely related to nicotine, but as far as anyone knows, lobeline is not metabolized to conitine and should not cause a false positive test. Nor should any of the other components have any effect on standard workplace drug screening tests.

Dosage: According to the British Pharmaceutical Codex, 50 to 200 milligrams of dried herb three times a day is the recommended dose for asthma, chronic bronchitis, and spastic colon. The recommended dose for tincture (1:8, 60 percent ethanol) is .4 to 1.6 milliliters up to three times a day.

Summary: Lobeline has not proven to be very effective in smoking cessation, and even modest doses may cause some nausea. Large doses can be very toxic. Use of the nicotine patch is associated with a much higher smoking cessation rate and is preferred. Similarly, there are many prescription medications for asthma and stomach cramps that are both safer and more effective. Lobelia should not be used by pregnant women.

References:

Philipov S, Istatkova R, Ivanovska N, Denkova P, Tosheva K, Navas H, et al. Phytochemical study and anti-inflammatory properties of *Lobelia laxiflora L.* Z Naturforsch [C] 1998;53(5-6):311-7.

Subarnas A, Tadano T, Nakahata N, Arai Y, Kinemuchi H, Oshima Y, et al. A possible mechanism of antidepressant activity of beta-amyrin palmitate isolated from *Lobelia inflata* leaves in the forced swimming test. Life Sci 1993;52(3):289-96.

Teng L, Crooks PA, Dwoskin LP. Lobeline displaces [3H]dihydrotetrabenazine binding and releases [3H]dopamine from rat striatal synaptic vesicles: comparison with d- amphetamine. J Neurochem 1998;71(1):258-65.

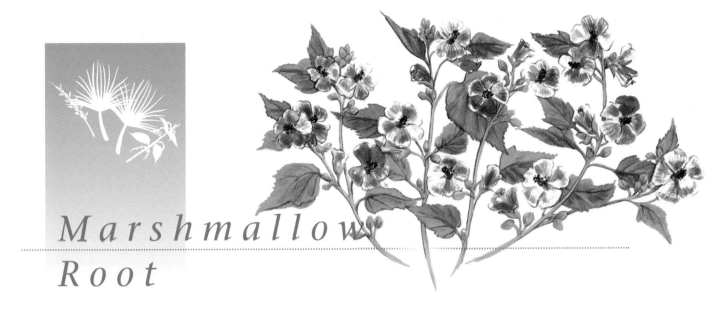

Marshmallow Root

Name: *Althaea officinalis* L. (Malvaceae), commonly called marshmallow, marsh mallow, or sweetweed. In French, it is *Guimauve officinale;* in German, *Eibisch* or *Weisse Malve.*

Source: Remedies are made from the dried peeled roots, usually collected in Autumn, when the plant is at least two years old.

History: The Romans raised this herb to eat, but the Greeks used it as a medication. Emperor Charlemagne believed in its healing properties and promoted its use in Europe during the Ninth Century. During the Middle Ages it was used (unsuccessfully) to treat venereal disease.

Traditional Claims: Demulcent and emollient

Commission E Recommendations: Extracts of the leaves are recommended for irritation of the mouth and throat. Extracts of the root are recommended for mild stomach upset.

Proven Effects: The main constituent of the herb is mucilage. Mucilage is a type of material produced by plants for storing energy. Technically, mucilage is a type of sugar. Pectins and starches also fall into this class. When the roots are soaked in water they swell and form a soothing gel, which may explain the popularity of ointments made with this product. When the gel passes through the gastrointestinal tract it has the effect of calming the intestines (although very large amounts can produce exactly the opposite effect). For that reason, European physicians still prescribe this herb to treat gastroenteritis, ulcer disease, and even colitis. The practice makes sense, but like so many of the other remedies endorsed by Commission E, the practice has not been validated in clinical trials.

Concerns: None

Warnings: None

Drug Testing: None of the components, either of the leaves or roots, should interfere with standard workplace urine drug screening tests.

Dosage: The recommended dosage is 6 grams of root or equal preparations. As a syrup, a single dose is 10 grams.

Summary: Emollients made from the roots have been safely used for hundreds, if not thousand of years, and the rationale for taking leaf extract internally makes a good deal of sense. Toxicity appears to be nil but, then again, so is the evidence for effectiveness.

References:

Nosal'ova G, Strapkova A, Kardosova A, Capek P, Zathurecky L, Bukovska E. [Antitussive action of extracts and polysaccharides of marsh mallow (*Althea officinalis L., var. robusta*)]. Pharmazie 1992;47(3):224-6.

Schulz H, Albroscheit G. High-performance liquid chromatographic characterization of some medical plant extracts used in cosmetic formulas. J Chromatogr 1988;442:353-61.

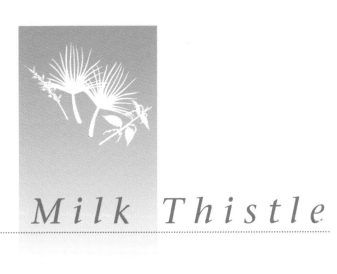

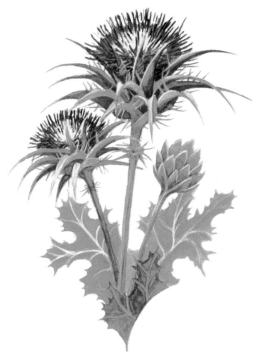

Milk Thistle

Name: *Silybum marianum,* L. Gaertner (Compositae), also *Carduus marianus L.,* commonly called milk thistle. In French, it is *Chardon Marie*; in German, it is *Mariendistel*.

Source: Milk thistle is in the same family as the daisy and artichoke. It grows wild in Europe and was first brought to the United States by European colonists. It is now grown commercially on both coasts of the United States. Because mature plants are covered with sharp spines, milk thistle was, and to some extent still is, planted as a barrier to keep out intruders. An extract made from milk thistle is referred to as silymarin, but silymarin actually contains three different flavonoid isomers (mirror images) called silybin, silydianin and silychristin. Silychristin is the most active of the three molecules, but most herbal remedies contain a mixture of all three isomers. The highest concentrations of silychristin are found in the seeds and roots.

History: The name is thought to derive from the appearance of the leaves, which have white veins. In the Middle Ages it was believed the veins carried the milk of the Virgin Mary. The ancient Greek physician Dioscorides first recommended milk thistle as a treatment for snake bite, but by the time of Pliny, in the second century A.D., mixtures of plant juice and honey were prescribed for liver and gallbladder disease, and that practice continues to this day. During the Middle Ages, milk thistle was also used in place of ergot, to cause the uterus to contract.

Traditional Claims: Milk thistle is used as a cholagogue and emmenagogue.

Commission E Recommendations: Milk thistle is used to treat dyspeptic complaints, and for supportive treatment in chronic inflammation of the liver and in cirrhosis of the liver.

Proven Effects: In animal studies, silymarin protects liver cell membranes against an assortment of toxins probably by preventing or inhibiting membrane peroxidation. In addition to being an antioxidant, the results of other animal studies suggest that silymarin can prevent stomach ulcers and decrease total cholesterol, while, at the same time, increasing good cholesterol (HDL), protect against DNA damage, increase protein synthesis in liver cells, and decrease the activity of substances that are known to promote tumor growth. Not surprisingly, many patients with liver disease have begun medicating themselves with silymarin extracts. In the most recent trial, where silymarin was given to alcoholic patients with cirrhosis, no improvement could be documented. Some clinical reports from Mexico and South America suggest that silymarin helps patients with mushroom poisoning to recover more quickly, and the results of other clinical trials suggest that milk thistle extracts do help prevent the liver from damage by external toxins, and speed recovery after infection with several types of hepatitis virus.

Concerns: None. This is a very old remedy, and there are no reports of toxicity in the modern medical literature. Not enough patients have been treated in clinical trials to be certain about this plant's clinical effectiveness, but no untoward side effects have ever been observed in any of the trials, even though efforts were made to detect them.

Warnings: None

Drug Testing: None of the flavonoids present in milk thistle is likely to have an effect on standard urine drug screening tests.

Dosage: A range of dosages have been evaluated in clinical trials. In one study of patients with type A and type B hepatitis, 140 mg of silymarin was given three times a day. In a separate study, 60 patients with mushroom poisoning were treated with 20 mg/kilogram/day (In a 150 pound individual that would amount to approximately 400 mg three times a day). The effective dosage is probably somewhere in between. Commission E recommends 12-15 grams of ripe seeds per day, or 200-400 mgs per day in an extract containing at least 70 percent silymarin.

Summary: The results of reasonable clinical trials suggest that patients with hepatitis, whether a result of drug toxicity or viral infection, are likely to benefit from using silymarin. Reports of toxicity from using milk thistle extract are non-existent. Only products made from the ripe seeds can be expected to be of any benefit.

References:

Alarcon de la Lastra AC, Martin MJ, Motilva V, Jimenez M, La Casa C, Lopez A. Gastroprotection induced by silymarin, the hepatoprotective principle of *Silybum marianum* in ischemia-reperfusion mucosal injury: role of neutrophils. Planta Med 1995;61(2):116-9.

Flora K, Hahn M, Rosen H, Benner K. Milk thistle (*Silybum marianum*) for the therapy of liver disease. Am J Gastroenterol 1998;93(2):139-43.

Krecman V, Skottova N, Walterova D, Ulrichova J, Simanek V. Silymarin inhibits the development of diet-induced hypercholesterolemia in rats. Planta Med 1998;64(2):138-42.

Pares A, Planas R, Torres M, Caballeria J, Viver JM, Acero D, et al. Effects of silymarin in alcoholic patients with cirrhosis of the liver: results of a controlled, double-blind, randomized and multicenter trial [see comments]. J Hepatol 1998;28(4):615-21.

Sierralta A, Jeria ME, Figueroa G, Pinto J, Araya JC, San Juan J, et al. [Mushroom poisoning in the IX region. Role of Amanita gemmata]. Rev Med Chil 1994;122(7):795-802.

Skottova N, Krecman V, Walterova D, Ulrichova J, Kosina P, Simanek V. Effect of silymarin on serum cholesterol levels in rats. Acta Univ Palacki Olomuc Fac Med 1998;141:87-9.

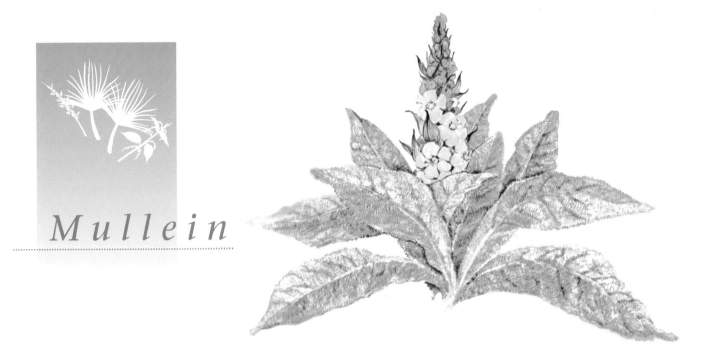

Mullein

Name: *Verbascum thapsus*, Schrad (Scrophulariaceae), commonly called mullein, hare's beard, cow's lungwort, donkey's ears, flannel dock, and Beggar's blanket. In French, it is *Moléne*, *Bouillon-blanc*, or *Bonhomme*; in German, *Gross Köigskerze*.

Source: A perennial with yellow flowers that grows throughout Europe and Asia Minor. Remedies are made from the flowers. A closely related plant, commonly known as orange mullein is also used by herbalists.

History: The name comes from the latin *mollis* meaning soft, because the large leaves have a velvety texture. In medieval times the stems were dried, dipped in tallow, and used to make torches. Juice from the plant was used to treat hemorrhoids and to cure gout. Today's users make a tea from the flowers, but in the past, flowers were picked and left to rot for several months before their juice was pressed out and bottled.

Traditional Claims: Flowers were used as a demulcent, expectorant, diuretic, sedative. Roots were used to treat cramps and diarrhea.

Commission E Recommendations: Expectorant

Proven Effects: In laboratory experiments, extracts of mullein, lemon balm, and artichoke, which all contain caffeic acid and its derivatives, exhibit the same hepatoprotective effects. Mullein is one of the plants used in folk medicine to treat tumors. Tumor growth involves the production of abnormal proteins. Extracts from the same three plants inhibit protein biosynthesis. They do so by inhibiting the actions of a substance that builds proteins (elongation factor eEF-2). Extracts from other plants, particularly aloe, seem to have the same effect. Other extracts of muellin's flowers have antiviral activity (in particular against influenza A and B as well as herpes simplex viruses). Muellin also contains a kind of saponin (saikosaponins) that is known to be a potent anti-inflammatory agent. Saponins are well known respiratory irritants, which probably accounts for the popularity of muellin as in expectorant, at least in Europe.

Concerns: Allergic skin reactions have been observed in some agricultural workers, but otherwise, toxicity of any sort appears to be extremely rare.

Warnings: None

Drug Testing: Nothing in mullein: is likely to cause a false positive workplace urine test.

Dosage: Commission E recommends a dose of 3-4 grams of dried herb per day, either brewed in a tea or in capsule form.

Summary: Many years of experience in Europe suggest that muellin-containing remedies are good expectorants. But new laboratory studies raise the possibility that this herb has antitumor and antiviral activity. Unfortunately, clinical trials are entirely lacking. But since there are no reports of serious toxicity, using this herb should not expose consumers to any serious risk, and it might be a very effective treatment in mild cases of upper respiratory infection.

References:

Bermejo Benito P, Abad Martinez MJ, Silvan Sen AM, Sanz Gomez A, Fernandez Matellano L, Sanchez Contreras S, et al. In vivo and in vitro anti-inflammatory activity of saikosaponins. Life Sci 1998;63(13):1147-56.

Galasinski W, Chlabicz J, Paszkiewicz-Gadek A, Marcinkiewicz C, Gindzienski A. The substances of plant origin that inhibit protein biosynthesis. Acta Pol Pharm 1996;53(5):311-8.

Klimek B. 6'-0-apiosyl-verbascoside in the flowers of mullein (Verbascum species). Acta Pol Pharm 1996;53(2):137-40.

Miyase T, Horikoshi C, Yabe S, Miyasaka S, Melek FR, Kusano G. Saikosaponin homologues from Verbascum spp. The structures of mulleinsaponins I-VII. Chem Pharm Bull (Tokyo) 1997;45(12):2029-33.

Romaguera C, Grimalt F, Vilaplana J. Occupational dermatitis from Gordolobo (Mullein). Contact Dermatitis 1985;12(3):176.

Zgorniak-Nowosielska I, Grzybek J, Manolova N, Serkedjieva J, Zawilinska B. Antiviral activity of Flos verbasci infusion against influenza and Herpes simplex viruses. Arch Immunol Ther Exp 1991;39(1-2):103-8.

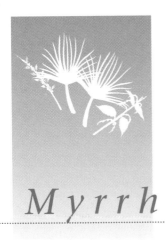

Myrrh

Name: *Commiphora myrrha* Engl. (Burseraceae), *Commiphora molmol* Engl. Myrrh is also obtained from at least two or three more distinct plants with a confusing variety of names. Commonly called Myrrh, Commiphora resin, Heerabol Myrrh or Somalian Myrrh. In French, it is *Myrrhe;* in German, it is *Myrrha.*

Source: Myrrh is the name applied to the resin extracted from the stems of a related group of small trees or bushes that grow mainly in Somalia. The resin is obtained by cutting the stems and collecting the thick yellow liquid that drains from them. As the liquid dries it hardens into a reddish-brown, somewhat sticky, solid. The resin contains water-soluble gums, alcohol-soluble resins, and an essential oil. Depending on where the trees are grown, the dried resin may contain anywhere from two to eight percent of a volatile oil. Myrrh comes from the same family (Burseraceae) as the other famous resin, frankincense.

History: Myrrh was, of course, one of the gifts carried by the Three Wise Men to the Christ Child but, in fact, myrrh was used long before the Bible was ever written. According to Greek mythology, Myrrha, the daughter of the King of Cyprus, took up Aphrodite's challenge, and had a child by her own father. The child was Adonis, the darling of the earth and heavens. Myrrha's father became outraged when he found out how he had been duped. He would have killed Myrrha had she not already been changed into a tree by the other gods who were trying to protect her! Dioscoriades mentions myrrh in his herbal, and so did Pliny the Elder (23-79 AD). Even before the birth of Christ, wine makers in the Middle East knew that by adding myrrh to wine they could prevent it from being ruined by bacteria. In the 10th Century, Arab and European physicians alike firmly believed that chewing on the resin could prevent travelers from catching the plague (it didn't). Culpepper's Herbal, written in 1790, recommended applying myrrh to wounds in order to help prevent infection (along with using it to induce labor, kill worms, treat cough, freshen the breath and cure deafness!). Myrrh is still used as a breath fresher today.

Traditional Claims: Expectorant, antispasmodic, disinfectant, astringent, and for treatment of bad breath.

Commission E Recommendations: As a topical treatment of mild inflammation of the oral and pharyngeal mucosa.

Proven Effects: Myrrh's ability to relieve pain is explained by the presence of two molecules called sesquiterpene lactones (furanoeudsema-1,3-diene and curzarene). The results of studies with experimental animals have shown that both of these molecules bind to brain opiate receptors. In other words, they activate some of the same brain circuits that are activated by drugs like morphine and heroin. In experimental animals, myrrh's ability to relieve pain is completely blocked by giving the narcotic antagonist naloxone (the drug used to treat narcotic overdoses). Of the two lactones, furanoeudesma-1,3-diene is far the most potent, but only very small amounts are contained in the resin. Myrrh also contains another, completely unrelated sesquiterpene lactone called T-cardinol. Laboratory studies have shown that T cardinol relaxes smooth muscle, and shares common mechanisms of action with some drugs that are widely used to treat high blood pressure (calcium blocking agents). Both the intestines and larger blood vessels have smooth muscle in their walls. If the smooth muscle contained in blood vessels relaxes, the vessel dilates and blood pressure drops. If the smooth muscle in the intestine relaxes, the normal propulsive movement of the intestine ceases. Constipation is the result. One side effect of most of the calcium blockers used to treat high blood pressure is, in fact, constipation. The fact that T-cardinol has the ability to relax smooth muscle probably explains why Middle Eastern physicians have, for thousands of years, used myrrh resin to treat diarrhea and upset stomach. The practice persists today. Physicians in Somalia still treat severe diarrheal disease with four to six grams of crushed resin in a liter of water. Unfortunately, neither the analgesic effects, nor the antidiarrheal effects, have ever been evaluated in a real clinical trial.

Concerns: Contact dermatitis can be a problem, especially for those exposed to myrrh on a regular basis. In Hong Kong, dermatitis is almost an occupational disease for traditional healers, especially those who specialize in setting broken bones ("bonesetter's herb dermatitis"). Skin disease in these herbalists has been traced to the practice of rubbing a secret blend of herbs on the skin overlying broken bone. They do so because they believe it speeds the healing process. The secret blend they use is composed of a mixture of different herbs, but scientists believe that most of the problem comes from the myrrh that is included in the blend. Skin rashes have also been reported after the use of a myrrh-containing solution sold in China (Tieh Ta Yao Gin - it also contains Angelica and Aloe) that is used to treat bruises and muscle aches. Similar skin rashes have been reported in patients who apply myrrh-containing products to healing wounds.

Warnings: There are no reports of any serious medical complications from the use of myrrh.

Drug Testing: None of the components in the resin are likely to be absorbed through the skin, but even if they are, they would be unlikely to result in a false positive workplace drug test.

Dosage: Commission E recommends a myrrh tincture, applied undiluted, three times a day to the irritated skin. It can also be used as a rinse or gargle; 5-10 drops of the tincture in a glass of water, as needed. The Commission also recommends dental powders containing not more than 10% of the resin.

Summary: Modern laboratory studies confirm what traditional herbalists have known for thousands of years; myrrh contains molecules that can relieve muscles and joint pain, can help cure stomach upset and diarrheal illness. Whether myrrh is better or worse than more conventional allopathic medicines is not known - there have never been any clinical trials. The idea of using myrrh gargle to relieve throat pain seems sensible enough, and would certainly be associated with minimal risk. After all, this particular remedy has been in use for several thousand years and the first report of serious toxicity has yet to be published. Applying myrrh, or myrrh-containing solutions to aching joints, alone or in combination with other herbs, may also be a reasonable thing to do, but effectiveness has never been validated in a clinical trial, and long term use is definitely associated with an increased risk of developing contact dermatitis.

References:

Al-Suwaidan SN, Gad el Rab MO, Al-Fakhiry S, Al Hoqail IA, Al Maziad A, Sherif AB. Allergic contact dermatitis from myrrh, a topical herbal medicine used to promote healing. Contact Dermatitis 1998;39(3):137.

Andersson M, Bergendorff O, Shan R, Zygmunt P, Sterner O. Minor components with smooth muscle relaxing properties from scented myrrh (*Commiphora guidotti*). Planta Med 1997;63(3):251-4.

Claeson P, Andersson R, Samuelsson G. T-cadinol: a pharmacologically active constituent of scented myrrh: introductory pharmacological characterization and high field 1H- and 13C-NMR data. Planta Med 1991;57(4):352-6.

Lee TY, Lam TH. Myrrh is the putative allergen in bonesetter's herbs dermatitis. Contact Dermatitis 1993;29(5):279.

Michie CA, Cooper E. Frankincense and myrrh as remedies in children. J R Soc Med 1991;84(10):602-5.

Miller JM, Goodell HB. Frankincense and myrrh. Surg Gynecol Obstet 1968;127(2):360-5.

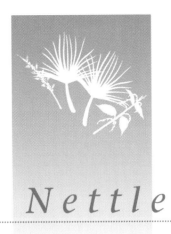

Nettle

Name: *Urtica dioica* L., (Urticaceae), commonly called the Stinging Nettle, or Urtica in English. A closely related herb, *Urtica urens* L., also called the Small Nettle, or Annual Nettle contains essentially the same ingredients. In German, it is *Brennesselkraut* or *Brennesselblatter*.

Source: Nettles grow along roadsides and unpopulated areas all across Europe and North America. Products sold commercially are made from dried crushed plants.

History: At one time, the nettle was cultivated as a source of fiber. Soft pliable fibers, nearly a yard in length, can be extracted from the plants. The name "nettle" comes from the an old English word meaning "to twist." In ancient Greece nettles were used as an antidote for hemlock poisoning and to treat venomous insect stings. According to ancient folklore, throwing a handful of nettles on a fire during a storm would prevent the house from being hit by lightning. The phrase "to grasp the nettle," meaning to do something difficult or unpleasant, derives from the old folk belief that someone suffering from a fever could be cured by uprooting a nettle plant with his/her bare hands. Even touching a nettle, let alone pulling on one, can be a painful experience. Hairs on the plant secrete formic acid. Concentrated doses can produce intense itching and even painful blisters. Young nettles do not produce formic acid, and they can be substituted for spinach in salads. Since nettles are rich in Vitamins A and C, substituting nettles for spinach or other leafy vegetable makes sense, provided you can tell young plants from old. Nettle seeds were once thought to be an aphrodisiac, which may have been at least partly true, since recent studies suggest the plant may be useful in treating prostate enlargement.

Traditional Claims: Diuretic and galactogenic (increase milk production). Nettle leaves have also been used either internally or topically to treat aching joints. Products made with the roots are said to be beneficial in treating the symptoms of prostate enlargement.

Commission E Recommendations: Nettle is used for irrigation therapy, rheumatism, urinary infection or inflammation, and the treatment of kidney stones or gravel.

Proven Effects: All parts of the plant contain flavonoids, specifically glycosides of quercetin (isoquercitrin and rutin), along with substantial amounts of chlorophyll. Nettles were once cultivated as a source for chlorophyll. Compounds found in root extracts called lignans bind with human sex hormone binding globulin (SHBG), and this interaction is thought to account for the improvement seen when nettles are given to men with benign prostate enlargement. At least in animal studies, nettle root extracts can prevent experimentally induced prostate enlargement. Other laboratory studies have shown that extracts of the leaf inhibit prostaglandin and leukotriene production - in other words, they are anti-inflammatory agents. Studies on white blood cells taken from healthy human volunteers showed that nettle extracts can prevent those cells from making and releasing inflammatory substances, such as tumor necrosis factor. Studies have also shown that another nettle component, called lectin, stimulates white blood cells, and that it may help boost the immune response. Even though nettles are widely recommended for treating seasonal allergies, evidence from clinical trials suggest that they don't provide much of a benefit. When ninety-eight allergy sufferers took part in a double-blind randomized study comparing the effects of a freeze-dried preparation of stinging nettles with placebo on allergic rhinitis, only sixty-nine individuals even bothered to complete the study, and the improvement they reported, though real, was extremely modest.

Concerns: Nettle extract may very well reduce some of the symptoms experienced by men with prostate enlargement, but under no circumstances should anyone ever begin treating symptoms of prostate disease without first seeing a physician and making sure that the symptoms are, in fact, due to prostate enlargement, and not something worse (cancer) or different (hyperactive bladder). Effects on blood sugar are another concern. Though poorly documented, there is some evidence that nettles may cause blood sugar levels to decrease. There is no evidence that anyone has ever suffered a hypoglycemic reaction, but users who develop symptoms such as headache, weakness, irritability or confusion, might well be having a hypoglycemic reaction.

Warnings: Taking nettles, or saw palmetto, or any other drug to treat the symptoms of prostate disease, without first knowing that the problem is, in fact, prostate disease, is a very bad idea.

Drug Testing: Nettle extracts are not known to interfere with routine workplace urine drug screening tests.

Dosage: The daily dose of dried herb and leaf is 8 to 12 grams per day. When the root is being used to treat prostate enlargement, the dose is only half that amount. If fresh leaves are being used, put two to three tablespoons in a cup of boiling water and allow the mixture to sit for 10 minutes. Use one tablespoon of the resulting liquid up to four times a day.

Summary: There is convincing laboratory evidence that nettle supplements can boost immunity and reduce inflammation. Clinical studies are, however, mostly lacking, and the one large trial that was done, comparing nettles to placebo in treating allergic symptoms, showed only very modest improvement. Mounting evidence also suggests that nettle extract may very well improve the symptoms of prostate enlargement, but the long-term toxicity of nettle-containing products has never been studied in animals, let alone in man.

References:

Galelli A, Truffa-Bachi P. *Urtica dioica* agglutinin. A superantigenic lectin from stinging nettle rhizome. J Immunol 1993;151(4):1821-31.

Hirano T, Homma M, Oka K. Effects of stinging nettle root extracts and their steroidal components on the Na+,K(+)-ATPase of the benign prostatic hyperplasia. Planta Med 1994;60(1):30-3.

Lichius JJ, Muth C. The inhibiting effects of *Urtica dioica* root extracts on experimentally induced prostatic hyperplasia in the mouse. Planta Med 1997;63(4):307-10.

Musette P, Galelli A, Chabre H, Callard P, Peumans W, Truffa-Bachi P, et al. *Urtica dioica* agglutinin, a V beta 8.3-specific superantigen, prevents the development of the systemic lupus erythematosus-like pathology of MRL lpr/lpr mice. Eur J Immunol 1996;26(8):1707-11.

Schottner M, Gansser D, Spiteller G. Lignans from the roots of *Urtica dioica* and their metabolites bind to human sex hormone binding globulin (SHBG). Planta Med 1997;63(6):529-32.

Mittman P. Randomized, double-blind study of freeze-dried *Urtica dioica* in the treatment of allergic rhinitis. Planta Med 1990;56(1):44-7.

Lutomski J, Speichert H. [Stinging nettle in medicine and nutrition]. Pharm Unserer Zeit 1983;12(6):181-6.

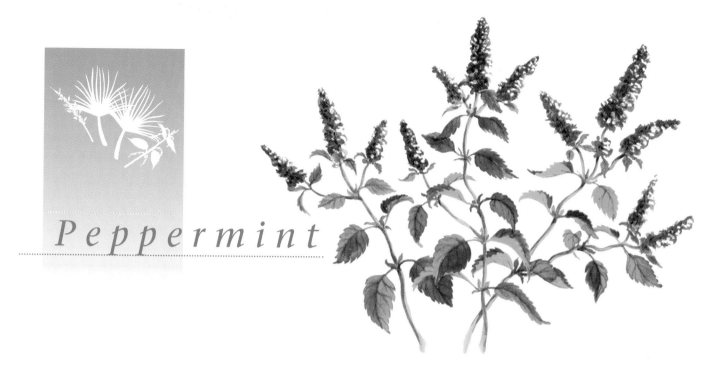

Peppermint

Name: *Mentha x piperita* L. (Labiatae), commonly called, Peppermint. In French, it is *Menthe poivrée*; in German, *Pfefferminze, Pfefferminzol,* and *Pfefferminzbläter*

Source: M. Piperitia is a hybrid that can be grown in most temperate climates. It was produced by crossing *Mentha aquatica* L. and *Mentha spicata* L. The entire plant is machine harvested just before it blooms and then allowed to dry. All parts of the plant contain an essential oil largely made up of menthol (up to 85 percent). Dried leaves are used to make teas. Steam distillation is used to extract the essential oil.

History: Peppermint was grown in ancient Egypt. Romans chewed the leaves to prevent bad breath, and used extracts to flavor wines and foods. It was believed that scattering dried leaves around granaries would keep away rats and mice. For unexplained reasons, peppermint did not reach Europe until the seventeenth century when an English botanist found the plant growing in a field of spearmint, outside of London, in a town named Mitcham. At one time, peppermint was thought to be an aphrodisiac.

Traditional Claims: Carminative, spasmolytic and choleretic (a substance that stimulates production of bile).

Commission E Recommendations: Peppermint is used to treat biliary spasm, gallbladder disorders and gastrointestinal spasm.

Proven Effects: Peppermint oil calms intestinal spasm, both in the laboratory and in double-blind, controlled clinical trials. This herb seems to be especially effective in patients with severe cases of irritable bowel syndrome. At the cellular level, calcium is a key element in muscle contraction, both in the muscles of the intestine and in the muscles that control the diameter of blood vessels. Calcium blocking agents are used to treat patients with high blood pressure because they prevent calcium from entering the cells, and when calcium levels in muscle cells drop, the muscle in the walls of the blood vessels relax, thereby lowering blood pressure. Many patients treated with calcium blockers become severely constipated because the medicines also relax the muscles in the intestines, which means that the bowel doesn't contract with enough force. In the case of patients with irritable bowel syndrome, calcium blockade turns out to be a benefit, not an undesired side effect. Peppermint oil is said to stimulate the gallbladder to contract, but its effect in humans has not really been studied. In Europe, a standardized herbal combination called Enteroplant, consisting of peppermint oil (90 mg) and caraway (50 mg) in an enteric coated capsule, is very popular for the treatment of mild stomach upset, and its effectiveness has been proven in at least one clinical trial. Other researchers have identified what seems to be a totally unrelated action; in a controlled trial, peppermint oil applied to the skin was just as good as acetaminophen or aspirin at relieving symptoms of tension headaches.

Concerns: Peppermint oil should not be applied to mucous membranes. It can cause severe burning. Patients with irritable bowel disease should probably be using enteric coated capsules of the oil because the chances are many of the beneficial components of the oil will be destroyed in the stomach.

Warnings: A very large dose (2 to 9 grams of the oil taken at one time) can cause acute renal failure. Patients with known gallbladder disease, especially gallstones, should not use peppermint. It might force small gallstones into the bile ducts and that could result in obstruction.

Drug Testing: None of the components of the essential oil should interfere with standard workplace urine drug screening tests.

Dosage: Infusions made from 2 to 3 grams of dried leaf can be used three times a day. Alternatively, 2 to 3 milliliters of a 1:5, 45 percent ethanol tincture can also be taken three times a day or 6 to 12 drops of essential oil up to three time a day; oil may be applied to the skin, either for the relief of headache or to treat muscle pain. When used on the skin, the preparation should contain between five and 20 percent essential oil. Nasal oils, used to treat colds in Europe, usually contain 1 to 5 percent oil.

Summary: Peppermint can be safely used to relieve a variety of gastrointestinal symptoms, reduce pain from muscle sprains, and possibly even help patients with tension headaches. Huge doses of peppermint oil cause serious toxicity, but peppermint oil, in traditionally-used doses, is a safe, time-proven remedy.

References:

Gobel H, Schmidt G, Soyka D. Effect of peppermint and eucalyptus oil preparations on neurophysiological and experimental algesimetric headache parameters. Cephalalgia 1994;14(3):228-34; discussion 182.

May B, Kuntz HD, Kieser M, Kohler S. Efficacy of a fixed peppermint oil/caraway oil combination in non-ulcer dyspepsia. Arzneimittelforschung 1996;46(12):1149-53.

Pittler MH, Ernst E. Peppermint oil for irritable bowel syndrome: a critical review and meta-analysis. Am J Gastroenterol 1998;93(7):1131-5.

Hills JM, Aaronson PI. The mechanism of action of peppermint oil on gastrointestinal smooth muscle. An analysis using patch clamp electrophysiology and isolated tissue pharmacology in rabbit and guinea pig. Gastroenterology 1991;101(1):55-65.

Liu JH, Chen GH, Yeh HZ, Huang CK, Poon SK. Enteric-coated peppermint-oil capsules in the treatment of irritable bowel syndrome: a prospective, randomized trial. J Gastroenterol 1997;32(6):765-8.

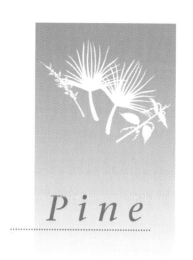

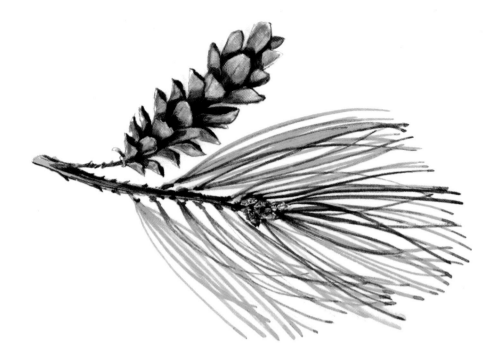

Pine

Name: *Pinus sylvestris* L., (Pinaceae), commonly called pine. In French, it is *Pin sylvestre*; in German, it is *Wald-Kiefer* or *Föhre*. Essential oil is also obtained from *P. palustris* and other *Pinue* species.

Source: Pine trees can be found growing in light sandy soils around the world. The resin from *Pinus palustris* is used to make turpentine. The essential oil obtained from the needles is usually added to liniments used to treat muscle sprains, while the sprouts, collected in spring from *P. silvestris,* are used to treat cough and respiratory infections. Pine bark, particularly that of *P. silvestris* contains a clinically promising antioxidant called pycnogenol.

History: Pine oils have been used as liniments, and for bathing, since ancient times. Homeopaths, in particular, recommended external application of the oil as a treatment for symptoms of arthritis.

Traditional Claims: Pine is used to increase secretions, as a mild antiseptic and to increase circulation.

Commission E Recommendations: The Commission recommends pine oil as an internal treatment for inflammation of the upper and lower respiratory tract, and externally for rheumatic and neuralgic complaints. It recommends using the sprouts for essentially the same conditions.

Proven Effects: Turpentine is not prescribed by allopathic physicians. Although Commission E recommends both the essential oil and the sprouts for upper respiratory infections, these recommendations have never been validated in a clinical trial. Pycnogenol (classified chemically as a procynanadin), found in the bark, has been studied extensively in the laboratory where it has been found to be an effective antioxidant/free radical-scavenger. But, in addition to its antioxidant activity, it stimulates nitric oxide production (ginkgo biloba does the same thing), an effect which could counteract many of the deleterious actions of the stress hormones, epinephrine and norepinephrine. Nitric oxide also stops platelets from sticking to each other and prevents the oxidation of low-density lipoprotein (LDL) cholesterol, two actions which could protect against atherogenesis and thrombus formation. Even the sawdust remaining after pine trees are processed in lumber mills seems to be of some value in preventing heart disease. A chemical called sitosterol is extracted from the residue and converted into sitostanol, a compound that prevents the absorption of cholesterol from the gastrointestinal tract. Sitostanol is the active ingredient in the cholesterol-lowering margarine sold in Europe that will soon be introduced in the United States.

Concerns: The essential oil can be very irritating when applied to mucous membranes.

Warnings: Very large doses of turpentine can cause seizure and even coma, although the few case reports in the literature suggest that most overdose victims recover.

Drug Testing: None of the components of the essential oil should interfere or interact in any way with standard workplace urine drug screening tests.

Dosage: Commission E recommends a daily dose of 2 to 3 grams of fresh or dry pine sprouts for respiratory infections. Alternatively, several drops of pine oil can be placed in hot water and inhaled. For sprains and muscle aches, a few drops of the oil should be rubbed into the tender area.

Summary: Pycnogenol may yet turn out to be one of the most important food supplements, at least in terms of preventing coronary artery disease. Small doses of inhaled pine oil vapors may make cold and flu sufferers feel better, and it is certainly safe. None of the other claims for this herb have been validated in clinical trials.

References:

Fitzpatrick DF, Bing B, Rohdewald P. Endothelium-dependent vascular effects of Pycnogenol . J Cardiovasc Pharmacol 1998;32(4):509-15.

Noda Y, Anzai K, Mori A, Kohno M, Shinmei M, Packer L. Hydroxyl and superoxide anion radical scavenging activities of natural source antioxidants using the computerized JES-FR30 ESR spectrometer system. Biochem Mol Biol Int 1997;42(1):35-44.

Troulakis G, Tsatsakis AM, Tzatzarakis M, Astrakianakis A, Dolapsakis G, Kostas R. Acute intoxication and recovery following massive turpentine ingestion: clinical and toxicological data. Vet Hum Toxicol 1997;39(3):155-7.

Miettinen T, Pekka P, Gyllinga H, Vanhannen M, Vartiaianen E. Reduction of serum cholesterol with sitostanol-ester margarine in a mildly hypercholesterolemic population. N Engl J Med 1995;333:1308-1312.

Virgili F, Kim D, Packer L. Procyanidins extracted from pine bark protect alpha-tocopherol in ECV 304 endothelial cells challenged by activated RAW 264.7 macrophages: role of nitric oxide and peroxynitrite. FEBS Lett 1998;431(3):315-8.

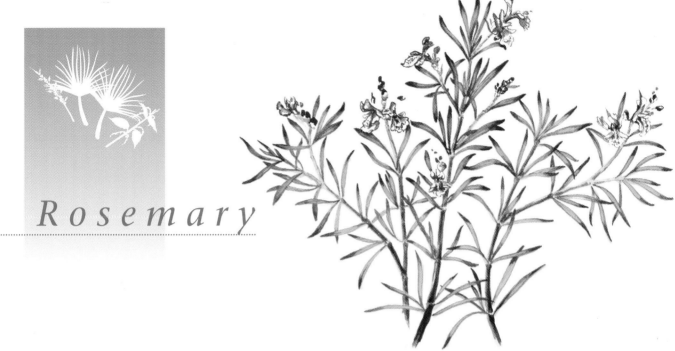

Rosemary

Name: *Rosmarinus officinalis* L. (Labiatae), commonly called rosemary, also Rosa maria, and dew-of-the-sea. In French, it is *Romarin;* in German, *Rosmarin* and *Rosmarinblätter.*

Source: A perennial plant with pale blue flowers that blooms from May to August. The dried leaves and flowers are used to produce an essential oil.

History: The Latin name of the plant means "dew-of-the-sea," probably because the plants generally grow well by the seashore. Rosemary was used as incense by the ancient Romans. According to legend, Mary sheltered the baby Jesus under a rosemary bush. Rosemary was used in Roman burial rites, and that practice continued well into the Middle Ages when branches of the plant were placed in the coffin. It was believed, quite wrongly, that oil of rosemary could be used to treat patients infected with plague. A sprig of rosemary placed in the button hole is supposed to bring good luck and improve memory.

Traditional Claims: Stomachic, carminative and cholagogue. Ointments made from the oil were, and still are, used to treat sprains and bruises.

Commission E Recommendations: Rosemary is used for circulatory disorders, dyspepsia (upset stomach) and rheumatism.

Proven Effects: Menthol and other aromatic vapors have long been used to treat upper respiratory tract infections. In laboratory studies, inhalation of these oils has been shown to reduce the frequency and intensity of coughing - at least in experimental animals. In clinical trials with the active component of these oils, a monoterpene, asthmatic patients showed objective improvement, and chemical tests disclosed that the inflammatory process had been inhibited at the molecular level (the arachandonic acid cascade had been inhibited). Even more importantly, recent studies suggest that rosemary has potent antioxidant and antitumor effects. Beef from cattle that have been fed with rosemary contains fewer carcinogens than those that have not been treated (the process of broiling converts some molecules into weak carcinogens). Whether these effects translate into real benefits for humans remains to be seen. Rosemary oil is increasingly being used by aromatherapists, but whether such use really confers any benefits is not known. Use of rosemary oil as an inhalant stems from a very old belief that stimulation of the olfactory nerves causes reflex stimulation of respiration and circulation. Commission E still suggests that adding rosemary oil to a hot bath will improve the circulation even though control trials have never been undertaken.

Concerns: None

Warnings: None

Drug Testing: There is no evidence that any component of rosemary, or rosemary oil, interacts with standard workplace urine drug screening tests.

Dosage: Teas can be made from the dried flowers by soaking one teaspoon in a cup of boiling water for 10-15 minutes. The average daily dose is 4-6 grams of herb.

Summary: Rosemary is a very tasty herb that no kitchen, or kitchen garden should be without. Laboratory evidence suggests that rosemary is a good antioxidant, and that regular use may help prevent tumor growth. The fact that rosemary feedings reduce the amount of carcinogens produced by broiling meat is interesting and encouraging. Other medical claims may or may not be true. In the absence of clinical trials there is no way to know, but since this herb is so inherently nontoxic, there is no reason not to try it.

References:

Aruoma OI, Halliwell B, Aeschbach R, Loligers J. Antioxidant and pro-oxidant properties of active rosemary constituents: carnosol and carnosic acid. Xenobiotica 1992;22(2):257-68.

Chan MM, Ho CT, Huang HI. Effects of three dietary phytochemicals from tea, rosemary and turmeric on inflammation-induced nitrite production. Cancer Lett 1995;96(1):23-9.

Juergens UR, Stuber M, Schmidt-Schilling L, Kleuver T, Vetter H. Anti-inflammatory effects of euclyptol (1.8-Cineole) in bronchial asthma: inhibition of arachidonic acid metabolism in human blood monocytes ex vivo. Eur J Med Res 1998;3(9):407-12.

Mace K, Offord EA, Harris CC, Pfeifer AM. Development of in vitro models for cellular and molecular studies in toxicology and chemoprevention. Arch Toxicol Suppl 1998;20:227-36.

Minnunni M, Wolleb U, Mueller O, Pfeifer A, Aeschbacher HU. Natural antioxidants as inhibitors of oxygen species induced mutagenicity. Mutat Res 1992;269(2):193-200.

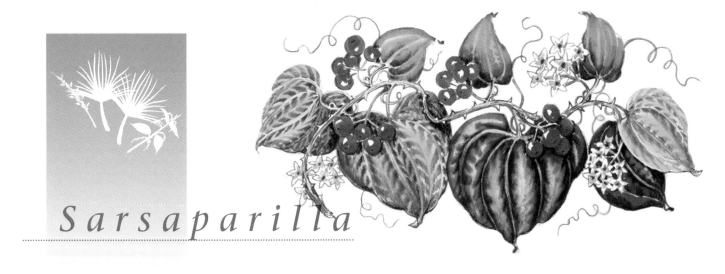

Sarsaparilla

Name: *Smilax aristolochiaefolia* Mill., S. *febrifuga Kunth,* S. *Ornata* Hook and *S regelii* Killip et Morton, (Liliaceae), commonly called Mexican, Ecuadoran and Honduran sarsaparilla.

Source: From the dried roots and rhizomes of various *Smilax* species grown in South America.

History: Europeans began to use this herb almost as soon as the first explorers returned from South America. During the 1800s, sarsaparilla was thought to be an excellent treatment for syphilis. As Professor Varro Tyler points out in his *Honest Herbal,* knowledge of this fact casts a slightly different light "on the white-hatted cowboy hero" who always strode into the bar in the Saturday afternoon B movie, asking for a glass of sarsaparilla! The herb is now mainly used as a flavoring in the manufacture of soft drinks, and as an ingredient in body building supplements.

Traditional Claims: Anti-inflammatory, antirheumatic, diuretic and diaphoretic. It is also used to treat skin disease, especially psoriasis.

Commission E Recommendations: Sarsaparilla is not on the approved list. The Commission had concerns over stomach irritation, secondary to the high content of saponins, substances that are known to be irritating to the stomach lining. The commission was also concerned about the danger of using sarsaparilla with heart medications. Sarsaparilla is mildly diuretic, which means it could cause the body to lose potassium, and that might increase the chances of digitalis causing a toxic reaction. The Commission's monograph, published in 1990, also cited the near total absence of clinical trials that would be needed to reach any intelligent conclusion.

Proven Effects: Extracts contain flavonoids (isoengetitin, isoastilbin and astilbin), saponins (sarasapogenin, smilagenin, and parillin) and many of the same sterols, including beta sitosterol, found in soy beans. Clinical trials are essentially nonexistent, but there is good laboratory evidence that extracts are anti-inflammatory and probably antioxidant. The expected range of effects for such a combination of ingredients would not be unlike the effects of fenugreek.

Concerns: As the editors of the American edition of the Commission E reports suggest, there is very little evidence that saponins cause gastric distress, and Commission E concerns in this regard may be exaggerated.

Warnings: If, in fact, sarsaparilla does act as a diuretic, then potassium loss could occur. Patients taking medications for heart disease should check with their physicians before trying this product.

Drug Testing: There are no reports that any of the components found in sarsaparilla extract interact or interfere with routine workplace urine drug screening tests.

Dosage: Dried root, 2 to 4 grams two to three times per day as a decoction; liquid extract (1:1, 50 percent ethanol), 2 to 4 milliliters two to three times a day.

Summary: Concerns about the toxicity of this agent are probably excessive. On the other hand, there is so little clinical data that it is difficult to be sure just what benefits might be recognized by taking sarsaparilla. Soft drinks made with sarsaparilla extract may be quite tasty, but they will not cure syphilis!

References:

Ageel AM, Mossa JS, al-Yahya MA, al-Said MS, Tariq M. Experimental studies on antirheumatic crude drugs used in Saudi traditional medicine. Drugs Exp Clin Res 1989;15(8):369-72.

Grunewald KK, Bailey RS. Commercially marketed supplements for bodybuilding athletes. Sports Med 1993;15(2):90-103.

Lee H, Lin JY. Antimutagenic activity of extracts from anticancer drugs in Chinese medicine. Mutat Res 1988;204(2):229-34.

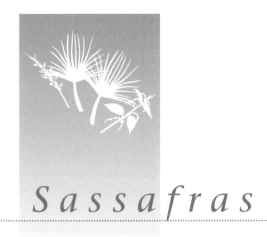

Sassafras

Name: *Sassafras albidum* (Nuttall) Nees (Lauraceae), commonly called sassafras.

Source: From the leaves, stems, and bark of a tree that grows mainly in the Eastern United States. A pleasant smelling essential oil is obtained by steam distillation of the bark. The main constituent of the oil (80 percent) is safrole. Safrole is a phenylpropene, and is closely related to the molecules that give cinnamon and anise their distinctive aromas. But unlike the related oils, safrole has been classified by the Food and Drug Administration (FDA) as a probable carcinogen.

History: Until safrole was classified as a carcinogen, sassafras oil was used as a soft drink flavoring. Powdered bark still is used to thicken Cajun gumbo. Native American Indians used a decoction made from the bark to treat infected wounds. Safrole was first banned in 1960. Then, in 1976, the FDA clarified its initial ruling and also banned the sale of sassafras bark and leaves for herbal teas. Health food stores continue to sell sassafras, but with labeling that indicates it is for external use only. Safrole-free extracts have been produced to use as flavoring, but in animal experiments they also enhance tumor growth.

Traditional Claims: Carminative, anodyne, and diaphoretic.

Commission E Recommendations: The Commission has never issued a report on sassafras.

Proven Effects: In the absence of any clinical studies, it is impossible to guess just what clinical benefits might be derived from using this herb. After safrole, the other main components of the oil are camphor (3.2 percent), methyleugenol (1.1 percent), and an assortment of sesquiterpenes, the best known of which is parthenolide, the molecule found in feverfew that relieves the pain of migraine headaches. Sassafras might have some of the same effects as feverfew but that possibility has never been investigated. Methyleugenol is clove oil, a commonly used dental anesthetic, which may mean that sassafras might be used for that purpose as well. The oil may also have some anti-inflammatory effects - several widely used anti-inflammatory medications (Sulindac™ and Indocin™ to name just two) are produced starting from the safrole molecule. Anecdotes suggest that the oil can be used to kill headlice. However, the oil can be very irritating to the skin.

Concerns: In spite of concerns that massive amounts of safrole might end up in teas made with sassafras (up to 200 milligrams per cup), modern measurement suggests that the actual concentrations are closer to 5 milligrams. Nonetheless, safrole is clearly a carcinogen in experimental animals, and safrole-containing products should not be used on a regular basis.

Warnings: Safrole is used by some underground chemists as a starting material to make "ecstasy," and related designer amphetamines. While there may be some doubt about the carcinogenicity of low levels of safrole, exposure to high concentrations could be very dangerous.

Drug Testing: There are no published reports, but the configuration of the safrole molecule is not that different from that of some designer amphetamines, and use of sassafras could conceivably cause a false positive workplace screening test for abused drugs. Of course, even if a false positive screening test did occur, confirmation would disclose that it was safrole, and not MDA or MDMA.

Dosage: The safe dose for oral sassafras is not known.

Summary: Sassafras contains a known carcinogen. Teas brewed with powdered bark would contain very small amounts of that carcinogen, and would probably be safe for occasional use. Unfortunately, there is no way to know for sure. External use of the oil is probably not much safer, since severe skin irritation can result. If head lice is the problem, use something else.

References:

Carlson M, Thompson RD. Liquid chromatographic determination of safrole in sassafras-derived herbal products. J AOAC Int 1997;80(5):1023-8.

Kapadia GJ, Chung EB, Ghosh B, Shukla YN, Basak SP, Morton JF, et al. Carcinogenicity of some folk medicinal herbs in rats. J Natl Cancer Inst 1978;60(3):683-6.

Kapadia GJ, Paul BD, Chung EB, Ghosh B, Pradhan SN. Carcinogenicity of *Camellia sinensis* (tea) and some tannin-containing folk medicinal herbs administered subcutaneously in rats. J Natl Cancer Inst 1976;57(1):207-9.

Segelman AB, Segelman FP, Karliner J, Sofia RD. Sassafras and herb tea. Potential health hazards. Jama 1976;236(5):477.

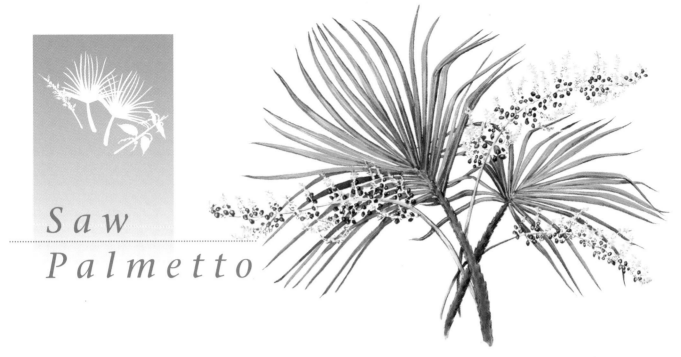

Saw Palmetto

Name: The botanical name for the dwarf palm or saw palmetto, is *Serenoa repens* (Arecaceae). A related variety, containing the same active ingredients, is called *Sabal serrulata*. Extracts of *Serenoa repens* are sold in Europe under various brand names (LESSr™, Permixon™, Sereprostat™). In German, it is *Sabalfrüchte*.

Source: The active ingredient comes from an oil extracted from berries at the tops of trees. Saw palmetto is a palm that grows mainly along the southern Atlantic coast of the United States. There are large commercial plantations in Florida, many near Cape Canaveral. A closely related palm grows in southern Europe and in northern Africa. The berries contains small amounts of a volatile oil rich in fatty acids (caproic, caprylic, capric, lauric, palmitic, and oleic acids). In addition, the berries contain beta-sitosterol and ferulic acid. In Europe, products sold to treat prostate enlargement contain at least 85 percent purified oils.

History: For many years the berries were used as a diuretic and as a treatment for the symptoms of urinary tract infections. They were not very effective, and by 1950 *Serenoa* had been dropped from the National Formulary. Even though physicians lost interest in the plant, claims that it could cause women's breasts to grow have been circulating for years. Strangely enough, the claims may contain an element of truth (see below). It is also claimed, without very much evidence, that *Serenoa* is an aphrodisiac. The results of modern laboratory studies suggest that the opposite may be the case.

Traditional Claims: Diuretic

Commission E Recommendations: Saw Palmetto is used to treat diminished urination associated with BPH Stages 1 and 2, and prostate adenoma.

Proven Effects: More than half of men age 50 and older experience some symptoms related to enlargement of the prostate gland. *Serenoa* has two separate and apparently unrelated effects on the cells of the prostate that reduce symptoms by making the gland smaller; *Serona* is an anti-inflammatory but it also blocks a key enzyme that promotes prostate gland enlargement. The prostate gland wraps around the urethra. Hormonal changes associated with aging cause the gland to enlarge. Enlargement, in itself, would not be that great a problem, but the gland is surrounded by a tight shell. As the individual cells grow, they run up against the tight covering, and pressure within the gland increases. The urethra gets compressed, and the result is well known to many middle-aged men: frequency, urgency, difficulty in starting to urinate, and the feeling that the bladder is not really being emptied. Until recently, the problem could only be solved by surgery. But in the early 1990s, effective medications became available. The first, called Finasteride (Proscar™) works by blocking an enzyme that converts testosterone to dihydrotestosterone (DHT). DHT, it turns out, is the hormone that makes the individual cells grow too much. Blocking DHT prevents the growth and allows the prostate to return to normal size. The problem with this approach is that it may take a year to see any results. Evidence suggests that *Serenoa* blocks DHT in much the same fashion as Proscar™. Other studies have shown that *Serenoa* has anti-inflammatory effects, at least within the prostate, and that could help reduce prostate size as well. The anti-inflammatory effect may explain why many men report improvements in far less time than 12 months. In controlled studies, a dose of 160 mg twice a day significantly reduced symptoms and caused minimal side effects. Results were nearly as good as those achieved with the new generation of prostate drugs (called alpha1-blockers, Cardura™, Flomax™, and Hytrin™ are the best known). Using the herbal approach may result in some substantial cost savings. Drugs like Cardura™ cost more than a dollar a tablet, and must be taken for life. Costs for Proscara™ are even higher, well over $2 per day. The diuretic effects of *Serenoa*, if any, have never been tested in a clinical trial.

Concerns: The same researchers who found that *Serenoa* blocked the conversion to DHT, also found that *Serenoa* interfered with the actions of testosterone. Blocking testosterone is not a good thing in general, and could be a very bad thing, especially for the libido. Instead of being an aphrodisiac, saw palmetto could be an anti-aphrodisiac! Actually, the situation is even worse. Beta-sitosterol, which is also present in the oil from the berries, behaves like a very weak female sex hormone (estrogen). That may explain the claims of some women who say that taking the extract made their breasts grow. In theory, they may be correct.

Warnings: Extracts of saw palmetto appear to be very safe products. Reports of toxicity are limited to the occasional stomach upset. The real cause for concern has nothing to do with the herb, but with the disease it is being used to treat. Cancer of the prostate can mimic the symptoms of benign prostatic hypertrophy (BPH). Only a physician can determine whether it is BPH causing the symptoms or some other disorder. A simple examination and blood test (for PSA, "prostate specific antigen") is all that is required. Once the possibility of cancer has been ruled out, the choice of treatment should be up to the patient.

Drug Testing: There are no reports suggesting that any of the components of the standardized oil could crossreact or cause a false positive in a workplace testing program.

Dosage: Commission E recommends 1 to 2 grams a day of the dried berries or 320 milligrams per day of the extract. Most of the controlled trials done in Europe utilized the 320 milligram per day dose.

Summary: There is good evidence that regular use can relieve the symptoms of BPH. Any man with symptoms of BPH needs first to be examined by a physician to make sure that the symptoms are not due to cancer. Once cancer is ruled out, saw palmetto may provide an effective and much cheaper treatment, although a concomitant decline in libido might come along with relief of the prostate symptoms. However, some of the new prostate drugs, such as Cardura™, even though more expensive, may provide relief much more quickly.

References:

Gerber GS, Zagaja GP, Bales GT, Chodak GW, Contreras BA. Saw palmetto (*Serenoa repens*) in men with lower urinary tract symptoms: effects on urodynamic parameters and voiding symptoms. Urology 1998;51(6):1003-7.

Herbal supplements. Is saw palmetto good for the prostate? Harv Health Lett 1998;23(7):6.

Monograph: *serenoa repens*. Altern Med Rev 1998;3(3):227-9.

Powers JE. That pesky prostate and the saw palmetto. S D J Med 1997;50(12):453-4.

Van Berkel GJ, Quirke JM, Tigani RA, Dilley AS, Covey TR. Derivatization for electrospray ionization mass spectrometry. 3. Electrochemically ionizable derivatives. Anal Chem 1998; 70(8):1544-54.

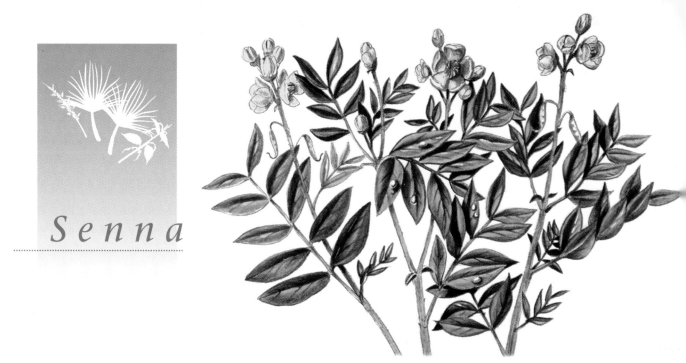

Senna

Name: *Senna alexandrina* Miller, or *Cassia senna* L. [*C. Acutifolia* Delile], (Fabaceae), commonly called Senna, but also Alexandrian Senna Pods, Khartoum senna, and Tinnevelly senna. In German it is *Sennesfrüchte*

Source: Senna is prepared from the dried leaves or fruits from either *Cassia senna* or *C. Angustifolia*. *Cassia senna* is a small shrub that grows in Somalia and on the Arabian peninsula. *C. Angustifolia* is native to India and Pakistan, but is now grown commercially in California. Senna pods are sold separately from leaves and fetch a greater price. Both parts of the plant contain the same active ingredients, but more of the active ingredient is contained in the pods than in the leaves.

History: Senna has been in use at least since the ninth century, when Arabian physicians first began treating constipation with preparations made from *Senna* leaves and the pods.

Traditional Claims Senna is used as a laxative.

Commission E Recommendations: Laxative.

Proven Effects: Like aloe, senna contains molecules called anthroquinones (Sennoside A and Sennoside B). In their natural state, when still in the plant, these molecules are tightly bound to a sugar molecule. The presence of the sugar molecule makes the complex inert, and prevents the molecule from being absorbed in the stomach and small intestine. But when the anthraquinone-sugar complex finally gets to the large intestine, bacteria in the gut remove the sugar molecule. Once that happens, the unbound anthraquinone (now called rheinanthrone) reacts with cells on the wall of the large intestine causing the cells to transport water and electrolytes into the intestinal tract. The latest data suggest that the senna works by increasing production of nitric oxide, a local neurotransmitter within the intestinal wall.Whatever the molecular mechanism, the resulting increase in volume stimulates the walls of the colon, causing it to contract. Bowel movements usually occur 6-10 hours after aloe or senna are taken.

Concerns: Senna does not produce nearly as much cramping as aloe, and not nearly as much of the active ingredients are absorbed into the bloodstream. For that reason,senna does not change the color of the urine. Still, some is absorbed, and small amounts still might appear in mother's milk, so nursing mothers should use another product. The biggest cause for concern is that long-term exposure, at least in laboratory animals, caused tumors of the colon, liver, and kidneys. Worse still, epidemiologic studies of long-term users suggest that they do, in fact, develop colon cancer at a higher rate than the general population. The colon cancer rate for individuals who develop melanosis coli (see below) is even higher.

Warnings: Chronic use of any laxative can deplete the body of potassium, and low levels of potassium can cause dangerous irregularities in the way the heart beats. Chronic use can result in a benign condition called melanosis coli. Brownish pigment accumulates in the wall of the large intestine, where it apparently does no harm, although doctors consider it a marker for laxative abuse. Even though the pigment disappears if senna is discontinued, chronic senna users appear to develop bowel cancer at a higher rate than the rest of the community. Virtually every scientific body that has reviewed the problem recommends that none of the anthrone-containing laxatives be used for more than 10 days.

Drug Testing: Using senna will not change the color of urine and will not interfere with standard workplace urine tests.

Dosage: Ground leaves can be taken in capsules, but whatever form of the drug that is used, it should state the anthrone content. The average daily dose is between 10 and 60 milligrams. Tea can be made from Tinnevelly senna fruit, or senna leaf, by adding one level teaspoonful of product to boiling water, letting it steep for 10 minutes, and then pouring it through a strainer before drinking.

Summary: Used occasionally, senna is a perfectly good laxative, safely taken by millions of people every day. Long-term use increases the risk for dangerous electrolyte depletion and the risk for colon cancer. Persistent constipation, unresponsive to senna, is a very good reason to visit your doctor.

References:

Brusick D, Mengs U. Assessment of the genotoxic risk from laxative senna products. Environ Mol Mutagen 1997;29(1):1-9.

de Witte P, Lemli L. The metabolism of anthranoid laxatives. Hepatogastroenterology 1990;37(6):601-5.

Franz G. The senna drug and its chemistry. Pharmacology 1993;47 Suppl 1:2-6.

Izzo AA, Sautebin L, Rombola L, Capasso F. The role of constitutive and inducible nitric oxide synthase in senna- and cascara-induced diarrhoea in the rat. Eur J Pharmacol 1997;323(1):93-7.

Mereto E, Ghia M, Brambilla G. Evaluation of the potential carcinogenic activity of Senna and Cascara glycosides for the rat colon. Cancer Lett 1996;101(1):79-83.

Morton J. The detection of laxative abuse. Ann Clin Biochem 1987;24(Pt 1):107-8.

Siegers CP, von Hertzberg-Lottin E, Otte M, Schneider B. Anthranoid laxative abuse—a risk for colorectal cancer? Gut 1993;34(8):1099-101.

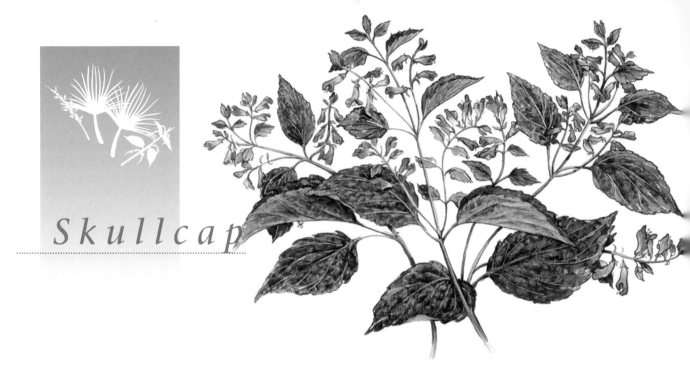

Skullcap

Name: *Scutellaria lateriflora* L. (Lamiaceae), commonly called skullcap, mad dog, mad weed, and hooded willow herb.

Source: A perennial plant with purple flowers, it blooms in the U.S. from July to September. It is usually found growing by ditches and river banks, wherever there is a damp environment. Closely related varieties grow in Europe and Asia (*S. Baicalensis* Georrgi). Remedies are made from the roots of the plant.

History: During the 1700s, American physicians used the herb to treat rabies, which is why it is sometimes known as "mad dog." Skullcap was also used to treat tetanus and seizures. Its common name, skullcap, comes from the fact that it was often given to inmates of mental asylums who were required to wear skullcaps. Traditional Chinese herbalists have used skullcap to treat neonatal jaundice and to speed convalescence.

Traditional Claims: Nervine, sedative, and antispasmodic.

Commission E Recommendations: Skullcap is not on the Commission's approved list. In fact, it is not mentioned at all.

Proven Effects: Until fairly recently, most researchers considered this herb to be devoid of medicinal value. Studies utilizing more sensitive techniques now suggest a number of possible benefits. There is, for example, some laboratory evidence that an as yet uncharacterized component blocks the effects of some of the stress hormones (adrenalin). Skullcap contains a number of different flavonoids, and some of them possess antibiotic and anti-inflammatory properties, at least in the laboratory. One kind of flavonoid, trihydroxyflavone, is a very effective free radical scavenger. These same flavonoids also show promise as a treatment to prevent the closure of coronary arteries that have been opened with balloon angioplasty (restenososis). Studies of patients being treated for lung cancer have shown that adding skullcap extract to the treatment regime partially prevents the immune depression that accompanies chemotherapy. Adding skullcap may also decrease the amount of tumor necrosis factor (a hormone that causes cell death, and that is believed to be one of the chief causes of wasting seen in cancer patients) circulating in the bloodstream. However, claims that skullcap calms the stomach, lowers blood pressure, and acts as a tranquilizer have never been evaluated in clinical trials.

Concerns: Ten years ago, there were reports suggesting that skullcap caused liver damage. The results of later studies suggested that the toxicity probably occurred because herb wholesalers had been substituting germander root for skullcap. The explanation is probably correct, because the latest research studies show that skullcap extract protects the livers of experimental animals exposed to a range of liver toxins.

Warnings: Provided that skullcap, and not germander, is in the extract, there would seem to be little cause for concern. Consumers must carefully read the label, and buy only from producers with trusted brand names.

Drug Testing: None of the components in skullcap should crossreact or interfere with any of the standard workplace urine drug screening tests.

Dosage: Traditional herbalists recommend an infusion made with one teaspoon of dried herbs steeped in one cup of boiling water for 20-30 minutes, two to three times a day.

Summary: There is reasonable scientific evidence that skullcap strengthens the immune response and decreases the inflammatory response, at least in patients undergoing chemotherapy. Whether it provides the same effects to people with colds and the flu is not known (skullcap is often combined with echinacea in cold medications). Providing that skullcap, and not something masquerading as skullcap is being taken, there would seem to be little harm in using this product.

References:

Gabrielska J, Oszmianski J, Zylka R, Komorowska M. Antioxidant activity of flavones from *Scutellaria baicalensis* in lecithin liposomes. Z Naturforsch [C] 1997;52(11-12):817-23.

Kimura Y, Yokoi K, Matsushita N, Okuda H. Effects of flavonoids isolated from scutellariae radix on the production of tissue-type plasminogen activator and plasminogen activator inhibitor-1 induced by thrombin and thrombin receptor agonist peptide in cultured human umbilical vein endothelial cells. J Pharm Pharmacol 1997;49(8):816-22.

Kimura Y, Matsushita N, Okuda H. Effects of baicalein isolated from *Scutellaria baicalensis* on interleukin 1 beta- and tumor necrosis factor alpha-induced adhesion molecule expression in cultured human umbilical vein endothelial cells. J Ethnopharmacol 1997;57(1):63-7.

Lin CC, Shieh DE, Yen MH. Hepatoprotective effect of the fractions of Ban-zhi-lian on experimental liver injuries in rats. J Ethnopharmacol 1997;56(3):193-200.

Smol'ianinov ES, Gol'dberg VE, Matiash MG, Ryzhakov VM, Boldyshev DA, Litvinenko VI, et al. [Effect of Scutellaria baicalensis extract on the immunologic status of patients with lung cancer receiving antineoplastic chemotherapy]. Eksp Klin Farmakol 1997;60(6):49-51.

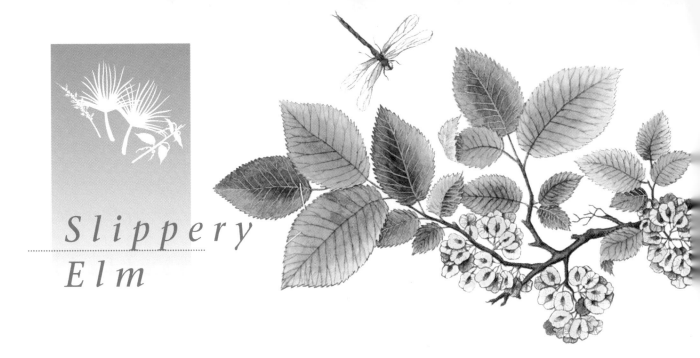

Slippery Elm

Name: Ulmus rubra L. (Ulmaceae). Also Ulmus rubra and campestris L., and other closely related varieties. Commonly called, red elm or sweet elm. In French, it is *Orme champétre or Ormeau*; in German, *Feld-Ulme or Rüster*.

Source: A fairly tall deciduous tree with rough bark that flowers in February and March. It grows throughout Europe and Asia Minor. Medications are made from the dried inner bark.

History: Extracts of the inner bark are effective laxatives, which probably explains the "slippery" in the plant's name. When the bark is mixed with water a thick mucilage forms. The mucilage has both nutritive and healing effects and has been used for hundreds of years, both as a medication and as a food supplement, for convalescent patients.

Traditional Claims: Demulcent, emollient, purgative, and for irritation of both upper and lower gastrointestinal tract.

Commission E Recommendations: The Commission has no opinion on this herb.

Proven Effects: The main constituent of the bark is mucilage, composed of water soluble sugars (polysaccharides). Taken orally, it is said to relieve gastrointestinal distress. Applied externally, it is said to be useful for soothing wounds. None of these claims have ever been validated in a controlled clinical trial, but the results of modern research studies suggest that traditional herbalists were correct. Something in the bark acts as a nitric oxide inhibitor, which means that bark extracts should have an anti-inflammatory effect. Nitric oxide also plays an important role in controlling gastrointestinal function. If slippery elm alters nitric oxide production, that could explain traditional claims that the herb relieves gastrointestinal symptoms.

Concerns: None. This is an extremely safe herb with no reports of significant toxicity.

Warnings: None.

Drug Testing: Bark extracts contain mainly polysaccharide sugars. They should have no effect on workplace urine drug screening tests.

Dosage: Powdered bark (1:10) in hot water, taken as often as needed. It may also be used as a poultice for topical applications.

Summary: Slippery elm bark is a very old and very safe remedy. Anecdotal reports of herbalists suggest that powdered bark in hot water will soothe the throat and stomach. Even though the claims are unsupported by clinical trials, the latest laboratory studies suggest that the herbalists were correct.

References:

Jun CD, Pae HO, Kim YC, Jeong SJ, Yoo JC, Lee EJ, et al. Inhibition of nitric oxide synthesis by butanol fraction of the methanol extract of *Ulmus davidiana* in murine macrophages. J Ethnopharmacol 1998;62(2):129-35.

Kim JP, Kim WG, Koshino H, Jung J, Yoo ID. Sesquiterpene O-naphthoquinones from the root bark of *Ulmus davidiana*. Phytochemistry 1996;43(2):425-30.

Ye G, Cao Q, Chen X, Li S, Jia B. *Ulmus macrocarpa* for the treatment of ulcerative colitis—a report of 36 cases. J Tradit Chin Med 1990;10(2):97-8

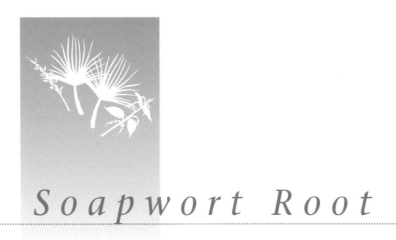

Soapwort Root

Name: *Saponaria officinalis* L. (Caryophyllaceae), commonly called Soapwort, Bouncing Bet, Fuller's herb, burisewort, and sheepweed. In French, it is *Saponaire officinale* or *Savonniére*. In German, it is *Rote Seifenwurzel* and *Seifenkraut*.

Source: Remedies are made from the dried roots of the plant which grows wild along the roadside and fields in Europe and America.

History: The herb got its name in 1548 when a British herbalist named William Turner first described it in his book, *The Names of Herbs.* It was probably used as a detergent by the ancient Romans. Extracts were used during the Middle Ages to clean wool before it was dyed.

Traditional Claims: Antirheumatic, diuretic, depurative and expectorant.

Commission E Recommendations: Soapwort is used to treat catarrh of the upper respiratory tract.

Proven Effects: Controlled clinical trials have never been done. Some interesting laboratory studies with one of the chemicals found in the roots, called saporin 6 (SO6), suggests that it inhibits tumor growth, particularly of leukemic cells. Commission E recommends that the roots can be used as an expectorant. Soapwort contains saponins and some saponins, to a greater or lesser degree, cause respiratory tract and gastrointestinal tract irritation. Sometimes, respiratory tract irritation can be helpful because it causes a more forceful cough and aids in sputum production. Whether this remedy is any better than any other over-the-counter (OTC) cough syrup is not known.

Concerns: Excessive saponin intake can lead to stomach upset.

Warnings: There are no known warnings, other than the fact that truly massive doses of soapwort can damage cell DNA (which is why soapwort is of interest to cancer researchers).

Drug Testing: There are no studies, but it seems unlikely that anything in soapwort could interfere with standard workplace urine screening tests. Adding soapwort as an adulterant would not be a good idea either, since it would make the urine foam. The presence of foam in a urine specimen would immediately alert the testing laboratory that the specimen had been adulterated!

Dosage: Commission E recommends 1.5 grams per day of the root, either plain or in a tea.

Summary: Soapwort is a traditional herbal remedy used as an expectorant. It is on the Commission E approved list, but its effectiveness has never been studied in a modern clinical trial. On the other hand, there are no reports of toxicity or drug interactions, and there seems to be no reason soapwort could not be used as an alternative to standard OTC cough syrups.

References:

Gasperi-Campani A, Zauli G, Roncuzzi L, Valvassori L, Vitale L, Gaggioli L, et al. Differential activity of saporin 6 on normal and leukemic hemopoietic cells. Exp Hematol 1989;17(7):755-9.

Sidhu GS, Oakenfull DG. A mechanism for the hypocholesterolaemic activity of saponins. Br J Nutr 1986;55(3):643-9.

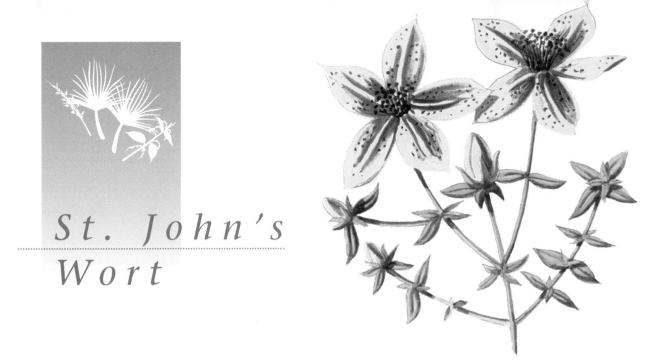

St. John's Wort

Name: *Hypericum perforatum,* L. (Hypericaceae), commonly called St. John's wort, and Fairy herb. In French, it is *Herbe de la St-Jean,* and *Millepertuis perforé;* in German, *Johanniskraut.*

Source: Products containing St. John's wort are made from the dried flowering tops and upper parts of the plant. They must be harvested just before, or just as, flowering begins. Flowers are harvested from the wilds during July-August, mainly in eastern Europe, although it is now grown commercially in South America. Hypericum contains a number of different, unrelated compounds, many of which possess important biological activity (naphthodianthrones, flavonoids, phloroglucinols and xanthones). These molecules are not distributed evenly throughout the plant, so depending on the source of the raw materials, hypericum formulations will contain variable amounts of each. Products are usually standardized for their content of a molecule called hypericin. Unfortunately, it is now clear that hypericin is not the molecule responsible for the antidepressant effect, so even "standardized" formulas may sometimes prove ineffective.

History: The common name for Hypericum, St. John's wort, comes from the fact that the herb flowers around the time of St. John's Day (June 24). Its flowers are golden yellow, but they also contain a red pigment that is said to symbolize the blood of St. John. Hypericum was first used to drive away witches and evil spirits, but the antidepressant properties of the herb were recognized early on. *Culpeper's Complete Herbal and English Physician*, published in 1826, claimed that a tincture made from wine and hypericum flowers could ward off melancholy and insanity.

Traditional Claims: Diuretic, sedative, astringent and antidepressant.

Commission E Recommendations: St. John's wort is used internally to treat anxiety, depression, and dyspepsia (upset stomach). Externally, it is used for contusion injuries, first degree burns and muscle pain.

Proven Effects: Laboratory studies of hypericum extract have shown that something in this plant prevents the reuptake of neurotransmitters (serotonin, norepinephrine and dopamine). Since reuptake is the way the brain terminates the activity of those neurotransmitters, inhibition of reuptake leads to exaggerated effects. Cocaine, for example, works in exactly the same way, by preventing dopamine reuptake. Modern antidepressant drugs, such as Prozac™, prevent the reuptake of serotonin. Their antidepressant effects are thought to be due, at least in part, to increased levels of serotonin in certain parts of the brain. The active molecule contained in hypericum extract is now known to be a substance called hyperforin, and not the red pigment hypericin. Well-controlled studies of outpatients with mild or moderate depression have shown that hypericum extracts are superior to placebo and about as effective as standard antidepressants. Claims for other actions have never been validated in believable clinical trials.

Concerns: The biggest concern for consumers using this herb might just be getting what they pay for. In August, 1998, reporters from the *Los Angeles Times* bought 10 different brands of St. John's wort and had them analyzed at an independent laboratory. Only three of the ten brands tested contained the amount advertised on the label (see the table below). In three cases, the hypericin content was less than half the amount stated. The findings of the survey only serve to emphasize the need for consumers to deal with reputable companies with established names. In the absence of serious government oversight, the reputation is about the only assurance consumers can rely upon. The only real medical concern is photosensitivity. Grazing animals that eat St. John's wort have had phytotoxic reactions, and several HIV positive patients treated with intravenous hypericin in very large doses (hypericin has antiviral properties), also developed severe sunburns. Anecdotal reports suggest that sunburn and severe phytotoxic reactions may be more common than had previously been thought, especially with very high doses of the extract, but there is still very little information in the literature. Otherwise, serious adverse effects due to St. John's wort appear to be quite rare. Dry mouth, dizziness, constipation, other gastrointestinal symptoms and confusion have been reported, but rarely. In trials, fewer than 2 percent of patients stopped taking the herb because of adverse effects.

Hypericin Content (milligrams) and Cost, for 10 Brands of St. John's Wort tested by *LOS ANGELES TIMES*

Spot Testing of Retail St. John's Wort

Brand Name	Claimed Potency Mg./Pill	Tested Potency Mg./Pill	% of Label Claim	Cost cents/pill	Hypercin Costs cents/mg.
Enzymantic Therapy	0.90	0.71	78.9	22	31
Futurebiotics	1.05	0.53	50.5	25	47
Jarrow Formulas	0.90	0.69	76.7	17	25
Kira	0.90	0.79	87.8	30	38
Nature's Herb's	0.35	0.46	131.4	17	37
Nature's Resource	0.30	0.42	140.0	15	36
Pure Source	0.90	0.20	22.2	12	60
Safeway Select	0.90	0.81	90.0	20	25
Sundown Herbals	0.45	0.09	20.0	11	122
Trader Joe's	0.90	0.74	82.2	9	12

The tested potency (milligrams of hypercin per pill) represents the average of three samples. The margin of error is approximately +/-5%. The testing, using a spectrophotometric method known as DAC-91, was done by Flora Research, an analytical firm in San Juan Capistrano.
Source: *Los Angeles Times*, August 31, 1998

Warnings: Depression is the most common psychiatric disorder, with a peak onset at age 50. Depression is not a disorder to be taken lightly. St. John's wort may be "nature's Prozac," but anyone suffering from real symptoms of depression should only be taking medication - natural or otherwise - under a doctor's supervision. Fair-complected users should avoid excessive sun exposure and wear a sun block while taking this herb.

Drug Testing: St. John's wort extract does contain some pigments that could, in theory, interfere with workplace urine drug screening tests, but such an occurrence has not been reported.

Dosage: Commission E recommends a daily dose of 2 to 4 grams of crude drug containing 0.2 to 1 mg of total hypericin. Commercially available products in the United States generally contain on the order of 300 mg. The recommended dose for depression, at least in Europe, is 900 mg per day as a starting dose, though in milder cases, doses as low as 300 mg per day may be sufficient.

Summary: St. John's wort is an antidepressant, comparable in strength to prescription antidepressants such as Elavil™ and Triavil™. As such, it should only be taken after consulting with a physician. The biggest problem with using this herb may be getting a reliable supply. Tests show that the contents of many supplements do not match what is on the label. Cheaper may not be better, and consumers may want to stay with more established brands. Even buying well-known names may not be enough, since the products are standardized for hypericin content, and we now know that a completely different compound, hyperforin, is the active ingredient. Since hypericin is not the active ingredient, a product containing exactly the stated amount of hypericin could, conceivably, be less potent than another product containing the same amount of hypericin, but less hyperforin! An industry-wide standard is badly needed.

Reference:

Chatterjee SS, Bhattacharya SK, Wonnemann M, Singer A, Muller WE. Hyperforin as a possible antidepressant component of hypericum extracts. Life Sci 1998;63(6):499-510.

Erdelmeier CA. Hyperforin, possibly the major non-nitrogenous secondary metabolite of *Hypericum perforatum L*. Pharmacopsychiatry 1998;31 Suppl 1:2-6.

Garrett BJ, Cheeke PR, Miranda CL, Goeger DE, Buhler DR. Consumption of poisonous plants (Senecio jacobaea, Symphytum officinale, Pteridium aquilinum, *Hypericum perforatum*) by rats: chronic toxicity, mineral metabolism, and hepatic drug-metabolizing enzymes. Toxicol Lett 1982;10(2-3):183-8.

Heiligenstein E, Guenther G. Over-the-counter psychotropics: a review of melatonin, St John's Wort, valerian, and kava-kava. J Am Coll Health 1998;46(6):271-6.

Miller AL. St. John's Wort (*Hypericum perforatum*): clinical effects on depression and other conditions. Altern Med Rev 1998;3(1):18-26.

Muller WE, Singer A, Wonnemann M, Hafner U, Rolli M, Schafer C. Hyperforin represents the neurotransmitter reuptake inhibiting constituent of hypericum extract. Pharmacopsychiatry 1998;31 Suppl 1:16-21.

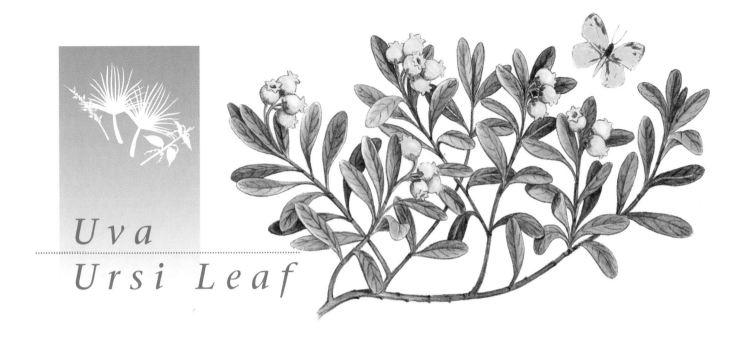

Uva Ursi Leaf

Name: *Arctostaphylos uva ursi* (L.) Sprengel (Ericaceae), commonly called Bearberry (*Arctostaphylos* is Greek for bearberry). In French, it is *Rasin d'ours* or *Busserole;* in German, *Bärentraube* and, *Bärentraubenblätter.*

Source: Remedies are made from the dried leaves. The plant is a trailing perennial ground cover that resembles cranberry. Even though it is the berries that attract bears, they are not thought to have any medicinal value. Only the leaves are used as medicines. Uva ursi grows in most temperate climates. It probably came originally from northern Asia.

History: The Greeks and Romans used this shrub to treat urinary tract symptoms, and the practice continued well on into the Middle Ages. As herbal remedies have become more popular, there has been renewed interest in using uva ursi to treat an assortment of urinary tract afflictions.

Traditional Claims: Urinary tract anti-inflammatory

Commission E Recommendations: Uva ursi is used to treat inflammation of the urinary tract.

Proven Effects: The active ingredients are thought to be a molecule called arbutin, and a related compound called hydroquinone, along with tannins and flavonoids. If the urine happens to be alkaline, arbutin and hydroquinone assume an active form that can prevent the growth of bacteria. This means that to get the maximal effect, bicarbonate, or something similar, has to be taken along with the uva ursi. There is also some evidence that uva ursi extracts might help to dissolve or prevent uric acid kidney stones. Unfortunately, the vast majority (>85 percent) of kidney stones are made of calcium, not uric acid. Even more unfortunate is the fact that there are no clinical trials to back up any of these claims.

Concerns: Human toxicity studies are nonexistent. The leaves contain large quantities of tannins (10-20 percent), and tannins, taken in large amounts for long periods, are thought to be carcinogens. Hydroquinone is also classified as a carcinogen, at least in laboratory animals, so long-term use could present some risk. Commission E, which recommends uva ursi for "inflammatory disease of the urinary tract," advises that it should not be given to pregnant or lactating women, and also recommends that it not be given to children under the age of 12.

Warning: So little is known about the toxicology of this herb that use for more than a week, more than a few times per year, makes very little sense.

Drug Testing: There is no evidence that any of the compounds present in this herb will interfere with standard workplace urine drug screening tests.

Dosage: Commission E recommends a dose of three grams of dried herb (containing 400-800 milligrams of hydroquinone derivatives) up to four times a day.

Summary: Historical evidence suggests uva ursi may be an effective treatment for some urinary tract infections, and that it may possibly prevent uric acid kidney stones. However, clinical trials proving such a benefit have never been carried out, and the plant contains too many known carcinogens to use on a regular basis, which is what would be required to prevent kidney stone formation. Even if uva ursi is effective in acute infections, safer medications are available.

References:

Grases F, Melero G, Costa-Bauza A, Prieto R, March JG. Urolithiasis and phytotherapy. Int Urol Nephrol 1994;26(5):507-11.

Matsuda H, Tanaka T, Kubo M. [Pharmacological studies on leaf of *Arctostaphylos uva-ursi* (L.) Spreng. III. Combined effect of arbutin and indomethacin on immuno-inflammation]. Yakugaku Zasshi 1991;111(4-5):253-8.

Matsuda H, Higashino M, Nakai Y, Iinuma M, Kubo M, Lang FA. Studies of cuticle drugs from natural sources. IV. Inhibitory effects of some Arctostaphylos plants on melanin biosynthesis. Biol Pharm Bull 1996;19(1):153-6.

Ritch-Krc EM, Thomas S, Turner NJ, Towers GH. Carrier herbal medicine: traditional and contemporary plant use. J Ethnopharmacol 1996;52(2):85-94.

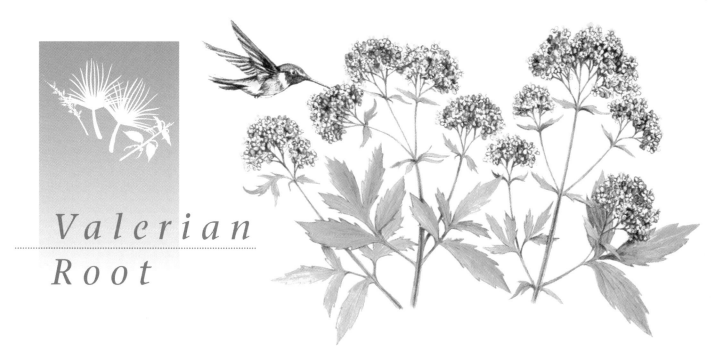

Valerian Root

Name: *Valeriana officinalis* L. (Valerianaceae). The name derives from the Latin word *valere* (to be in health). Related subspecies include *V. exalata, V. nitida, V. edulis, and V. wallichii,* commonly called Valerian, or sometimes Valeriana. In French, it is *Valériane officinale* or *Herbe aux chats;* in German, *Baldrianwurzel* or *Baldrian*.

Source: Valerian will grow in any temperate climate. Dozens of different subspecies and varieties are recognized. Valerian's active ingredients are found in a volatile oil extracted from its roots. The oil contains a chemical called bornyl acetate, along with smaller amounts of valerenic acid, acetoxyvalerenic acid and valerenal, collectively known as valepotriates. A group of related molecules with sedative properties, called sesquiterpenes, are also found in the oil. The essential oil content varies widely from subspecies to subspecies. Concentrations of bornyl acetate can vary from less than one percent to more than 33 percent, depending on the variety of plant. The three valepotriates, the compounds considered most likely to be responsible for Valerian's sedative effects, are found together only in *V. Officinalis*. Herbal drug manufacturers usually adjust their products to contain a standardized amount of the valepotriates, and then set the price accordingly. Commercial products made with *V. Edulis* are common, but they do not contain all three valepotriates or any sesquiterpenes. They may, therefore, be less effective.

History: Even before the Middle Ages, valerian was used as a sedative, and as treatment for stomach upset. In the 1800s, valerian was prescribed in much the same way tranquilizers and sleeping pills are today. During World War I, valerian was the main drug used to treat victims of "shell-shock." In the 1950s, when synthetic tranquilizing drugs (first the barbiturates, then the benzodiazepines) were introduced, valerian went out of fashion. Chinese and Indian herbalists, along with European homeopaths, continued prescribing valerian. Today, it is still widely used as a sedative in both Russia and Germany. American physicians have largely abandoned valerian in favor of Valium™ and Librium™.

Traditional Claims: Neruine, sedative.

Commission E Recommendations: Use for restlessness, sleeping disorders based upon nervous conditions.

Proven Effects: Valerian is a mild, sleep-inducing, sedative. Studies designed to prove these claims scientifically are few and far between, but the few studies that have been done support that notion. The largest of the sleep studies involved 128 volunteers with insomnia. Each took

400 mg of valerian extract, or placebo, 30 minutes before going to bed. The time required to fall asleep, and the number of times participants woke during the night, was reduced. The improvement was most marked in women, and in people under the age of 40. Other controlled studies have produced similar results. The problem is, there have been so few studies done with valerian.

Concerns: There are very few concerns with valerian use. The United States Pharmacopeia, which cautions against the use of any botanical product for more than two weeks, admits that in the case of valerian, there is a "lack of reported harmful side effects." Even massive overdoses seem to produce little toxicity. In Hong Kong, where valerian products are extremely popular and widely available, and where suicide attempts with valerian are not uncommon, not much happens. With appropriate medical treatment, almost all cases recover without any residual effects. Users do not need to be concerned about valerian's nasty smell. It does not mean that the valerian has gone bad; only that one of the components of valerian oil develops an unpleasant aroma with storage.

Warnings: Buyers need to beware of what they are purchasing. Sesquiterpene content in commercial preparations can vary by a factor of ten, and if the product is made just from *V. Edulis*, the sesquiterpene content is usually nil. Since no one is quite sure what part of the oil produces the positive effects, buying a product missing one of valerian's active ingredients does not seem to make much sense. Manufacturers in the United States are not required to provide any data on the purity of their herbal products, and content may vary considerably from batch to batch, and from manufacturer to manufacturer. Make sure you are dealing with a reputable manufacturer. Also, don't expect to get much benefit from valerian teas. Valerian's active ingredients are found in the oil, and do not dissolve in water. Finally, valerian is a sedative. That means it should not be combined with other sedatives, and definitely should not be taken with alcohol.

Drug Testing: None of the molecules present in valerian is known to cause any interference with workplace drug tests. But sedative drugs can cause impairment. If you take valerian, and then drive, and are stopped by the police, you can still be charged with "driving under the influence" (DUI), even though you have not been drinking alcohol. Nor is using valerian tincture a good excuse for flunking a Breathalyzer test. Valerian tinctures do contain alcohol, but not enough alcohol to raise blood levels above legal limits,even if you use many times the recommended dose; that argument has already been tried in court, and it does not work.

Dosage: Valerian is sold in teas, tinctures, tablets and capsule forms, and the dosage varies depending on the manufacturer. Recommended doses range from 200 to 1,000 mg of *V. Officinalis* root, 30 to 60 minutes before retiring.

Summary: Valerian appears to be a reasonably effective, very safe, and economically priced sedative. Taken in reasonable doses, toxicity is not a problem, but buyers need to make sure that they are getting *V. Officinalis*. and not *V. Edulis*. Valerian may be a natural product, but it is a sedative and can cause impairment. It should only be taken at bedtime.

References:

Cavadas C, Araujo I, Cotrim MD, Amaral T, Cunha AP, Macedo T, et al. In vitro study on the interaction of *Valeriana officinalis L.* extracts and their amino acids on GABAA receptor in rat brain. Arzneimittelforschung 1995;45(7):753-5.

Cott J. NCDEU update. Natural product formulations available in Europe for psychotropic indications. Psychopharmacol Bull 1995;31(4):745-51.

Kammerer E. [Phytogenic sedatives-hypnotics—does a combination of valerian and hops have a value in the modern drug repertoire?]. Z Arztl Fortbild (Jena) 1993;87(5):401-6.

Leuschner J, Muller J, Rudmann M. Characterisation of the central nervous depressant activity of a commercially available valerian root extract. Arzneimittelforschung 1993;43(6):638-41.

Lindahl O, Lindwall L. Double-blind study of a valerian preparation. Pharmacol Biochem Behav 1989;32(4):1065-6.

Wagner J, Wagner ML, Hening WA. Beyond benzodiazepines: alternative pharmacologic agents for the treatment of insomnia. Ann Pharmacother 1998;32(6):680-91.

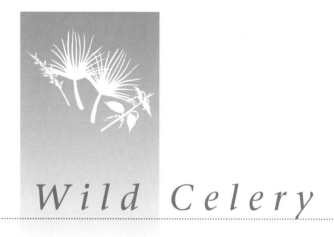

Wild Celery

Name: *Apium graveolens* L. (Umbelliferae), commonly called Wild Celery. In French, it is called *Céleri Ache Odorante*; in German, *Sellerie*.

Source: Dried ripe fruits of plants that are mainly cultivated in India and Eastern Europe.

History: Wild celery was popular with the Romans even though it has a rather bitter taste. Italian gardeners in the Middle Ages began to cultivate the variety that is eaten today. Traditional herbalists used it to treat gout and arthritic symptoms.

Traditional Claims: Diuretic, carminative, appetite stimulant, tonic and aphrodisiac.

Commission E Recommendations: Positive benefits are not clear, and because of the danger of photosensitization, this herb is not recommended by the Commission.

Proven Effects: The characteristic smell of celery is due to a chemical called 3-n-butyl phthalide. In laboratory studies, treatment with this compound, and with whole celery seed oil, prevents the growth of tumors in animals exposed to carcinogens. It is not known whether this benefit carries over to humans. The same compound is thought to account for celery's ability to calm the stomach. Diuretic effects are probably from mannitol, a sugar produced in the celery plant. In large doses, mannitol causes the kidneys to increase urine production. Clinical trials in humans are nonexistent.

Concerns: If wild celery plants become infected with certain types of fungi, they begin to produce substances called psoralens (furanocoumarins). These chemicals absorb ultraviolet light. Field workers who handle the plants become extremely sensitive to light and can experience severe sunburns. The same phenomenon sometimes happens with parsley. In theory, psoralens could become incorporated in commercial products, though there are no reports of that occurring.

Warnings: Violent allergic reactions (anaphylaxis) have been reported. Similar violent reactions are possible with carrot and mugwort. As strange as it may seem, there is an association between sensitivity to different pollens and sensitivity to some edible vegetables. These seem to fall into groups. There is, for example, an association between ragweed pollen allergy and hypersensitivity to watermelon, melon, cucumber and banana. Individuals who are allergic to birch pollen may also be allergic to hazelnut, apple, carrot, potato, and kiwi. Individuals who are allergic to mugwort pollen may have violent allergic reactions to celery, carrot, spices, nuts, mustard and

Leguminoseae vegetables. The explanation appears to be that the pollens and the vegetables contain molecules which closely resemble each other and which can trigger the same allergic reactions. Anyone who has had skin tests showing that they are allergic to mugwort should not be using celery root oil.

Drug Testing: None of the components of celery seeds should interfere with standard workplace urine drug screening tests.

Dosage: Bring to boil one teaspoon of seeds in 1/2 cup of water, let stand a few minutes, and then strain. Use up to three times a day.

Summary: Use of this herb is not recommended by Commission E. There is tantalizing evidence that something in celery seeds may prevent, or at least retard tumor growth. However, this has never been proven in humans. In fact, there have been no clinical trials. The possibility of severe allergic reaction exists, especially for individuals who have allergies to mugwort, and possibly to carrots as well.

References:

Atta AH, Alkofahi A. Anti-nociceptive and anti-inflammatory effects of some Jordanian medicinal plant extracts. J Ethnopharmacol 1998;60(2):117-24.

Caballero T, Martin-Esteban M. Association between pollen hypersensitivity and edible vegetable allergy: a review. J Investig Allergol Clin Immunol 1998;8(1):6-16.

Zheng GQ, Kenney PM, Zhang J, Lam LK. Chemoprevention of benzopyrene-induced forestomach cancer in mice by natural phthalides from celery seed oil. Nutr Cancer 1993;19(1):77-86.

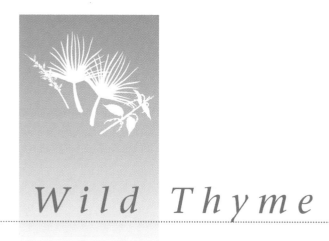

Wild Thyme

Name: *Thymus serpyllum* L. Fries (Labiatae) commonly called wild thyme. In French, it is *Serpolet á feuilles étroites*; in German, *Feld-Thymian* or *Kleiner Kostets*. Hundreds of related (some distantly) plants are referred to by the same name, making the situation for consumers quite confusing. Products sold in the United States often contain the dried leaves of related plants, such as *Thymus pulegioides* L., and *T. Praecox* subsp. *articus*. *Thymus vulgaris* L., also called garden thyme or common thyme, grows robustly in American and European gardens. In French, it is called *Thym cultivé*; in German, *Garten-Thymian*.

Source: Wild thyme (*Thymus serpyllum*)is native to Europe and does not grow in the United States. *T. Vulgaris,* also known as English thyme or garden thyme, is native to the Western Mediterranean but now grows in American gardens. Extracts of the flowers of wild thyme are used as an expectorant. Garden thyme is used mainly as a culinary herb, but infusions made from its leaves have traditionally been used to treat upset stomach and have been applied locally to treat healing wounds.

History: Legend has it that thyme grew from the tears shed by Helen of Troy. Thyme was a component of the embalming compounds used by the ancient Egyptians. It was probably introduced into Europe by the Romans. In the Middle Ages, the plant was associated with death and was planted around graves.

Traditional Claims: Wild thyme is used as an antiseptic, antispasmodic, expectorant, astringent, and digestive aid. Garden thyme was also used as a deodorant and vermifuge.

Commission E Recommendations: The Commission recommends wild thyme for inflammation of the upper respiratory tract. Garden thyme is also recommended for treating the symptoms of bronchitis, whooping cough, and upper respiratory tract infections.

Proven Effects: Wild thyme contains most of the same ingredients as garden thyme, but in lower concentrations. The essential oil extracted from the flowers of *T. vulgaris* contains thymol, a powerful antiseptic, widely used by dentists. Thyme essential oil (3%) has been used as a preservative in the pharmaceutical and cosmetic industries for many years. There is good evidence that thyme oil, in common with the essential oils of anise seed, cinnamon leaf, red thyme, and tea tree, can be used as a treatment to kill body lice (pediculus humanus). The oils are dissolved in alcohol, applied in the evening and rinsed off in the morning. In the laboratory, aqueous extracts of thyme prevent the growth of *H. pylori*, a bacteria that is known to play a role in the occurrence of peptic ulcer disease. Very few clinical studies have ever been undertaken, and thyme's usefulness in respiratory infections has never been validated. Thyme oil is used widely by aroma therapists, who have published at least one controlled trial, the results of which suggest that thyme oil can be used to help grow hair! A randomized, double-blind, controlled trial of seven months duration involved 43 balding men who massaged essential oils (thyme, rosemary, lavender, and cedarwood) into their scalps daily, and 43 others who rubbed in a placebo-containing oil. The participants were photographed on a regular basis, and the pictures were reviewed by two dermatologists for evidence of hair growth. (The dermatologists did not know which men were using placebo and which were using the essential oils). No side effects occurred and, by the end of the study, half of the men treated with the oil had grown significantly more hair than the controls.

Concerns: Reports of side effects are so rare as to be of no concern.

Warnings: Thymol in large quantities can be toxic. Users should not exceed the recommended dose.

Drug Testing: There is no evidence that any of the components of the essential oil interfere with standard workplace drug tests.

Dosage: For cough, Commission E recommends a tea made from 1 to 2 grams of the dried thyme leaves, several times a day as needed. Alternatively, 1-2 grams of fluidextract of garden thyme can be taken up to three times a day. For treating healing sores and ulcers, the Commission recommends compresses made from a 5 percent infusion of thyme. The recommended dose of wild thyme is 6 grams per day of the dried flowers.

Summary: Thyme has been used as a cough suppressant for centuries. Even though clinical trials proving its effectiveness have never been published, the experience of European herbalists suggests that thyme is certainly safe and probably effective. The results of laboratory tests suggest that application of oil would be a safe way to treat lice infestations. Whether the oil can also be used to grow hair remains to be seen! Large amounts of oil can be toxic.

References:

Hay IC, Jamieson M, Ormerod AD. Randomized trial of aromatherapy. Successful treatment for alopecia areata [In Process Citation]. Arch Dermatol 1998;134(11):1349-52.

Manou I, Bouillard L, Devleeschouwer MJ, Barel AO. Evaluation of the preservative properties of *Thymus vulgaris* essential oil in topically applied formulations under a challenge test. J Appl Microbiol 1998;84(3):368-76.

Tabak M, Armon R, Potasman I, Neeman I. In vitro inhibition of Helicobacter pylori by extracts of thyme. J Appl Bacteriol 1996;80(6):667-72.

Veal L. The potential effectiveness of essential oils as a treatment for headlice, Pediculus humanus capitis. Complement Ther Nurs Midwifery 1996;2(4):97-101.

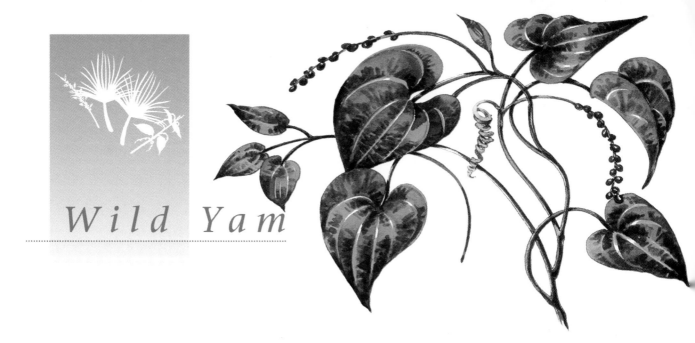

Wild Yam

Name: *Discorea villosa* L. (Dioscoreaceae), commonly called yams. Hundreds of different species are included under this heading. The important edible ones include *D. alata* and *D. escfulenta* (grown in Southeast Asia), *D. routandatra* and *D. cayenensis* (grown in Africa). The varieties grown in Mexico, which are of most commercial importance, are *D. composita*, *D. mexicana* and *D. floribunda*.

Source: The yam is a very important food, but its commercial importance derives from the fact that the molecules contained in the yams can be used by chemists to synthetically produce hormones such as testosterone and estrogens. After yams are harvested, they are chopped into small pieces and allowed to ferment for several days. They are then soaked in acid and the chemicals to be used for making hormones, called sapogenins, are extracted. Many different sapogenins exist, but the two most important ones are called diosgenin and yamogenin. Other plants rich in sapogenins are fenugreek and sisal.

History: Remedies containing saponins are generally thought to be effective expectorants, and have been used for that purpose for hundreds of years, although control clinical trials are largely lacking, as are studies that would prove claims that saponins increase the body's ability to absorb important nutrients. The herb itself was never the focus of much interest until quite recently, when it was suggested that the saponins contained in yams could prevent heart disease and relieve some of the symptoms of menopause.

Traditional Claims: Expectorant

Commission E Recommendations: The Commission never offered an opinion on this herb.

Proven Effects: Saponins combine with cholesterol in the intestines and prevent it from being absorbed, resulting in lower blood cholesterol concentrations. This effect has been demonstrated in the laboratory and in clinical trials. Whether long-term treatment with yams is anywhere near as effective (or safe) as treatment with some of the prescription "statin" type drugs, such as Zocor™ and Mevacor™, is not known. Although there is considerable anecdotal evidence suggesting that this herb has a positive effect on menopausal symptoms and osteoporosis, these claims have never been evaluated in a controlled trial. Accounts in the popular press often repeat the mistaken notion that the active ingredients in birth control pills come from the wild yam. Actually, yams contain substances (diosgenin, a steroidal saponin) that are used by the drug industry as building blocks from which sex hormones can be manufactured. The latest evidence suggests that, like soy, diosgenin may have its own inherent estrogenic effects and act as a true phytoestrogen. In the complete absence of clinical trials, it is impossible to tell.

Concerns: Saponins in large quantities can irritate the stomach, but otherwise, oral preparations, whether of yam, horse chestnut, or fenugreek, appear to be relatively harmless.

Warnings: None

Drug Testing: None of the components of this herb should have any effect on standard workplace urine drug screening tests

Dosage: Yams were never evaluated by Commission E and the effective dose, either for treatment of elevated cholesterol, or for use as a phytoestrogen, is not really known. Large doses are likely to cause stomach upset.

Summary: The recent excitement about this herb may well be warranted. Components of these plants can lower cholesterol and may help prevent heart disease. Whether they can also relieve hot flashes and prevent osteoporosis is not known with certainty. As a group, all of the saponin-containing plants seem to be nontoxic. Consumers might also want to consider adding other saponin-containing plants, such as asparagus, spinach, green beans and tomatoes, to their diets.

References:

Marquet F, Abou el Fadil F, Boubia B, Guffroy C, Pansu D, Descroix-Vagne M. Selection of cholesterol absorption inhibitors devoid of secondary intestinal effects. Reprod Nutr Dev 1997;37(6):691-707.

Tian RH, Ohmura E, Matsui M, Noharas T. Abutiloside A, a 26-acylamino-3 beta, 16 alpha-dihydroxy-5 alpha- cholesta-22-one glycoside from *Solanum abutiloides*. Phytochemistry 1997;44(4):723-6

Wilkins AL, Miles CO, De Kock WT, Erasmus GL, Basson AT, Kellerman TS. Photosensitivity in South Africa. IX. Structure elucidation of a beta- glucosidase-treated saponin from *Tribulus terrestris*, and the identification of saponin chemotypes of South African T. terrestris. Onderstepoort J Vet Res 1996;63(4):327-34.

Yamada T, Hoshino M, Hayakawa T, Ohhara H, Yamada H, Nakazawa T, et al. Dietary diosgenin attenuates subacute intestinal inflammation associated with indomethacin in rats. Am J Physiol 1997;273(2 Pt 1):G355-64.

Zava DT, Dollbaum CM, Blen M. Estrogen and progestin bioactivity of foods, herbs, and spices. Proc Soc Exp Biol Med 1998;217(3):369-78.

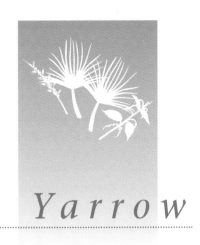

Yarrow

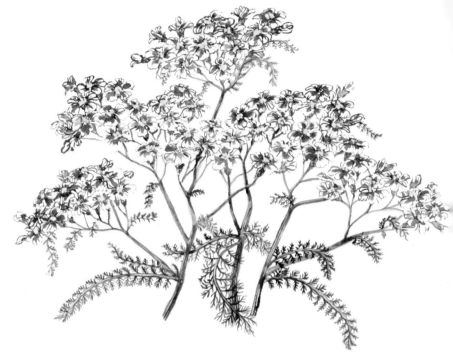

Name: *Achillea millefolium* L. (Compositae), commonly called yarrow or milfoil. Also known as woundwort, carpenter's weed, and devil's plaything. In French, it is *Millefeuille;* in German, *Schafgarbe.*

Source: Yarrow is a very common plant that grows in pastures around the world, especially if the soil is well drained. Remedies are made from the dried flowers and stems collected just as the plant is flowering. There are a number of closely related subspecies.

History: According to legend, Achilles made poultices with this plant to treat soldiers who had been wounded in battle. For thousands of years, yarrow has been applied to open wounds to stop the bleeding and to accelerate healing. Scandinavians, on the other hand, used yarrow in place of hops to make beer. In the 16th century, Germans added the seed to wine as a preservative. According to folklore, it also helped women predict the future.

Traditional Claims: Antiseptic, digestive, antibacterial and anti-inflammatory.

Commission E Recommendations: Internally for loss of appetite. Hot soaks for the treatment of pelvic discomfort are also recommended.

Proven Effects: Depending on how the essential oil of this plant is extracted, the content of active ingredients will vary. However, large quantities of sesquiterpene lactones (achillicin) are present and thought to be the active agents. The results of some studies suggest that yarrow is a good anti-inflammatory agent, but these laboratory findings have never been validated in a clinical trial. The results of other experimental studies suggest that achillicin can help stop bleeding and that it also calms the stomach. There are no clinical trials.

Concerns: Skin allergy to all members of the Compositae family are relatively common (arnica, artichoke, chamomile, coltsfoot, dandelion) and occasionally the rashes may be quite severe. They subside when the plant is withdrawn from the diet.

Warnings: None

Drug Testing: None of the components of yarrow should have any effect on routine workplace urine drug screening tests.

Dosage: Commission E recommends a daily dose of 4.5 grams of dried herb, or three teaspoons per day of juice pressed from the fresh plant. For use in a sitz bath, soak 100 grams of yarrow in 5 gallons of warm water.

Summary: The way to control bleeding is with pressure, and the practice of applying plants to control bleeding would be a bad idea (except, perhaps, in the case of an isolated survivalist who knew his plants!). Still, yarrow might be useful for a mildly upset stomach and there is no evidence to suggest that occasional use leads to toxicity.

References:

Chandler RF, Hooper SN, Hooper DL, Jamieson WD, Flinn CG, Safe LM. Herbal remedies of the Maritime Indians: sterols and triterpenes of *Achillea millefolium L.* (Yarrow). J Pharm Sci 1982;71(6):690-3.

Davies MG, Kersey PJ. Contact allergy to yarrow and dandelion. Contact Dermatitis 1986;14(4):256-7.

Hausen BM, Breuer J, Weglewski J, Rucker G. alpha-Peroxyachifolid and other new sensitizing sesquiterpene lactones from yarrow (*Achillea millefolium L.*, Compositae). Contact Dermatitis 1991;24(4):274-80.

Taran DD, Saratikov AS, Prishchep TP, Vengerovskii AI. [The wound-healing properties of the essential oils of yarrow and Yakut wormwood and khamazulen in napalm burns]. Voen Med Zh 1989(8):50-2.

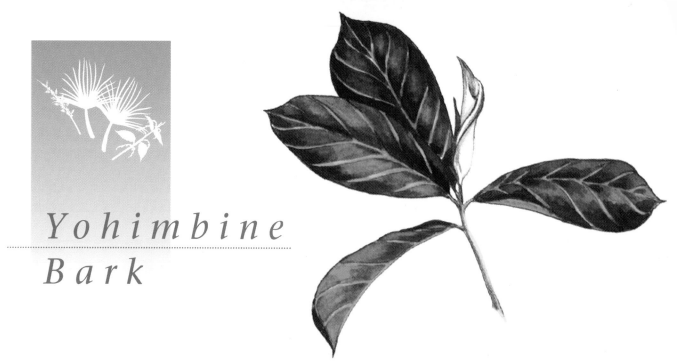

Yohimbine Bark

Name: *Pausinystalia yohimbe* (K. Shumann) Pierre ex Beille and also sometimes *Corynanthe yohimbi* Schumann (Rubiaceae), commonly called yohimbine, yohimbe bark and yohimbehe cortex. Prescription drugs containing yohimbine include Aphrodyne™, Dayto Himbin™, Prohim™, Yocon™, Yohimex™, and Yovital™. In German, it is *Yohimberinde*.

Source: The dried bark of the trunk and branches of *Pausinystalia yohimbe* Pierre ex Beille, a tree native to west Africa. Smaller amounts can be extracted from the roots of *Rauwolfia serpentina L* Benth (Apocynaceae), better known as the source of the antihypertensive drug reserpine.

History: Shavings of the inner bark, boiled in water for half an hour, have traditionally been used as an aphrodisiac. In modern times, yohimbine has been used to treat male sexual dysfunction.

Traditional Claims: Yohimbine is used as an aphrodisiac.

Commission E Recommendations: Yohimbine is not on the list of approved herbs. It is used as an aphrodisiac.

Proven Effects: Yohimbine rapidly enters the brain and stimulates the brain centers controlling blood pressure and heart rate. Yohimbine is classified as an alpha-2-adrenergic antagonist. Drugs in this group decrease sympathetic nervous system activity, and increase the activity of the parasympathetic nervous system. One consequence of these actions is increased blood flow to the penis and improved erectile function. Another consequence is dilated pupils. In addition to the effects on penile blood flow, yohimbine has other actions that may also improve male sexual performance. Its structure closely resembles the structure of the neurotransmitter serotonin, and those of hallucinogenic drugs such as LSD, psilocin, and DMT. Users of yohimbine sometimes report nervousness and anxiety, so it is safe to assume that the drug causes some sort of central nervous system stimulation, and perhaps even sexual arousal. Yohimbine's effects on the brain are the object of considerable interest in Europe, where two closely related chemical derivatives of yohimbine (almitrine and raubasine) are being used as an experimental treatment for stroke.

Concerns: Drugs that increase the activity of the parasympathetic nervous system cause the pupils to dilate, and may make it difficult to focus. In theory, yohimbine might cause urinary retention, although there are no clinical reports suggesting that is, in fact, a problem. With higher doses, mood elevation, nervousness and insomnia are almost certain to occur, and profuse sweating is also likely. Nausea and vomiting occur when yohimbine is given by injection, but such an occurrence would be very unlikely after taking the recommended oral dose.

Warnings: Even modest doses of yohimbine will increase heart rate and blood pressure, so patients with high blood pressure should not take this drug, nor should anyone with kidney disease (elevated blood pressure can cause further kidney damage). Package inserts for prescription yohimbine also carry warnings against use by patients with ulcer disease, by women (pregnant or not), and by anyone taking mood-modifying drugs or antidepressants, such as Prozac™ and Paxil™.

Drug Testing: No studies have been done, but yohimbine's structure is so like that of other hallucinogens, a false positive screening test would not be surprising. The screening tests for LSD are particularly prone to giving false positive results. And since the eyes of yohimbine users will be dilated anyway, they may well be mistaken for drug users, particularly if they have been stopped by police for possible DUI. If a urine test is done at work, make sure the laboratory knows you are taking yohimbine. The best way to avoid a DUI charge is not to drive while you are taking this product.

Dosage: The recommended dose for Yocon™ and other prescription-only yohimbine formulations is one 5.4 milligram tablet three times a day. Herbal food supplements containing powdered yohimbine may be standardized to contain whatever yohimbine content the manufacturer thinks is desirable. Some of the supplements may contain twice the amount found in the prescription formulations.

Summary: According to a very recent study published in the *Journal of Urology*, "The benefit of yohimbine medication for erectile dysfunction seems to outweigh its risks. Therefore, yohimbine is believed to be a reasonable therapeutic option for erectile dysfunction that should be considered as initial pharmacological intervention." Just be careful about drug tests, and remember that patients with high blood pressure or heart disease should not be taking these products, nor should yohimbine be taken at the same time as other mood-altering agents.

References:

Benzi G. Pharmacological features of an almitrine-raubasine combination. Activity at cerebral levels. Eur Neurol 1998;39 (Suppl 1):31-8.

Cassells NP, Craston DH. The effects of commonly used adulterants on the detection of spiked LSD by an enzyme immunoassay. Sci Justice 1998;38(2):109-17.

Ernst E, Pittler MH. Yohimbine for erectile dysfunction: a systematic review and meta-analysis of randomized clinical trials. J Urol 1998;159(2):433-6.

Li SW. Stroke and functional rehabilitation: the Chinese experience. Eur Neurol 1998;39(Suppl 1):26-30.

Nasser AM, Court WE. Stem bark alkaloids of *Rauvolfia caffra*. J Ethnopharmacol 1984;11(1):99-117.

Commission E Recommendations

E uropeans take a very different approach to the use of herbal medicine than Americans. In the United States, the sale of food supplements, provided their labeling does not make obvious medical claims, is basically unregulated. Manufacturers may imply that a particular product "supports prostate health," but they cannot claim that their version of saw palmetto will relieve the symptoms of prostate enlargement, and they cannot provide consumers with any sort of detailed information about how that product works - even if that information is quite valid. They cannot, for example, provide a package insert stating that the ability of valerian to induce sleep has been validated in controlled clinical trials since there have been no validated studies.

The Food and Drug Administration (FDA) has not done much to improve the situation. Industry-led efforts at reform have been generally rebuffed. Many reasonable people think some of these products could be sold as over-the-counter drugs (OTC). Such a classification would allow more informative labeling and ensure better quality control. That approach is unacceptable to the FDA, which still insists on proof of safety and effectiveness before an herbal remedy may be sold as an OTC product. Whether such an approach is entirely rational in the case of drugs like hops and valerian, which have been safely used for more than a thousand years, is debatable. Many of these products are currently being sold in countries with sophisticated health surveillance systems where toxic reactions would be quickly noted if, in fact, they were occurring.

The use of herbal medicines is much better regulated within the European community, especially in Germany than in the U.S. In 1976, the German legislature passed a law known as AMG 76. Under that law, the German government required a review of all medicine (not just herbal) for sale within that country. Expert committees were appointed to review different groups and types of drugs. These committees worked within the Federal Health Agency, the German equivalent of our Department of Health and Human Services.

A total of 16 different commissions were formed, and each was designated by an initial. Commission B1 reviewed drugs used in cardiology and nephrology, Commission B2 reviewed drugs used in rheumatology, and so on. Commission E was tasked with a review of "phytotherapy," or herbal medicines. Commission E had 24 members, all well-respected health professionals and researchers. Evidence of safety and effectiveness for a total of 360 different herbs was reviewed and the findings published as official government documents called "monographs." These have recently been translated into English and published as *The Complete German Commission E Monographs, Therapeutic Guide to Herbal Medicines,* edited by Mark Blumenthal, and published by the American Botanical Council.

American physicians will probably not be very impressed. For one thing, the references used by the experts to form their opinions are not included in the monographs, and much of the wording is more vague than anything written about prescription drugs. But for the moment, there is "no other game in town." Consumers really have nowhere else to go. The FDA refuses to provide information and manufacturers are not allowed to!

This chapter contains a summary of Commission E recommendations. It is unedited, and it lists a number of herbs that were not discussed in this book. Their inclusion does not constitute an endorsement or recommendation, merely the recognition that people are experimenting with these products. Some reliable, unbiased information, even if it is not as complete, is better than none at all. Chapter 7 is divided into two parts. First the suggested use for the herbs are listed, by herb, alphabetically. This same information is restated in the second part of the chapter, which lists the Commission's recommended herbs by ailments and diseases.

Commission E's terminology has been retained, even though some readers may find the list of diseases confusing. The Commission still uses terms, such as catarrh that long ago disappeared from the vocabularies of American physicians. In hopes of clarifying the situation somewhat, explanations are provided in parenthesis after the more confusing terms.

Part A: Herbs and Their Applications

Agrimony
Diarrhea
Gastrointestinal Tract Inflammation
Inflammation, Oral or Pharyngeal
Skin Injury or Irritation (external)
Sore Throat

Aloe
Constipation

Angelica Root
Abdominal Bloating
Dyspepsia
Flatulence
Gastrointestinal Tract Spasm
Loss of Appetite
Peptic Discomforts

Anise Seed
Catarrh, Upper Respiratory Tract (external)
Dyspepsia
Respiratory Catarrh (external)
Upper Respiratory Catarrh (external)

Arnica Flower
Bone Dislocations (external)
Bruises and Contusions (external)
Edema, Post-traumatic Injury (external)
Furunculosis (boils) (external)
Hematoma (external)
Insect Bites (external)
Joint Pain (external)
Oral or Pharyngeal Inflammation (external)
Phlebitis (external)
Rheumatic Muscle Pain (external)
Sore Throat (external)

Artichoke Leaf
Dyspepsia

Asparagus Root
Kidney Stones and Gravel (irrigation therapy)
Urinary Tract Infection or Inflammation (irrigation therapy)

Autumn Crocus
Familial Mediterranean Fever
Gout

Belladonna
Biliary Spasm
Gastrointestinal Pain
Gastrointestinal Tract Spasm

Bilberry Fruit
Diarrhea
Gastrointestinal Tract Inflammation
Oral or Pharyngeal Inflammation
Sore Throat

Birch Leaf
Kidney Stones and Gravel
(irrigation therapy)
Rheumatic Ailments (secondary)
Urinary Tract Infection or Inflammation
(irrigation therapy)

Bitter Orange Peel
Loss of Appetite
Dyspepsia

Black Cohosh Root
Dysmenorrhea
Menopausal Symptoms
Premenstrual Syndrome (PMS)

Blackberry Leaf
Diarrhea
Gastrointestinal Tract Inflammation
Oral or Pharyngeal Inflammation
Sore Throat

Blackthorn Berry
Oral or Pharyngeal Inflammation
Sore Throat

Blessed Thistle Herb
Loss of Appetite
Dyspepsia

Bogbean Leaf
Loss of Appetite
Dyspepsia

Boldo Leaf
Dyspepsia
Gastrointestinal Tract Spasm
Gastrointestinal Tract Inflammation

Bromelain
Sinusitis
Swelling, Post-operative or Post-traumatic, especially of the nasal and paranasal sinuses

Brewer's Yeast
Acne
Furunculosis (boils)
Loss of Appetite

Buckthorn Bark
Constipation

Buckthorn Berry
Constipation

Bugleweed
Breast Pain (mastodynia)
Nervous System Disorder
Thyroid, Mild Overactive

Butcher's Broom
Circulatory Disorders
Hemorrhoids
Itching
Leg Cramps
Swelling, Legs
Swelling, Post-operative or Post-traumatic
Venous Insufficiency (secondary usage)

Calendula Flower
Oral or Pharyngeal Inflammation
Sore Throat
Ulcus Cruris (external)
Wounds, Poorly Healing (external)

Camphor
Hypertension
Muscle Pain (external)
Respiratory Catarrh
Rheumatism (external)
Upper Respiratory Tract Catarrh

Caraway Oil
Abdominal Bloating
Dyspepsia
Flatulence
Gastrointestinal Tract Spasm

Caraway Seed
Abdominal Bloating
Dyspepsia
Gastrointestinal Tract Spasm

Cardamom Seed
Dyspepsia

Cascara Sagrada Bark
Constipation

Cayenne (Paprika)
Muscle Spasms of Shoulders, Arm
and Spine (external)

Celandine Herb
Biliary Spasm
Gastrointestinal Tract Spasm

Centaury Herb
Loss of Appetite
Dyspepsia

Chamomile Flower, German
Ano-genital Irritation (external)
Bad Breath (external)
Gargle/Mouthwash (external)
Gastrointestinal Tract Inflammation
Gastrointestinal Tract Spasm
Gums, Inflamed (external)
Oral or Pharyngeal Inflammation
(external)
Mucous Membrane, Irritation (external)
Respiratory Infection, Chronic
(inhalations)
Skin Bacterial Infections (external)
Skin Injury or Irritation (external)

Chaste Tree Fruit
Lactation, Poor
Menopausal Symptoms
Menstrual Disorders
Premenstrual Syndrome (PMS)

Chicory
Loss of Appetite
Dyspepsia

Cinchona Bark
Abdominal Bloating
Loss of Appetite
Dyspepsia

Cinnamon Bark
Abdominal Bloating
Loss of Appetite
Dyspepsia
Flatulence
Gastrointestinal Tract Spasm

Cinnamon Bark, Chinese
Abdominal Bloating
Loss of Appetite
Dyspepsia
Flatulence
Gastrointestinal Tract Spasm

Cloves
Anesthesia, Topical (external)
Oral or Pharyngeal Inflammation
(external)
Mouthwash (external)
Sore Throat (external)

Coffee Charcoal
Diarrhea
Gastrointestinal Tract Inflammation
Oral or Pharyngeal Inflammation
Sore Throat

Cola Nut
Fatigue, Mental and Physical

Coltsfoot Leaf
Catarrh, Upper Respiratory Tract
Cough
Hoarseness
Oral or Pharyngeal Inflammation
Sore Throat

Comfrey Herb and Leaf
Bruises and Contusions (external)
Sprains (external)

Comfrey Root
Bruises and Contusions (external)
Ligaments, Pulled (external)
Muscles, Pulled (external)
Sprains (external)

Condurango Bark
Loss of Appetite

Coriander Seed
Loss of Appetite
Dyspepsia

Couch Grass
Kidney Stones and Gravel
(irrigation therapy)
Urinary Tract Infection of Inflammation
(irrigation therapy)

Dandelion Herb
Abdominal Bloating
Loss of Appetite
Dyspepsia
Flatulence

Dandelion Root with Herb
Loss of Appetite
Biliary Dyskinesia
Dyspepsia
Diuretic

Devil's Claw Root
Loss of Appetite
Dyspepsia
Locomotor System, Degenerative
Disorder (supportive therapy)

Dill Seed
Dyspepsia

Echinacea Pallida Root
Colds and Flu
Influenza

Echinacea Purpurea Herb
Colds and Flu
Influenza
Respiratory Infection, Chronic
Skin Ulcers (external)
Urinary Tract Infection or Inflammation
Wounds, Poorly Healing (external)

Elder Flower
Colds and Flu

Eleuthero (Siberian Ginseng) Root
Convalescence (as a tonic)
Debility (as a tonic)
Fatigue (as a tonic)
Mental Concentration (as a tonic)

Ephedra
Asthma
Bronchospasm
Colds and Flu
Upper Respiratory Tract Diseases

Eucalyptus Leaf
Catarrh, Upper Respiratory Tract
Respiratory Catarrh

Eucalyptus Oil
Catarrh, Upper Respiratory Tract
Respiratory Catarrh
Rheumatism (external)

Fennel Honey
Catarrh of the Upper Respiratory Tract
in children (not infants or toddlers)

Fennel Oil
Abdominal Bloating
Catarrh, Upper Respiratory Tract
Dyspepsia
Flatulence
Gastrointestinal Tract Disorder
Peptic Discomforts
Respiratory Catarrh

Fennel Seed
Abdominal Bloating
Catarrh, Upper Respiratory Tract
Dyspepsia
Flatulence
Gastrointestinal Tract Disorder
Respiratory Catarrh
Upper Respiratory Tract Catarrh

Fennel Syrup
Catarrh of the Upper Respiratory Tract
in children

Fenugreek Seed
   Loss of Appetite
   Local Inflammation
      (as a topical poultice)

Fir Needle Oil
   Catarrh, Upper Respiratory Tract
   Muscle Pain (external)
   Neuralgia (external)
   Respiratory Catarrh
   Rheumatism (external)

Fir Shoots, Fresh
   Catarrh, Upper Respiratory Tract
   Muscle Pain (external)
   Neuralgia (external)
   Respiratory Catarrh
   Rheumatism (external)

Flaxseed
   Bowel, Irritable
   Colon, Irritable
   Constipation, Chronic
   Diverticulitis
   Irritable Bowel Syndrome
   Local Inflammation (as a cataplasm)

Fumitory
   Biliary Spasm
   Gallbladder Disorders
   Gastrointestinal Tract Spasm

Galangal
   Loss of Appetite
   Dyspepsia

Garlic
   Geriatric Vascular Changes
   High Cholesterol/Hypercholesteremia
   Hyperlipidemia

Gentian Root
   Abdominal Bloating
   Dyspepsia
   Flatulence
   Loss of Appetite

Ginger Root
   Dyspepsia
   Motion Sickness

Ginkgo Biloba Leaf Extract
   Arterial Occlusive Disease
   Circulatory Disorders
   Depression (secondary)
   Dizziness
   Free Radical Deactivation
   Headache
   Memory Loss
   Mental Concentration
   Retinal Lesion and Edema
   Tinnitus (ringing in the ear)
   Vertigo

Ginseng Root
   Convalescence (as a tonic)
   Debility (as a tonic)
   Fatigue (as a tonic)
   Mental Concentration (as a tonic)

Goldenrod
   Kidney Stones and Gravel
      (irrigation therapy)
   Urinary Tract Inflammation
      (irrigation therapy)

Guaiac Wood
   Rheumatism (supportive therapy)

Gumweed Herb
   Catarrh, Upper Respiratory Tract
   Respiratory Catarrh

Haronga Bark and Leaf
   Dyspepsia
   Pancreatic Insufficiency

Hawthorn Leaf with Flower
   Cardiac Insufficiency
   Geriatric Vascular Changes

Hay Flower
   Arthritis (topical heat therapy)

Heart's Ease Herb
   Milk Scall in children (external)
   Seborrhea (external)

Hempnettle Herb
Catarrh, Upper Respiratory Tract

Henbane Leaf
Gastrointestinal Tract Spasm
Spasm, Gastrointestinal

Hops
Anxiety
Insomnia
Mood Disturbance
Restlessness
Sleep Disturbances

Horehound Herb
Abdominal Bloating
Loss of Appetite
Dyspepsia
Flatulence

Horse Chestnut Seed
Itching
Leg Cramps
Post-thrombic Syndrome
Swelling, Post-operative or Post-traumatic
Varicose Veins/Varicosis
Venous Insufficiency

Horseradish
Catarrh, Upper Respiratory Tract
Muscle Aches
    (external hyperemic treatment)
Respiratory Catarrh

Horsetail Herb
Edema, Post-traumatic
Kidney Stones and Gravel
    (irrigation therapy)
Urinary Tract Infection or Inflammation
    (irrigation therapy)
Wounds (external)

Iceland Moss
Loss of Appetite
Cough
Oral or Pharyngeal Inflammation
Sore Throat

Indian Snakeroot
Anxiety
Hypertension, Mild
Sympatheticotonia
Sinus Tachycardia

Ivy Leaf
Bronchitis, Chronic
Catarrh, Upper Respiratory Tract

Jambolan Bark
Diarrhea
Gastrointestinal Tract Inflammation
Oral or Pharyngeal Inflammation
Mucous Membrane Irritation
Skin Injury or Irritation (external)
Sore Throat

Java Tea
Kidney Stones and Gravel
    (irrigation therapy)
Urinary Tract Infection or Inflammation
    (irrigation therapy)

Juniper Berry
Dyspepsia

Kava Kava
Anxiety
Muscle Pain
Restlessness
Stress

Kidney Bean Pods (without seeds)
Dysuria

Knotweed Herb
Catarrh, Upper Respiratory Tract
Oral or Pharyngeal Inflammation
Sore Throat
Respiratory Catarrh

Lady's Mantle
Diarrhea

Larch Turpentine
 Catarrh, Upper Respiratory Tract
 Furunculosis (boils)
 Neuralgia
 Respiratory Catarrh
 Rheumatism

Lavender Flower
 Circulatory Disorders (Balneotherapy)
 Gastrointestinal Disorders
 Insomnia
 Mood Disturbance
 Nervous Stomach
 Restlessness
 Roehmheld Syndrome
 Sleep Disturbances

Lemon Balm
 Dyspepsia
 Insomnia
 Sleep Disturbances
 Gastrointestinal Complaints

Licorice Root
 Catarrh, Upper Respiratory Tract
 Duodenal Ulcers
 Gastrointestinal Ulcers
 Respiratory Catarrh

Lily-of-the-Valley Herb
 Cardiac Insufficiency, Mild
 Heart Insufficiency, Due to old age
 Cor pulmonale, Chronic

Linden Flower
 Colds and Flu
 Cough

Lovage Root
 Kidney Stones and Gravel
  (irrigation therapy)
 Urinary Tract Infection or Inflammation
  (irrigation therapy)

Mallow Flower
 Cough, Dry
 Oral or Pharyngeal Inflammation

Mouth Irritation
Mucous Membrane Irritation
Sore Throat

Mallow Leaf
 Cough, Dry
 Oral or Pharyngeal Inflammation
 Mucous Membrane Irritation
 Sore Throat

Manna
 Anal Fissures
 Constipation
 Hemorrhoids
 Rectum, Post-surgical Care of

Marshmallow Leaf
 Cough, Dry
 Oral or Pharyngeal Irritation
 Mucous Membrane Irritation

Marshmallow Root
 Cough, Dry
 Gastric Mucosa, Inflammation of
 Gastrointestinal Tract Inflammation
 Oral or Pharyngeal Irritation
 Mucous Membrane Irritation

Mate
 Fatigue, Mental and Physical

Mayapple Root and Resin
 Condyloma (external)

Meadowsweet
 Colds and Flu

Medicinal Yeast
 Acne
 Loss of Appetite
 Furunculosis (boils)

Milk Thistle Fruit
 Cirrhosis
 Dyspepsia
 Liver Disease

Mint Oil
Catarrh, Upper Respiratory Tract
Flatulence
Gallbladder Disorders
Gastrointestinal Disorders
Myalgia (external)
Neuralgia (external)
Respiratory Catarrh

Mistletoe Herb
Arthritis
Joint Inflammation, Degenerative
Malignant Tumors

Motherwort Herb
Cardiac Symptoms
Tachycardia
Thyroid, Overactive

Mullein Flower
Catarrh, Upper Respiratory Tract

Myrrh
Oral or Pharyngeal Inflammation
(external)

Nettles Herb and Leaf
Kidney Stones and Gravel
(irrigation therapy)
Rheumatism
Urinary Tract Infection or Inflammation
(irrigation therapy)

Niauli Oil
Catarrh, Upper Respiratory Tract
Respiratory Catarrh

Oak Bark
Ano-genital Irritation
Diarrhea
Gastrointestinal Tract Inflammation
Oral or Pharyngeal Inflammation
Skin Injury or Irritation (external)
Sore Throat

Oat Straw
Itching (external)
Seborrhea (external)
Skin Injury or Irritation (external)

Onion
Loss of Appetite
Atherosclerosis
Geriatric Vascular Changes

Orange Peel
Loss of Appetite

Paprika (Cayenne)
Muscle Spasm of shoulder, arm and spine
of adults and school age children
(external)

Parsley Herb and Root
Kidney Stones and Gravel
(irrigation therapy)
Urinary Disorders (irrigation therapy)

Passionflower Herb
Anxiety
Restlessness

Peppermint Leaf
Biliary Spasm
Gallbladder Disorders
Gastrointestinal Tract Spasm

Peppermint Oil
Biliary Spasm
Catarrh, Upper Respiratory Tract
Colon, Irritable
Gastrointestinal Disorders
Gastrointestinal Tract Inflammation
Oral of Pharyngeal Inflammation
Irritable Bowel Syndrome
Mucous Membrane Irritation
Muscle Pain (external)
Neuralgia (external)
Respiratory Catarrh

Peruvian Balsam
Bruises and Contusions (external)
Burns (external)
Frostbite (external)
Hemorrhoids (external)
Prostheses, Bruises Caused by (external)
Skin Ulcers (external)
Ulcers Cruris (external)
Ulcers, Skin (external)
Wounds, Poorly Healing (external)

Petasites Root
Cholelithiasis
Kidney Stones and Gravel
Spastic Pain of Urinary Tract

Pheasant's Eye Herb
Cardiac Insufficiency
Circulatory Disorders

Pimpinella Root
Catarrh, Upper Respiratory Tract
Respiratory Catarrh

Pine Needle Oil
Catarrh, Upper Respiratory Tract
Neuralgia (external)
Respiratory Catarrh
Rheumatism (external)

Pine Sprouts
Catarrh, Upper and Lower
    Respiratory Tract
Lower Respiratory Tract Catarrh
Muscle Pain (external)
Neuralgia (external)
Respiratory Catarrh

Plantain
Catarrh, Upper Respiratory Tract
Mucous Membrane Irritation
Oral and Pharyngeal Inflammation
Skin Injury or Irritation (external)
Respiratory Catarrh

Pollen
Loss of Appetite
Debility
Feebleness

Poplar Bud
Frostbite (external)
Hemorrhoids (external)
Skin Injury or Irritation (external)
Sunburn (external)

Potentilla
Diarrhea
Dysmenorrhea
Gastrointestinal Tract Inflammation
Oral or Pharyngeal Inflammation

Primrose Flower
Catarrh, Upper Respiratory Tract

Primrose Root
Catarrh, Upper Respiratory Tract
Respiratory Catarrh

Psyllium Seed, Black
Colon, Irritable
Constipation
Irritable Bowel Syndrome

Psyllium Seed, Blonde
Anal Fissures (secondary)
Bowel, Irritable
Colon, Irritable
Constipation
Diarrhea
Hemorrhoids (secondary)
Irritable Bowel Syndrome
Rectum, Post-surgical Care of (secondary)

Psyllium Seed Husk, Blonde
Anal Fissures (secondary)
Bowel, Irritable
Colon, Irritable
Constipation
Diarrhea
Hemorrhoids (secondary)
Irritable Bowel Syndrome

Pumpkin Seed
Bladder Irritation
Urination, Diminished Associated with
    BPH Stages 1 and 2
Urination, Diminished Associated with
    Prostate Adenoma

Radish
Biliary Dyskinesia
Catarrh, Upper Respiratory Tract
Cholelithiasis
Dyspepsia
Peptic Disorders
Respiratory Catarrh

Rhatany Root
Oral or Pharyngeal Mucosa Inflammation
    (external)

Rhubarb Root
Constipation

Rose Flower
Oral or Pharyngeal Mucosa Inflammation

Rosemary Leaf
Circulatory Disorders (external)
Dyspepsia
Rheumatism (external)

Sage Leaf
Dyspepsia
Nose and Throat Inflammation
(external)
Perspiration, Excessive

Sandalwood, White
Urinary Tract Infection or Inflammation
(secondary)

Sandy Everlasting
Dyspepsia

Sanicle Herb
Catarrh, Upper Respiratory Tract
Respiratory Catarrh

Saw Palmetto Berry
Urination, Diminished Associated with
BPH Stages 1 and 2
Urination, Diminished Associated with
Prostate Adenoma

Scopolia Root
Biliary Spasm
Gastrointestinal Tract Spasm
Spasm, Gastrointestinal
Urinary Spasm, for adults and children
over six-years-old

Scotch Broom Herb
Circulatory Disorders
Functional Heart Disease

Senega Snakeroot
Catarrh, Upper Respiratory Tract
Respiratory Catarrh

Senna Leaf
Constipation
Hemorrhoids (secondary)

Senna Pod
Constipation

Shepherd's Purse
Menorrhagia
Metrorrhagia
Nose Bleeds (external)
Skin Injury or Irritation
(external)

Soapwort Root, Red
Catarrh, Upper Respiratory Tract
Respiratory Catarrh

Soapwort Root, White
Catarrh, Upper Respiratory Tract
Respiratory Catarrh

Soy Lecithin
High Cholesterol
Hypercholesteremia

Soy Phospholipid
Loss of Appetite
Hepatitis
High Cholesterol
Hypercholesteremia
Liver Disease

Spiny Restharrow Root
Kidney Stones and Gravel
(irrigation therapy)
Urinary Tract Infection or Inflammation
(irrigation therapy)

Squill
Cardiac Insufficiency
Kidney Capacity Diminished

St. John's Wort
  Anxiety
  Bruises and Contusions
    (external)
  Burns
  Depression
  Dyspepsia
  Injuries (external)
  Nervous Unrest
  Muscle Pain (external)

Star Anise Seed
  Catarrh, Upper Respiratory Tract
  Dyspepsia
  Respiratory Catarrh

Stinging Nettle Herb and Leaf
  Kidney Stones and Gravel
    (irrigation therapy)
  Rheumatism
  Urinary Tract Infection or Inflammation
    (irrigation therapy)

Stinging Nettle Root
  Urination, Diminished Associated with
    BPH Stages 1 and 2
  Urination, Diminished Associated with
    Prostate Adenoma

Sundew
  Cough, Dry
  Coughing Fits

Sweet Clover
  Bruises and Contusions (external)
  Bruises, Superficial Effusion of Blood
    (external)
  Hematoma (external)
  Hemorrhoids
  Itching
  Leg Cramps
  Lymphatic Congestion
  Phlebitis
  Post-thrombic Syndrome
  Thrombophlebitis
  Venous Insufficiency

Thyme
  Catarrh, Upper Respiratory Tract
  Bronchitis
  Respiratory Tract Catarrh
  Whooping Cough

Thyme, Wild
  Catarrh, Upper Respiratory Tract
  Respiratory Catarrh

Tolu Balsam
  Catarrh, Upper Respiratory Tract
  Respiratory Catarrh

Tormentil Root
  Diarrhea
  Gastrointestinal Tract Inflammation
  Oral or Pharyngeal Mucosa Inflammation

Turmeric Root
  Dyspepsia

Turmeric Root, Javanese
  Peptic Disorders

Turpentine Oil, Purified
  Bronchial Secretion, Excessive
  Catarrh, Upper Respiratory Tract
  Neuralgia (external)
  Respiratory Catarrh
  Rheumatism (external)

Usnea
  Oral or Pharyngeal Mucosa Inflammation

Uva Ursi Leaf
  Urinary Tract Infection or Inflammation

Uzara Root
  Diarrhea

Valerian Root
  Anxiety
  Insomnia
  Restlessness
  Sleep Disturbances

Walnut Leaf
Perspiration, Excessive (external)
Skin Injury or Irritation (external)

Watercress
Catarrh, Upper Respiratory Tract
Respiratory Catarrh

White Dead Nettle Flower
Catarrh, Upper Respiratory Tract
Oral or Pharyngeal Irritation (external)
Leukorrhea
Respiratory Catarrh
Skin Injury or Irritation (external)
Thrush (external)

White Mustard Seed
Arthrosis Joint Pain (external)
Arthritis (external)
Catarrh, Upper Respiratory Tract
(external)
Respiratory Catarrh (external)

White Willow Bark
Fever
Headache
Rheumatism

Witch Hazel Leaf and Bark
Hemorrhoids
Mucous Membrane Irritation
Skin Injury or Irritation
Varicose Veins/Varicosis

Woody Nightshade Stem
Eczema, Chronic

Wormwood
Loss of Appetite
Biliary Dyskinesia
Dyspepsia

Yarrow
Loss of Appetite
Dyspepsia
Gastrointestinal Tract Spasm
Pelvic Cramps (as sitz bath)
Premenstrual Syndrome (PMS)
(as sitz bath)

Yeast, Brewer's/Hansen CBS 5926
Acne
Diarrhea

Part B. Ailments and Diseases
Note: The abbreviation F.C. means "fixed combinations."

Abdominal Bloating
Angelica Root
Caraway Oil
Caraway Seed
Chinchona Bark
Cinnamon Bark
Cinnamon Bark, Chinese
Dandelion Herb
Fixed Combinations (F.C.) of Peppermint
leaf and Caraway seed
F.C. Peppermint leaf and Fennel seed
F.C. Peppermint leaf, Caraway seed, and
Chamomile flower
F.C. Peppermint leaf, Caraway seed, and
Fennel seed
F.C. Peppermint leaf, Caraway seed,
Chamomile flower, and Bitter
Orange peel
F.C. Peppermint leaf, Caraway seed, and
Fennel seed, and Chamomile flower
F.C. Peppermint leaf, Fennel seed, and
Chamomile flower
F.C. Peppermint oil and Caraway oil
F.C. Peppermint oil and Fennel oil
F.C. Peppermint oil, Caraway oil, and
Chamomile flower
F.C. Peppermint oil, Caraway oil, and
Fennel oil
F.C. Peppermint oil, Caraway oil, Fennel
oil, and Chamomile flower
Fennel Oil
Fennel Seed
Gentian Root
Horehound Herb

Acne
Brewer's Yeast
Medicinal Yeast
Yeast, Brewer's/Hansen CBS 5926

Anal Fissures
Manna
Psyllium Seed, Blonde (secondary)
Psyllium Seed Husk, Blonde (secondary)

Anesthesia Topical
Cloves

Ano-genital Irritation
Chamomile Flower, German
Oak bark

Anxiety
Hops
Indian Snakeroot
Kava Kava
Passionflower Herb
St. John's Wort
Valerian Root

Appetite, Loss of
Angelica Root
Bitter Orange Peel
Blessed Thistle Herb
Bogbean Leaf
Brewer's Yeast
Centaury herb
Chicory
Cinchona bark
Cinnamon bark
Cinnamon bark, Chinese
Condurango bark
Coriander seed
Dandelion herb
Dandelion root with herb
Devil's Claw root
F.C. Angelica root, Gentian root, and
   Bitter Orange peel
F.C. Angelica root, Gentian root, and
   Fennel
F.C. Angelica root, Gentian root, and
   Wormwood
F.C. Angelica root, Gentian root,
   Wormwood, and Peppermint oil

F.C. Ginger root, Gentian root, and
   Wormwood
Fenugreek seed
Galangal
Gentian root
Horehound herb
Iceland Moss
Medicinal Yeast
Onion
Orange peel
Pollen
Soy Phospholipid
Wormwood
Yarrow
Yeast, Medicinal

Arterial Occlusive Disease
Ginkgo Biloba Leaf Extract

Arthrosis Joint Pain
White Mustard Seed (external)

Arthritis
Hay Flower (topical heat therapy)
Mistletoe Herb
White Mustard Seed (external)

Asthma
Ephedra

Atherosclerosis
Onion

Bad Breath
Chamomile Flower, German (external)

Biliary Dyskinesia (gallbladder pain)
Absinth
Dandelion Root with Herb
Radish
Wormwood

Biliary Spasm (gallbladder pain)
Belladonna
Celandine Herb
Fumitory
Peppermint Leaf
Peppermint Oil
Scopolia Root

Bladder Irritation
Pumpkin seed

Bone Dislocations
Arnica flower (external)

Bowel Irritable
Flaxseed
Peppermint oil
Psyllium seed, Black
Psyllium seed, Blonde
Psyllium seed husk, Blonde

Breast Pain
Bugleweed

Bronchial Secretion, Excessive
Turpentine oil, Purified

Bronchitis
Ivy leaf

Bruises and Contusions
Arnica flower (external)
Comfrey herb and leaf (external)
Comfrey root (external)
Peruvian Balsam (external)
St. John's Wort (external)
Sweet Clover (external)

Bruises, Superficial Effusion of Blood
Sweet Clover (external)

Burns
Peruvian Balsam (external)
St. John's Wort (external)

Cardiac Insufficiency (Heart failure)
Hawthorn Leaf with Flower
Lily-of-the-Valley Herb
Pheasant's Eye Herb
Squill

Cardiac Symptoms (Chest pain)
Motherwort Herb

Catarrh, Upper Respiratory Tract
(Productive cough)
Anise seed
Camphor
Coltsfoot leaf
Eucalyptus leaf
Eucalyptus Oil
F.C. Anise oil and Iceland Moss
F.C. Anise seed, Linden flower, and
    Thyme
F.C. Anise seed, Marshmallow root,
    Iceland Moss, and Licorice root
F.C. Anise seed, Marshmallow root,
    Primrose root, and Sundew
F.C. Camphor, Eucalyptus oil, and
    Purified Turpentine
F.C. Eucalyptus oil, Primrose root, and
    Thyme
F.C. Gumweed herb, Primrose root, and
    Thyme
F.C. Ivy leaf, Licorice root, and Thyme
F.C. Licorice root, Primrose root,
    Marshmallow root, and Anise seed
F.C. Marshmallow root, Fennel seed,
    Iceland Moss, and Thyme
F.C. Marshmallow root, Primrose root,
    Licorice root, and Thyme oil
F.C. Primrose root and Thyme
F.C. Primrose root, Marshmallow root,
    and Anise seed
F.C. Primrose root, Sundew, and Thyme
F.C. Sundew and Thyme
Fennel Honey
Fennel Oil
Fennel Seed
Fennel Syrup
Fir Needle oil
Fir Shoots, Fresh
Gumweed herb
Hempnettle herb
Horseradish
Ivy leaf
Knotweed herb
Larch Turpentine
Licorice root
Mint oil
Mullein flower
Nasturtium
Niauli oil

Catarrh, Upper Respiratory Tract (cont.)
  Peppermint oil
  Pimpinella root
  Pine needle oil
  Pine sprout
  Plantain
  Primrose flower
  Primrose root
  Radish
  Sanicle herb
  Senega Snakeroot
  Soapwort root, Red
  Soapwort root, White
  Star Anise seed
  Thyme
  Thyme, Wild
  Tolu Balsam
  Turpentine oil, Purified
  Watercress
  White Dead Nettle flower
  White Mustard seed (external)

Cholelithiasis (Gallstones)
  Bishop's Weed fruit (secondary)
  Petasites root
  Radish

Cholesterol, High
  Garlic
  Soy Lecithin
  Soy Phospholipid

Circulatory Disorders
  Butcher's Broom
  Camphor
  Ginkgo Biloba Leaf Extract
  Lavender flower
  Pheasant's Eye herb
  Rosemary leaf
  Scotch Broom herb

Cirrhosis Hepatic
  Milk Thistle fruit

Colds and Flu
  Echinacea Pallida root
  Echinacea Purpurea herb
  Elder flower

Ephedra
F.C. Anise oil, Fennel oil, Licorice root,
  and Thyme
F.C. Anise oil, Primrose root, and Thyme
F.C. Anise seed, Ivy leaf, Fennel seed, and
  Licorice root
F.C. Anise seed, Marshmallow root,
  Eucalyptus oil, and Licorice root
F.C. Eucalyptus oil, Primrose root, and
  Thyme
F.C. Gumweed herb, Primrose root, and
  Thyme
F.C. Ivy leaf, Licorice root, and Thyme
F.C. Marshmallow root, Fennel seed,
  Iceland Moss, and Thyme
F.C. Primrose root and Thyme
F.C. Star Anise seed and Thyme
F.C. Thyme and White Soapwort root
Linden flower
Meadowsweet

Colon, Irritable
  Flaxseed
  Peppermint oil
  Psyllium seed husk, Blonde
  Psyllium seed, Black
  Psyllium seed, Blonde

Condyloma (Warts)
  Mayapple Root and Resin (external)

Constipation
  Aloe
  Buckthorn bark
  Buckthorn berry
  Cascara Sagrada bark
  F.C. Senna leaf and Blonde Psyllium seed
    husk
  F.C. Senna leaf, Peppermint oil, and
    Caraway oil
  Flaxseed
  Manna
  Psyllium seed husk, Blonde
  Psyllium seed, Black
  Psyllium seed, Blonde
  Rhubarb Root
  Senna Leaf
  Senna Pod

Convalescence
  Eleuthero (Siberian Ginseng) Root
    (as a tonic)
  Ginseng Root (as a tonic)

Cor pulmonale, Chronic
(Heart failure secondary to lung disease)
  Lily-of-the-Valley Herb

Cough
  Coltsfoot leaf
  F.C. Licorice root, Primrose root,
    Marshmallow root, and Anise seed
  F.C. Primrose root, Marshmallow root,
    and Anise seed
  Iceland Moss
  Linden flower
  Mallow flower
  Mallow leaf
  Marshmallow leaf
  Marshmallow root
  Sundew

Cramps, Leg
  Butcher's Broom
  Horse Chestnut seed
  Sweet Clover

Cramps, Pelvic
  Yarrow (as sitz bath)

Debility (General weakness)
  Eleuthero (Siberian Ginseng) root
  Ginseng root (as a tonic)
  Pollen

Degenerative Disorder, Locomotor System
  Devil's Claw root

Degenerative Joint Inflammation
  Arnica Flower (external)
  Mistletoe Herb
  White Mustard Seed (external)

Depression
  Ginkgo Biloba Leaf Extract (secondary)
  St. John's Wort

Diarrhea
  Agrimony
  Bilberry fruit
  Blackberry leaf
  Coffee Charcoal
  Jambolan bark
  Lady's Mantle
  Oak bark
  Potentilla
  Psyllium seed husk, Blonde
  Psyllium seed, Blonde (secondary)
  Tormentil root
  Uzara root
  Yeast, Brewer's/Hansen CBS 5926

**Diminished Urination Associated
with BPH Stages 1 and 2** (Prostatism)
  Pumpkin Seed
  Saw Palmetto berry
  Stinging Nettle root

**Diminished Urination Associated
with Prostate Adenoma** (Prostate tumor)
  Pumpkin seed
  Saw Palmetto berry
  Stinging Nettle root

Dislocation, Bones
  Arnica Flower (external)

Diuretic (To increase urine production)
  Dandelion root with herb

Diverticulitis
  Flaxseed

Dizziness
  Ginkgo Biloba Leaf Extract

Dysmenorrhea (Painful menstruation)
  Black Cohosh root
  Potentilla

Dyspepsia (Upset stomach)
  Angelica root
  Anise seed
  Artichoke leaf
  Bitter Orange peel

Dyspepsia (Upset stomach) (cont.)

Blessed Thistle herb
Bogbean leaf
Boldo leaf
Caraway oil
Caraway seed
Cardamom seed
Centaury herb
Chicory
Cinchona bark
Cinnamon bark
Cinnamon bark, Chinese
Cloves
Coriander seed
Dandelion herb
Dandelion root with herb
Devil's Claw root
Dill seed
F.C. Angelica root, Gentian root, and
    Bitter Orange peel
F.C. Angelica root, Gentian root, and
    Caraway seed
F.C. Angelica root, Gentian root, and
    Wormwood
F.C. Angelica root, Gentian root,
    Wormwood, and Peppermint oil
F.C. Anise oil, Fennel oil, and Caraway oil
F.C. Anise seed, Fennel seed, and
    Caraway seed
F.C. Caraway oil and Fennel oil
F.C. Caraway oil, Fennel oil, and
    Chamomile flower
F.C. Caraway seed and Fennel seed
F.C. Caraway seed, Fennel seed, and
    Chamomile flower
F.C. Dandelion root with herb, Celandine
    herb, and Wormwood
F.C. Dandelion root with herb,
    Peppermint leaf, and Artichoke leaf
F.C. Ginger root, Gentian root, and
    Wormwood
F.C. Javanese Turmeric root, Celandine
    herb, and Wormwood
F.C. Javanese Turmeric root, Peppermint
    leaf, and Wormwood
F.C. Milk Thistle fruit, Peppermint leaf,
    and Wormwood
F.C. Peppermint leaf and Caraway seed

F.C. Peppermint leaf and Fennel seed
F.C. Peppermint leaf, Caraway seed, and
    Chamomile flower
F.C. Peppermint leaf, Caraway seed, and
    Fennel seed
F.C. Peppermint leaf, Caraway seed,
    Chamomile flower, and Bitter
    Orange peel
F.C. Peppermint leaf, Caraway seed,
    Fennel seed, and Chamomile flower
F.C. Peppermint leaf, Chamomile flower,
    and Caraway seed
F.C. Peppermint leaf, Fennel seed, and
    Chamomile flower
F.C. Peppermint oil and Caraway oil
F.C. Peppermint oil and Fennel oil
F.C. Peppermint oil, Caraway oil, and
    Chamomile flower
F.C. Peppermint oil, Caraway oil, and
    Fennel oil
F.C. Peppermint oil, Caraway oil, Fennel
    oil, and Chamomile flower
F.C. Peppermint oil, Fennel oil, and
    Chamomile flower
F.C. Turmeric root and Celandine herb
    Fennel oil
Fennel seed
Galangal
Gentian root
Ginger root
Haronga bark and leaf
Horehound herb
Juniper berry
Lemon Balm
Milk Thistle
Mistletoe herb
Radish
Rosemary leaf
Sage leaf
Sandy Everlasting
St. John's Wort
Star Anise seed
Turmeric root
Turmeric root, Javanese
Wormwood
Yarrow

Dysuria (Painful urination)
Kidney Bean pods (without seeds)

Eczema (Chronic skin disease)
Woody Nightshade stem

Edema, Post-traumatic
(Extremity swelling secondary to fluid accumulation, as in post mastectomy)
Arnica flower (external)
Horsetail herb

Familial Mediterranean Fever
Autumn Crocus

Fatigue, Mental and Physical
Cola nut
Eleuthero (Siberian Ginseng) Root (as a tonic)
Ginseng root (as a tonic)
Mate

Fever
White Willow Bark

Flatulence
Angelica root
Caraway oil
Cinnamon bark
Cinnamon bark, Chinese
Dandelion herb
F.C. Angelica root, Gentian root, and Wormwood
F.C. Peppermint leaf and Caraway seed
F.C. Peppermint leaf and Fennel seed
F.C. Peppermint leaf, Caraway seed, and Chamomile flower
F.C. Peppermint leaf, Caraway seed, and Fennel seed
F.C. Peppermint leaf, Caraway seed, Chamomile flower, and Bitter Orange peel
F.C. Peppermint leaf, Caraway seed, Fennel seed, and Chamomile flower
F.C. Peppermint leaf, Fennel seed, and Chamomile flower
F.C. Peppermint oil and Caraway oil
F.C. Peppermint oil and Fennel oil
F.C. Peppermint oil, Caraway oil, and Chamomile flower
F.C. Peppermint oil, Caraway oil, and Fennel oil

F.C. Peppermint oil, Caraway oil, Fennel oil, and Chamomile flower
F.C. Peppermint oil, Fennel oil, and Chamomile flower
Fennel oil
Fennel seed
Gentian root
Horehound herb
Mint oil

Flu and Colds
Echinacea Pallida root
Echinacea Purpurea herb
Elder flower
Ephedra
F.C. Anise oil, Fennel oil, Licorice root, and Thyme
F.C. Anise oil, Primrose root, and Thyme
F.C. Anise seed, Ivy leaf, Fennel seed, and Licorice root
F.C. Anise seed, Marshmallow root, Eucalyptus oil, and Licorice root
F.C. Eucalyptus oil, Primrose root, and Thyme
F.C. Gumweed herb, Primrose root, and Thyme
F.C. Ivy leaf, Licorice root, and Thyme
F.C. Marshmallow root, Fennel seed, Iceland Moss, and Thyme
F.C. Primrose root and Thyme
F.C. Star Anise seed and Thyme
F.C. Thyme and White Soapwort root
Linden flower
Meadowsweet

Free Radical Deactivation
Ginkgo Biloba Leaf Extract

Frostbite
Peruvian Balsam (external)
Poplar bud (external)

Furunculosis (Boils)
Arnica Flower (external)
Brewer's Yeast
Larch Turpentine
Yeast, Medicinal

Gallbladder Disorders
F.C. Dandelion root with herb,
   Celandine herb, and Wormwood
Fumitory
Mint oil
Peppermint leaf

Gargle or Mouthwash
Chamomile flower, German
Cloves

Gastric Mucosa, Inflammation of
Marshmallow root

Gastrointestinal Disorders
Agrimony
Angelica Root
Belladonna
Bilberry Fruit
Blackberry Leaf
Boldo Leaf
Caraway Oil
Caraway Seed
Celandine Herb
Chamomile Flower, German
Cinnamon Bark
Cinnamon Bark, Chinese
F.C. Dandelion root with herb,
   Celandine herb, and Artichoke leaf
Coffee Charcoal
Fennel Oil
Fennel Seed
Fumitory
Henbane Leaf
Jambolan Bark
Lavender Flower
Lemon Balm
Licorice Root
Marshmallow Root
Mint oil
Oak Bark
Peppermint Leaf
Peppermint Oil
Potentilla
Scopolia Root
Tormentil Root
Yarrow

Gastrointestinal Pain
Belladonna

Gastrointestinal Tract Inflammation
Agrimony
Bilberry fruit
Blackberry leaf
Boldo leaf
Chamomile flower, German
Coffee Charcoal
Jambolan bark
Marshmallow root
Oak bark
Peppermint oil
Potentilla
Tormentil root

Gastrointestinal Tract Spasm
Angelica root
Belladonna
Boldo leaf
Caraway oil
Caraway seed
Celandine herb
Chamomile flower, German
Cinnamon bark
Cinnamon bark, Chinese
F.C. Angelica root, Gentian root, and
   Caraway seed
F.C. Licorice root, Peppermint leaf, and
   German Chamomile flower
Fumitory
Henbane leaf
Peppermint leaf
Scopolia root
Yarrow

Gastrointestinal Ulcers
F.C. Licorice root and German
   Chamomile flower
F.C. Licorice root, Peppermint leaf, and
   German Chamomile flower
Licorice root

Geriatric Vascular Changes
Garlic
Hawthorn leaf with flower
Onion

Gout
   Autumn Crocus

Gums, Inflamed
   Chamomile flower, German

Headache
   Ginkgo Biloba Leaf Extract
   White Willow bark

Hematoma (Bruise)
   Arnica flower
   Sweet Clover

Hemorrhoids
   Butcher's Broom
   Manna
   Peruvian Balsam
   Poplar bud
   Psyllium seed husk, Blonde (secondary)
   Psyllium seed, Blonde (secondary)
   Senna leaf
   Sweet Clover
   Witch Hazel leaf and bark

Hepatic Cirrhosis
   Milk Thistle fruit

Hepatitis
   Soy Phospholipid

High Cholesterol/Hypercholesteremia
   Garlic
   Soy Lecithin
   Soy Phospholipid

Hoarseness
   Coltsfoot leaf

Hypercholesteremia
   Garlic
   Soy Lecithin
   Soy Phospholipid

Hyperemia
   Horseradish

Hyperlipidemia
   Garlic

Hypertension (High blood pressure)
   Camphor
   Indian Snakeroot

Inflammation, Gastrointestinal Tract
   Agrimony
   Bilberry fruit
   Blackberry leaf
   Boldo leaf
   Chamomile flower, German
   Coffee Charcoal
   Jambolan bark
   Marshmallow root
   Oak bark
   Peppermint oil
   Potentilla
   Tormentil root

Inflammation, Degenerative Joint
   Arnica Flower (external)
   Mistletoe Herb
   White Mustard Seed (external)

**Inflammation, Mouth, Oral,
Pharyngeal and Throat**
   Agrimony
   Arnica flower
   Bilberry fruit
   Blackberry leaf
   Blackthorn Berry
   Calendula flower
   Chamomile flower, German
   Cloves
   Coffee Charcoal
   Coltsfoot leaf
   Iceland Moss
   Jambolan bark
   Knotweed herb
   Mallow flower
   Mallow leaf
   Marshmallow leaf
   Marshmallow root
   Myrrh
   Oak bark
   Peppermint oil
   Plantain

Inflammation, Mouth, Oral, Pharyngeal and Throat (cont.)
Potentilla
Rhatany root (external)
Rose flower
Sage leaf (external)
Tormentil root
Usnea
White Dead Nettle flower (external)

Influenza
Echinacea Pallida root
Echinacea Purpurea herb
Elder flower
Ephedra
F.C. Anise oil, Fennel oil, Licorice root, and Thyme
F.C. Anise oil, Primrose root, and Thyme
F.C. Anise seed, Ivy leaf, Fennel seed, and Licorice root
F.C. Anise seed, Marshmallow root, Eucalyptus oil, and Licorice root
F.C. Eucalyptus oil, Primrose root, and Thyme
F.C. Gumweed herb, Primrose root, and Thyme
F.C. Ivy leaf, Licorice root, and Thyme
F.C. Marshmallow root, Fennel seed, Iceland Moss, and Thyme
F.C. Primrose root and Thyme
F.C. Star Anise seed and Thyme
F.C. Thyme and White Soapwort root
Linden flower
Meadowsweet

Injuries, Bruises
Arnica flower (external)
Comfrey herb and leaf (external)
Comfrey root (external)
Peruvian Balsam (external)
St. John's Wort (external)
Sweet Clover (external)

Injury or Irritation, Skin
Agrimony (external)
Chamomile flower, German
Jambolan bark (external)
Oak bark (external)

Oat straw (external)
Plantain (external)
Poplar Bud (external)
Shepherd's Purse (external)
Walnut Leaf (external)
White Dead Nettle flower
Witch Hazel leaf and bark

Insect Bites
Arnica flower

Insomnia
F.C. Passionflower herb, Valerian root, and Lemon Balm
F.C. Valerian root and Hops
F.C. Valerian root, Hops, and Lemon Balm
F.C. Valerian root, Hops, and Passionflower herb
Hops
Lavender flower
Lemon Balm
Valerian root

Irrigation, Mouth
Chamomile Flower, German
Cloves
Mallow flower

Irrigation Therapy
Asparagus root
Birch leaf
Couch Grass
Goldenrod
Horsetail herb
Java tea
Lovage root
Nettles Herb and Leaf
Parsley Herb and Root
Spiny Restharrow root
Stinging Nettle herb and leaf

Irritable Bowel Syndrome
Flaxseed
Peppermint oil
Psyllium seed, Black
Psyllium seed, Blonde
Psyllium seed husk, Blonde

Itching
  Butcher's Broom
  Horse Chestnut seed
  Oat straw
  Sweet Clover

Joint, Degenerative Inflammation
  Arnica Flower (external)
  Mistletoe Herb
  White Mustard Seed (external)

Joint Pain
  Arnica flower (external)
  F.C. Camphor, Eucalyptus oil, and
    Purified Turpentine oil (external)
  White Mustard Seed (external)

Kidney, Capacity Diminished
  Squill

Kidney Stones and Gravel
  Asparagus root
  Birch leaf
  Couch Grass leaf
  F.C. Birch, Goldenrod and Java tea
  Goldenrod
  Horsetail herb
  Java tea
  Lovage root
  Nettle Herb and Leaf
  Parsley herb and root
  Petasites root
  Spiny restharrow root
  Stinging Nettle herb and leaf

Lactation Poor
  Chaste Tree fruit

Leg Cramps
  Butcher's Broom
  Horse Chestnut seed
  Sweet Clover

Legs, Swelling
  Butcher's Broom

Leukorrhea (Vaginal discharge)
  White Dead Nettle flower

Ligaments, Pulled
  Comfrey Root (external)

Liver Cirrhosis
  Milk Thistle Fruit

Liver Disease
  Milk Thistle Fruit
  Soy Phospholipid

Locomotor System, Degenerative Disorder
  Devil's Claw root

Lymphatic Congestion
  Sweet Clover

Malignant Tumors
  Mistletoe herb

Mediterranean Fever, Familial
  Autumn Crocus

Memory Loss
  Ginkgo Biloba Leaf Extract

Menopausal Symptoms
  Black Cohosh root
  Chaste Tree fruit

Menorrhagia
(Excessive menstrual bleeding)
  Shepherd's Purse

Menstrual Disorders
  Chaste Tree Fruit

Mental Concentration
  Eleuthero (Siberian Ginseng) root
    (As a tonic)
  Ginkgo Biloba Leaf Extract (as a tonic)
  Ginseng Root (as a tonic)

Mental and Physical Fatigue
  Cola nut
  Eleuthero (Siberian Ginseng) Root
    (as a tonic)
  Ginseng root (as a tonic)
  Mate

Metrorrhagia
(Abnormal menstrual bleeding)
Shepherd's Purse

Milk Scall
Heart's Ease Herb

Mood Disturbance
Hops
Lavender Flower

Motion Sickness
Ginger Root

Mouth and Throat Inflammation
Agrimony
Arnica flower
Bilberry fruit
Blackberry leaf
Blackthorn Berry
Calendula flower
Chamomile flower, German
Cloves
Coffee Charcoal
Coltsfoot leaf
Iceland Moss
Jambolan bark
Knotweed herb
Mallow flower
Mallow leaf
Marshmallow leaf
Marshmallow root
Myrrh
Oak bark
Peppermint oil
Plantain
Potentilla
Rhatany root (external)
Rose flower
Sage leaf (external)
Tormentil root
Usnea
White Dead Nettle flower (external)

Mouthwash or Gargle
Chamomile flower, German
Cloves

Mucous Membrane Irritation
Chamomile flower, German
Jambolan bark
Mallow flower
Mallow leaf
Marshmallow leaf
Marshmallow root
Peppermint oil
Plantain
Witch Hazel leaf and bark

Muscle Pain
Arnica flower (external)
Camphor
Cayenne (external)
Comfrey Root (external)
Fir Needle oil
Fir Shoots, Fresh
F.C. Camphor, Eucalyptus oil, and
    Purified Turpentine
Horseradish
Kava Kava
Nasturtium
Paprika (external)
Peppermint oil (external)
Pine Sprouts (external)
St. John's Wort (external)

Muscle Spasm
Cayenne (external)
Paprika (external)

Muscles, Pulled
Comfrey Root (external)

Nervous Stomach
F.C. Licorice Root and German
    Chamomile flower
Lavender flower

Nervous System Disorder
Bugleweed

Neuralgia (Pain related to a specific nerve)
Fir Needle oil (external)
Fir shoots Fresh
Larch Turpentine
Mint oil (external)
Monkshood

Neuralgia (cont.)
Peppermint oil (external)
Pine needle oil (external)
Pine Sprouts (external)
Turpentine oil, Purified

Nose Bleeds
Shepherd's Purse (external)

Oral Inflammation
Agrimony
Arnica flower
Bilberry fruit
Blackberry leaf
Blackthorn Berry
Calendula flower
Chamomile flower, German
Cloves
Coffee Charcoal
Coltsfoot leaf
Iceland Moss
Jambolan bark
Knotweed herb
Mallow flower
Mallow leaf
Marshmallow leaf
Marshmallow root
Myrrh
Oak bark
Peppermint oil
Plantain
Potentilla
Rhatany root (external)
Rose flower
Sage leaf (external)
Tormentil root
Usnea
White Dead Nettle flower (external)

Pain, Gastrointestinal
Belladonna

Pain, Muscle
Arnica flower (external)
Camphor
Cayenne (external)
Comfrey Root (external)
Fir Needle oil

Fir Shoots, Fresh
F.C. Camphor, Eucalyptus oil, and
    Purified Turpentine
Horseradish
Kava Kava
Nasturtium
Paprika (external)
Peppermint oil (external)
Pine Sprouts (external)
St. John's Wort (external)

Pancreatic Insufficiency
Haronga Bark and Leaf

Pelvic Cramps
Yarrow (as sitz bath)

Perspiration, Excessive
Sage leaf
Walnut leaf

Phlebitis
(Vein irritation and inflammation)
Arnica flower (external)
Sweet Clover

Pharyngeal Inflammation
Agrimony
Arnica flower
Bilberry fruit
Blackberry leaf
Blackthorn Berry
Calendula flower
Chamomile flower, German
Cloves
Coffee Charcoal
Coltsfoot leaf
Iceland Moss
Jambolan bark
Knotweed herb
Mallow flower
Mallow leaf
Marshmallow leaf
Marshmallow root
Myrrh
Oak bark
Peppermint oil
Plantain

Pharyngeal Inflammation (cont.)
Potentilla
Rhatany root (external)
Rose flower
Sage leaf (external)
Tormentil root
Usnea
White Dead Nettle flower (external)

Physical and Mental Fatigue
Cola nut
Eleuthero (Siberian Ginseng) Root
  (as a tonic)
Ginseng root (as a tonic)
Mate

PMS
Black Cohosh root
Chaste Tree fruit
Yarrow

Post-operative Swelling
Bromelain
Butcher's Broom
Horse Chestnut seed

Post-traumatic Swelling
Bromelain
Butcher's Broom
Horse Chestnut seed

Post-thrombic Syndrome
Horse Chestnut seed
Sweet Clover

Premenstrual Syndrome
Black Cohosh root
Chaste Tree fruit
Yarrow

**Prostate Adenoma, Diminished
Urination Associated with**
Pumpkin seed
Saw Palmetto berry
Stinging Nettle root

Prostheses, Bruises Caused by
Peruvian Balsam (external)

Purgative (Laxative)
F.C. Senna leaf, Peppermint oil, and
  Caraway oil
Senna

Rectum, Post Surgical Care of
Manna (secondary)
Psyllium seed, Blonde (secondary)

Respiratory Catarrh (Productive cough)
(See Catarrh)

Respiratory Infection, Chronic
Chamomile flower, German
Echinacea Purpurea herb

Restlessness
F.C. Passionflower herb, Valerian root,
  and Lemon Balm
F.C. Valerian root, Hops, and Lemon
  Balm
F.C. Valerian root, Hops, and
  Passionflower herb
Hops
Kava Kava
Lavender flower
Passionflower herb
Valerian root

Retinal Lesion and Edema
Ginkgo Biloba Leaf Extract

Rheumatism
Arnica flower (external)
Birch leaf (secondary)
Camphor
Eucalyptus oil
Fir Needle oil
Fir Shoots, Fresh
Guaiac wood
Larch Turpentine
Nettle Herb and Leaf
Pine Needle oil (external)
Rosemary leaf
Stinging Nettle herb and leaf
Turpentine oil, Purified
White Willow bark

Seborrhea
Heart's Ease Herb (external)
Oat Straw (external)

Sinusitis
Bromelain

Skin, Bacterial Infections
Chamomile flower, German

Skin Injury or Irritation
Agrimony (external)
Chamomile flower, German
Jambolan bark (external)
Oak bark (external)
Oat straw (external)
Plantain (external)
Poplar Bud (external)
Shepherd's Purse (external)
Walnut Leaf (external)
White Dead Nettle flower
Witch Hazel leaf and bark

Skin Ulcers
Peruvian Balsam (external)
Echinacea Purpurea Herb (external)

Sleep Disturbances
F.C. Passionflower herb, Valerian root, and Lemon Balm
F.C. Valerian root and Hops
F.C. Valerian root, Hops, and Lemon Balm
F.C. Valerian root, Hops, and Passionflower herb
Hops
Lavender flower
Lemon Balm
Valerian root

Sleeplessness
F.C. Passionflower herb, Valerian root, and Lemon Balm
F.C. Valerian root and Hops
F.C. Valerian root, Hops, and Lemon Balm
F.C. Valerian root, Hops, and Passionflower herb

Hops
Lavender flower
Lemon Balm
Valerian root

Sore Throat
Agrimony
Arnica flower (external)
Bilberry fruit
Blackberry leaf
Blackthorn berry
Calendula flower
Cloves (external)
Coffee Charcoal
Coltsfoot leaf
Iceland Moss
Jambolan bark
Knotweed herb
Mallow flower
Mallow leaf
Marshmallow leaf
Oak bark

Spasm, Gastrointestinal Tract
Angelica root
Belladonna
Boldo leaf
Caraway oil
Caraway seed
Celandine herb
Chamomile flower, German
Cinnamon bark
Cinnamon bark, Chinese
F.C. Angelica root, Gentian root, and Caraway seed
F.C. Licorice root, Peppermint leaf and German Chamomile flower
Fumitory
Henbane leaf
Peppermint leaf
Scopolia root
Yarrow

Spasm, Muscle
Cayenne (external)
Paprika (external)

Spasm, Urinary
Scopolia root

Spasms
Cayenne (external)
Paprika (external)

Sprains
Comfrey herb and leaf (external)
Comfrey root (external)

Stress
Kava Kava

Sunburn
Poplar bud (external)

Swelling, Legs
Butcher's Broom

Swelling, Post-operative
Bromelain
Butcher's Broom
Horse Chestnut seed

Swelling, Post-traumatic
Bromelain
Butcher's Broom
Horse Chestnut seed

Sympatheticotonia
Indian Snakeroot

Tachycardia
Indian Snakeroot
Motherwort herb

Thrombophlebitis
Sweet Clover

Thrush
White Dead Nettle Flower (external)

Thyroid Overactive
Bugleweed
Motherwort herb

Tinnitus
Ginkgo Biloba Leaf Extract

Tonic
Eleuthero (Siberian Ginger) root
Ginkgo Biloba Leaf Extract
Ginseng root

Throat, Sore
Agrimony
Arnica flower (external)
Bilberry fruit
Blackberry leaf
Blackthorn berry
Calendula flower
Cloves (external)
Coffee Charcoal
Coltsfoot leaf
Iceland Moss
Jambolan bark
Knotweed herb
Mallow flower
Mallow leaf
Marshmallow leaf
Oak bark

Ulcers, Gastrointestinal
F.C. Licorice root and German
    Chamomile flower
F.C. Licorice root, Peppermint leaf, and
    German Chamomile flower
Licorice root

Ulcers, Skin
Peruvian Balsam (external)
Echinacea Purpurea Herb (external)

Ulcus Cruris
Calendula Flower (external)
Peruvian Balsam (external)

Urinary Disorders
Parsley herb and root

Urinary Tract Infection or Inflammation
Asparagus root
Birch leaf
Couch Grass
Echinacea Purpurea herb
F.C. Birch leaf, Goldenrod, and Java tea
F.C. Uva Ursi leaf, Goldenrod,
    and Java tea

Urinary Tract Infection or Inflammation (cont.)
Goldenrod
Horseradish
Horsetail herb
Java tea
Lovage root
Sandalwood, White (secondary)
Spiny Restharrow root
Stinging Nettle herb and leaf
Uva Ursi leaf (secondary)

Urinary Spasm
Scopolia root

Urination, Diminished Associated with BPH Stages 1 and 2
Pumpkin Seed
Saw Palmetto berry
Stinging Nettle root

Urination, Diminished Associated with Prostate Adenoma
Pumpkin seed
Saw Palmetto berry
Stinging Nettle root

Varicose Veins/Varicosis
Horse Chestnut seed
Witch Hazel leaf and bark

Vascular Changes, Geriatric
Garlic
Hawthorn leaf with flower
Onion

Venous Insufficiency
Butcher's Broom (secondary)
Horse Chestnut seed
Sweet Clover

Vertigo
Ginkgo Biloba Leaf Extract

Wounds, Poorly Healing
Calendula flower (external)
Echinacea Purpurea herb (external)
Horsetail herb (external)
Peruvian Balsam (external)

Whooping Cough
Thyme

Glossary

Achillicin: The active ingredient in yarrow (*Achillea millefolium*), so named because Achilles was said to have used poultices made with this herb to treat his wounded soldiers.

Adaptogen: A substance that strengthens body functions and increases the body's resistance to stress. The term was originally used to describe the effects of ginseng, but there are many other putative adaptogens.

Alkaloids: Until 1803, when morphine was first isolated from opium, it was mistakenly believed that chemicals in plant leaves had to be acids. Morphine turned out to be just the opposite - an alkaloid. Today when people speak of alkaloids, they are usually referring to mind-altering chemicals such as psilocybin that are also obtained from plants.

Allantoin: A chemical found in comfrey that is thought to explain that herb's ability to promote skin healing. High blood levels in humans are considered to be a sign of oxidative stress.

Allicin: The substance that gives garlic its distinctive smell.

Alliin: An odorless precursor compound that is converted into allicin, the compound that gives garlic its odor.

Almitrine: A molecule with a structure almost identical to that of yohimbine, currently under investigation as a treatment for stroke.

Aloin: The active ingredient in aloe, also called babrolin.

Allopathic medicine: The term that naturopathic and homeopathic physicians use to describe standard medical practice.

Alpha acids: Three different acids, humulone, cohumulone, and adhumulone, are contained in hops. Once in the body, they are converted into a compound that gives hops its sedative effects.

Alpha-tocopherol: Another name for vitamin E, nature's antioxidant.

Amentoflavone: Flavonoid found in St. John's wort that may account for that herb's antidepressant activity.

American ginseng: The common name for *Panax quinquefolius*.

Analgesic: A substance that relieves pain.

Anethole: The main constituent of the essential oils obtained from anise and fennel. It has both antioxidant and anti-inflammatory properties.

Annual: A plant that completes its life cycle (germination to flowering to seed production to death) in one year.

Anticholinergic: A drug that prevents a neurotransmitter called acetylcholine from attaching at its normal receptor site (called muscarinic receptor). The result is decreased sweating, decreased saliva production, temperature elevation, and facial flushing. Anticholinergic poisoning can be produced by atropine-containing plants, including deadly nightshade and *Datura stramonium* which is also known as Jamestown or jimsonweed, stinkweed, thorn-apple, and devil's apple, and henbane (*Hyoscyamus niger*) and *Scopolia carniolica*.

Anthroquinones: The molecules in senna (Sennosides A & B) and aloe that act as laxatives (aloin). They stimulate the intestines to secrete water and salts into the bowel, increasing bulk and stimulating bowel contraction. Long-term use may result in increased risk for cancer.

Antiemetic: A substance that prevents nausea and vomiting, i.e., ginger.

Antioxidants: Herbs or chemicals taken in hopes of preventing free radical-mediated tissue damage.

Antipyretic: A substance that is used to reduce fever. Aspirin is a very potent antipyretic. Herbalists use willow, elm and holly.

Antispasmodic: A substance that relieves cramps.

Aphrodisiac: A substance capable of stimulating sexual desire.

Apigenin: The active molecule in chamomile. It reacts with the same molecular receptors that react with Valium™ and other benzodiazepines.

Aperitive: A substance that increases appetite. Marijuana is notoriously good for this purpose. Herbalists suggest wormwood, yellow gentian, peppermint and caraway.

Arbutin: The active ingredient in uva ursi that has antibacterial actions.

Ascorbic acid: Vitamin C, an antioxidant.

Asian ginseng: The common name for *Panax ginseng.*

Astragalin: A type of flavonoid found in *Astragalus.* It is a potent antioxidant.

Babrolin: The active ingredient in aloe, also called aloin.

Bacteriostatic: A substance that prevents bacteria from growing.

Bakkenolide G: An anti-platelet compound found in coltsfoot.

Berberine: A molecule found in goldenseal, an herb often taken in hopes of masking illicit drug use. Laboratories can detect berberine and know from its presence that goldenseal has been used.

Beta-asarone: A carcinogen found in the variety of Calamus that grows in India, but not in the varieties grown in the United States.

Beta-sitosterol: The main sterol found in soya bean seeds. Used as a starting point for the manufacture of medical steroids. Its structure resembles that of cholesterol and its supplementation may prevent cholesterol absorption from the intestines. It also has anti-inflammatory properties.

Bisabolol: The molecule in chamomile that calms the stomach and imparts the characteristic blue color to the essential oil.

BMI. Body Mass Index. Defined as weight in kilograms divided by height in meters squared.

CAD: Coronary artery disease.

Caffeic acid: A chemical found in artichokes that protects the liver from toxins such as carbon tetrachloride.

Capsaicin: The chemical in chili peppers that makes them hot.

Carbenoxolone: A licorice derivative used to treat ulcers in Europe. It has not been approved for use in the United States.

Carotenoid: A naturally occurring antioxidant.

Capsanthine: The pigment that gives chilies their red color.

Carvone: The main constituent of spearmint oil.

Carminative: A substance used to combat flatulence. Cocaine was originally promoted for this purpose, but better informed herbalists recommend chamomile, peppermint, anise and valerian.

Catarrh: Inflammation of mucous membranes, especially of the respiratory tract, accompanied by excessive production of mucous and other secretions.

Catechins: Antioxidant flavonoids found in tea.

"Cerebral insufficiency": A term used by European physicians referring to a number of different, often completely unrelated, disorders leading to altered mentation. The definition is extremely vague and is not favored by American physicians.

CFSAN: "The Center for Food Safety and Applied Nutrition," the division of the FDA charged with regulating food supplements, and thus herbal medicines.

"Chinese White" ginseng: The name given to the American variety of ginseng, *Panax quinquefolius,* now grown commercially in China. It is generally considered to be of poor quality.

Cholagogue: A substance used to make the gallbladder contract and release bile. The body produces hormones that do this, and it is not clear whether any of the traditional medicines (chicory, thistle, mugwort) really do produce this effect.

Choleretic: See cholagogue.

Choreoathetosis: A movement disorder associated with some psychotropic drugs, and with the herbal remedy, kava.

Citronella: The chemical that imparts the distinctive smell to lemons.

Commission E: A panel of respected scientists appointed by the German government to review the safety and effectiveness of herbal remedies.

Coumesterol: The plant estrogen (phytoestrogen) found in dandelions.

COX: Abbreviation for cyclooxygenase inhibitor.

Cutaneous: Relating to the skin.

Cyclamin: A toxic component of horse chestnut. In India, concentrated horse chestnut extracts were added to water to paralyze the fish and make them easier to catch.

Cyclooxygenase: One of the key enzymes controlling the body's inflammatory response. This enzyme is responsible for producing some of the molecules that cause inflammation. Nonsteroidal anti-inflammatory drugs (NSAIDs) like Tylenol™ work by blocking the actions of cyclooxygenase.

Cytokines: A variety of soluble growth and activation factors released from different types of white blood cells involved in the immune response. These substances play a key role in setting off and controlling the immune response. Some well-known examples include tumor necrosis factor, interleukin-2, interleukin-4, interferon gamma, etc.

Daidzen: A common type of phytoestrogen found in soybeans.

Danthrone: A known carcinogen found in laxatives derived from plants in the lily family (aloes and senna). Its sale is banned in the United States.

Dementia: A general term for disease, like Alzheimer's, that causes disordered thought processes.

Demulcent: An oil substance that can be used to protect or soothe a mucous membrane.

Denatured: What occurs when a protein loses its normal structure. Tannins cure leather by "denaturing" the proteins present in rawhide.

Depurative: A substance used to purify the blood. It is another very ancient notion, dating from a time when it was believed that disease was due to impurities, or even "humors," circulating in the blood. Of course, specific toxins, like diphtheria, do cause disease. But they are treated with specific antitoxins, not depurative herbs.

Diaphoretic: Sweaty. Some herbs are said to make people sweat. These include borage, chamomile and cowslip. Also an archaic term used to describe drugs that induce sweating, thereby causing a fever to subside. Actually, patients often break out in a sweat when a fever is about to go away. Old herbalists confused cause and effect.

Dicoumorol: Substance found in sweet clover that counteracts the effects of Vitamin K and prevents normal blood coagulation. In the past, synthetic dicoumarol was used as a blood thinner, but it has been replaced with another similar molecule called warfarin.

Dihydromethysticin: A pyrone-type molecule, one of the two active ingredients in kava.

Dioecious: Male and female flowers are produced on different plants, as with the hemp plant.

Diosgenin: A saponin contained in fenugreek and wild yams that prevents cholesterol from being absorbed from the gastrointestinal tract.

Discorides: A first century Greek physician, author of *De Materia Medica*, which contained descriptions of over 500 medicinal plants.

Diuretic: An agent that leads to increased urine production, including such medications as Diuril™ and Lasix™. Herbalists recommend chervil, horsetail, sea buckthorn and silverweed.

Dropsy: An archaic term for chronic heart failure with swelling of the ankles and legs. Traditional herbalists often treated this condition with garlic.

DSHEA: "The Dietary Supplement Health and Education Act of 1994." This law, enacted by the 103rd Congress, allows herbal medicines to be sold as if they were foods, which means that information about safety and effectiveness is not required by the FDA.

Dysmenorrhea: Painful menstruation.

Dyspepsia: A general term for indigestion or upset stomach.

Echimidine: The most toxic of the pyrrolizidines alkaloids. Even small amounts can cause liver damage.

Edema: Abnormal accumulation of fluid in a tissue, as in swollen legs or feet. Edema fluid can accumulate anywhere in the body.

EGb 761: The ginkgo extract sold in Europe to treat "cerebral insufficiency."

Eleutherosides: The active ingredients in *E. senticosus*, a close relative to *Panax Ginseng*. The active ingredients in the latter are called ginsenosides.

Elongation factor eEF-2: A key factor in normal protein production, and also in abnormal tumor growth. Its actions are blocked by something contained in mullein.

Emetic: A substance that causes vomiting. The drug emetine acts on the vomiting centers of the brain to produce vomiting. Herbalists had in mind very bitter compounds that simply made one sick to the stomach.

Emmenagogue: Something to increase menstrual flow. The word dates from a time before the molecular biology of the menstrual cycle was even contemplated, let alone understood.

Emollient: A substance applied to the skin to reduce inflammation and irritation.

Enteroplant: An enteric coated combination of peppermint and caraway sold in Europe to treat mild stomach upset.

Enterolactone: A type of plant estrogen produced by bacteria living in the intestines where they digest lentils and certain fruits.

Escin: A saponin found in horse chestnut. It is useful in the treatment of venous insufficiency and chronic leg ulcers.

Estragole: A component of guarana that is thought to be psychoactive.

Eau des Carmes: A sleep-inducing remedy produced by the Carmelite nuns during the Middle Ages. It contained lemon rind, cinnamon, cloves, nutmeg and coriander in a white wine.

Expectorant: Cough remedies, herbal or otherwise, have two components: an antitussive agent that prevents coughing and an expectorate that helps to liquify lung secretions allowing them to be coughed up more easily. Traditional herbalists recommend cowslip, thyme and coltsfoot. Modern physicians would more likely recommend Robitussin™ mixtures.

FDA: Abbreviation for the "Food and Drug Administration," the U.S. federal agency charged with regulating prescription drugs.

Febrifuge: A substance that counteracts fever. Traditionally willow and chamomile. Modern physicians recommend aspirin.

Ferulic acid: A terpene alkaloid involved in the production of both vanillin and capsaicin.

Flavonoids: Compounds that occur naturally in plants. They are found in high concentrations in citrus fruits and vegetables, but also in teas and wine. The average American takes in 25 mg per day. Flavonoids are potent anti-inflammatory agents and antioxidants, and they may help prevent heart disease. Apigenin, found in chamomile, is the best known example.

Foam cells: Damaged white blood cells. Their formation is the first step in forming atherosclerotic blockages.

Furunculosis: Boils or skin abscesses.

Galactogenic: A substance that will increase a woman's ability to produce milk. Modern science has failed to identify any such compound. Traditional herbalists recommend fennel, basil, caraway and anise.

Galenic: A remedy produced from a plant.

Gamma linolenic acid: A key ingredient in fat metabolism. Humans produce this molecule from linoleic acid from plant materials in the diet.

Genistein: A common type of phytoestrogen found in soybeans and clover.

Genus: One or more closely related species of plants that share some important structural characteristic. The first word in the two-word botanical name, i.e. *Crataegus monogyna*, gives the genus.

Gingerols: The molecules in ginger that impart the pleasant aroma. Other components of the herb are probably responsible for the antiemetic effects.

Glycyrrhizic acid: The substance that gives licorice its sweet taste.

Gonadotropins: Hormones released by the brain that tell the ovaries and testes to produce sex hormones.

GRAS: "Generally recognized as safe," a classification used by the U.S. Food and Drug Administration.

H2-Blocker: The H stands for histamine. Drugs that block the type 2 histamine receptor prevent the stomach from producing acid and help ulcers heal.

Harpagoside: The active ingredient in devil's claw, thought to be responsible for the relief of arthritic pain provided by this herb.

Helenalin: A sesquiterpene lactone and potent anti-inflammatory found in the essential oil extracted from arnica.

Hemostatic: A substance used to control bleeding. Except in individuals with underlying medical disorders, such substances are not used. But a bleeding alcoholic might be given Vitamin K to help the clotting process. The traditional herbal remedies are St. John's wort and comfrey.

High Density Lipoprotein (HDL): Also known as good cholesterol. This form of cholesterol does not accumulate in blood vessels. Within certain limits, the higher the HDL level, the less the risk of heart disease.

Homeopathy: A system of medicine based on the belief that patients can be cured by giving minute amounts of substance which, if given in large amounts, would make them sick.

Hypericin: The red pigment found in flowers of St. John's wort, formerly thought to be the main active ingredient. Many commercial preparations are standardized to contain a fixed percentage of hypericin.

Hyperforin: The active ingredient in St. Johns wort. It prevents the reuptake of serotonin, sharing a common action with antidepressants such as Prozac™.

Hypnotic: Another name for a sleeping pill. Today, short acting benzodiazepines are the most widely prescribed. Herbalists would recommend chamomile, hawthorn and valerian.

Hypotensive: Literally, low blood pressure. Traditionalists use the word to describe herbs that reduce the blood pressure of patients suffering from high blood pressure. Modern physicians use the term to describe someone in shock with dangerously low blood pressure, and call the medicines used to treat high blood pressure "antihypertensives."

Intermittent claudication: Leg cramps due to inadequate blood supply. Ginkgo is sometimes used as a treatment.

Isoflavones: A naturally occurring plant component that shares many similarities with estrogen, the female sex hormone.

Kaempferol: A flavonoid antioxidant found in red wine.

Kawain: A pyrone, one of the two active ingredients in kava.

Lectin: A compound found in nettles that stimulates white blood cell production.

Leutolin: A flavonoid found in chasteberry and artichokes. It is an antioxidant with anti-inflammatory effects, and it also lowers cholesterol.

Lignans: A naturally occurring plant component that shares many similarities with estrogen, the female sex hormone.

Limonene: The active ingredient in peppermint.

Linoleic acid: A polyunsaturated fat that lowers cholesterol and helps prevent heart disease. Sunflower oil and grapeseed oil are good sources.

Lipid peroxidation: What occurs when certain fats, especially low density lipoprotein (LDL) reacts with free radicals. The resultant compound sets off atherosclerotic changes in blood vessels.

Lipoxygenase: One of the two key enzymes that control the body's inflammatory response. The other is called cyclooxygenase.

Lobeline: An alkaloid from lobelia that is still used by some for smoking cessation. Lobeline has mostly been replaced by the nicotine patch and antidepressants such as Zyban™.

Low density lipoprotein (LDL): Also known as "bad" cholesterol. When free radicals interact with LDL, the structure of LDL is changed in such a way as to promote atherosclerosis.

LOX: Abbreviation for lipoxygenase inhibitor.

Luteolin: A flavonoid found in chamomile.

Lupulin: A yellow granular powder found in hops that gives hops their sedative effects.

Lycopsamine: A pyrrazolidine alkaloid toxic to the liver.

Lymphedema: Swelling of an extremity due to obstructed flow of lymph. It may be secondary to infection or surgery, as in the arm swelling some women experience after mastectomy.

Mannitol: A sugar found in celery. Taken in large quantities, it increases the flow of urine (osmotic diuretic).

Mast Cell: A kind of white blood cell that contains histamine, the chemical that causes allergic reactions. Apigenin, contained in chamomile, blocks histamine release.

Melanosis coli: An accumulation of brownish pigment in the walls of the colon seen in chronic users of senna, cascara, and aloe laxatives. The condition itself is harmless and reversible, but its presence is associated with an increased risk of colon cancer.

Melatonin: A hormone produced in the brain that, among other things, seems to regulate the sleep/wake cycle. Melatonin is also produced by some plants, and its presence may explain some herbs' beneficial effects. Large amounts of melatonin may be found in feverfew and St. John's wort.

Methyleugenol: The substance that gives clove oil its aroma; used as a local anesthetic by dentists.

MPB (4-O-Methylpyridoxine): A dangerous neurotoxin found in the seeds of ginkgo biloba. MPB is not found in the leaves, which is why Western herbalists use only the leaves for herbal remedies.

Mucilage: A gelatinous substance contained in some plants (comfrey, sea weed) that is composed of a mixture of proteins and complex sugars.

Mydriatic: A substance that will cause the pupils to dilate, such as the drops your eye doctor uses to examine your eyes. Deadly night shade, henbane, and coca (cocaine) will also dilate the pupils.

NDGA: Abbreviation for nordihydroguaiarectic acid, a potent antioxidant found in chaparral, used as a food preservative until 1967 when concerns about carcinogenicity led the FDA to remove it from the list of approved chemical preservatives.

NSAIDs: Nonsteroidal anti-inflammatory drugs such as Advil™. Drugs with similar actions are contained in many herbs (devil's claw, for example).

Nervine: An archaic term for tranquilizer or sedative.

Neurotransmitter: A chemical that is released by a nerve ending and used to transmit messages from one nerve or cell to another.

Neurovegetative: A somewhat vague term used by European physicians to refer to a variety of neurologic disorders, especially those having to do with concentration and memory.

Nitric oxide: A kind of neurotransmitter. It causes blood vessels to dilate. Production is abnormal in patients with atherosclerosis.

OTC: Abbreviation for "over-the-counter" drug. An American drug classification for medications that can be bought without a doctor's prescription. Unlike herbal remedies, OTC products are strictly regulated by the government.

Parasympathetic nervous system: A portion of the autonomic nervous system controlled from the brainstem. Activation causes the pupils to constrict, decreases the amount of sweat and saliva produced, and slows the heart rate.

Parthenolide: A sesquiterpene lactone that is thought to be the component of feverfew that helps prevent migraine headaches.

Pectoral: Literally meaning on the chest. Herbalists use the word to describe remedies used to treat chest congestion, such as anise and coltsfoot.

Perennial: A plant that lives for two or more years.

Photosensitivity: Increased sensitivity to the sun's ultraviolet light that may result in severe sunburns. This is thought to happen in some users of St. John's wort.

Phytoestrogens: Substances found in plants that have many of the same effects as female sex hormones, especially soy proteins.

Phytotherapy: Using plants as medicines.

Polyvalent: Herbalists use the term to describe any remedy that cures more than one type of illness.

Proanthocyanidins: A type of tannin, found in green teas and other plants. Large amounts may be toxic; smaller amounts may protect against cancer and heart disease.

Procyanadins: Antioxidants found in grapeseed oil. Evidence suggests they may provide the same cardioprotective benefits as red wine.

Prostoglandins: Molecules containing 20 carbon atoms. The name derives from the fact that they were first identified in human semen and were presumed to come from the prostate gland. In fact, they are found in many tissues in man and animals. They act as hormones and, among other things, control blood pressure, smooth muscle contraction, and gastric acid secretion.

Probucol (Lorelcol™): A medicine used to treat elevated cholesterol by accelerating the breakdown of LDL cholesterol that also is an antioxidant.

Prolactin: A hormone produced by the pituitary gland that controls milk production.

Prooxidants: Substances that accelerate the process of oxidation. Some antioxidants, such as beta carotene and Vitamin A become prooxidants when excessive amounts are taken.

Prunetin: The plant estrogen contained in plums and cherries.

PSA (prostate specific antigen): A substance produced by cells in the prostate. Blood levels of PSA increase in patients with prostate cancer, but not in men with benign prostate enlargement.

Psoralens (Trisoralen™): These agents cause the skin to produce more melanin pigment, but they also sensitize the skin to sunlight. They are used to treat some skin diseases such as vitiligo and psoriasis.

Purgative: Synonym for laxative.

Pyrones: The active chemical constituents in kava (dihydromethysticin and kawain). These chemicals are depressants and act in much the same way as other minor tranquilizers.

Pyrrazolidine alkaloids: Liver toxins found in a variety of plants, especially members of the Boraginaceae (i.e., comfrey) and Compositae families.

Pyuria: The presence of white blood cells (pus) in the urine.

Quercetin: An antioxidant found in red wine and elder.

Quinic acid: A chemical found in artichokes that protects the liver from the effects of toxic chemicals.

Red ginseng: The common name given to ginseng that is steamed for several hours before drying. The process creates unique ingredients not found in air-dried ginseng.

Resorptive: An herb such as flax, or a mixture of herbs, applied topically to make bruises disappear.

Reuptake: The mechanism by which the neurotransmitters, like dopamine and serotonin, is terminated. Prozac™ selectively prevents the reuptake of serotonin. Cocaine prevents dopamine reuptake.

Rhizome: The stem portion of a plant that grows underground. Roots grow from its bottom and leaves from its top. Plants store food in the rhizome, which is why it is usually thickened. Ginger is produced from the plant's rhizomes, not its roots, as is goldenseal.

Rosmarinic acid: A component of lemon balm that causes sedation. It may also be an anti-inflammatory agent.

Rubefacient: A substance that, when applied externally, makes the skin red; generally, a counterirritant.

Rutin: A flavonoid antioxidant found in red wine, elder and hawthorn.

Safrole: A molecule found in sassafras, similar to the molecule that gives cinnamon its pleasant smell. Sassafras is no longer used in the U.S. because the FDA classified safrole as a carcinogen.

Saponin: A family of related molecules found in a wide variety of plants. When saponins are added to water and shaken, the water becomes frothy and forms a lather. The reason the lather forms is that saponin molecules reduce the surface tension of the water. Some saponins possess anti-tumor activity.

Saporin 6: A compound with anti-tumor activity found in the roots of soapwort.

Saikosaponins: A type of saponin with extremely potent anti-inflammatory effects that is found in mullein and related plants.

Shogaols: One of three types of molecules found in ginger, and thought to be responsible for ginger's antiemetic effects.

Siberian ginseng: Common name for *Eleutherococcus senticosus*, a plant closely related to, but different from, *Panax ginseng.*

Stolon: A shoot growing from the tip of a branch that eventually develops into a new plant.

Strobile: A cone-shaped fruit. In hops, the part of the flower that contains the active substances.

Superoxide dismutase (SOD): An antioxidant enzyme produced by the body. It cannot be taken as a supplement because it is destroyed in the stomach.

Spasmolytic: An herb or drug that relieves abdominal cramping, typically caraway, peppermint, or chamomile.

Stomachic: A term used by traditional herbalists to describe any herb or drug that "stimulates" the stomach, not just to make more acid, but to function more efficiently. Angelica is a typical stomachic herb.

Stomatitis: Inflammation of the oral cavity, from whatever cause.

Sesquiterpene lactones: The molecular structure of bisabolol, the active component of ginger, and the parthenolides found in feverfew. Molecules with a similar structure are also found in chamomile.

Substance P: A chemical found in some nerve endings responsible for transmitting pain. Capsicum relieves arthritic pain by depleting nerve supplies of Substance P, thereby preventing the transmission of pain signal.

Stupefacient: A drug that causes drowsiness or sleep.

Sympathomimetic: A chemical compound that stimulates the central nervous system in the same way as adrenalin (epinephrine).

Symphytine: One kind of alkaloid, a liver toxin.

Terpenoid: A type of alkaloid; the type of active ingredient found in some plants, such as valerian.

Tincture: A solution made by soaking herbs in alcohol; usually 10 or 20 grams of dried plant in 100 milliliters of alcohol.

Tisanes: Either a tea made from dried herbs drunk for medicinal purposes, or any mixture of herbs in liquid compounded for medicinal purposes.

Tonic: A mixture of herbs in solution, either with or without alcohol, taken in hopes of stimulating or restoring vigor, either to the person in general, or some part of the body, i.e., "a liver tonic," or a "blood tonic."

Transtorine: A naturally occurring antibiotic isolated from ma huang.

Valepotriates: The collective name for the compounds (bornyl acetate, valerenic acid and valerenal) thought to be responsible for the sedative effects of valerian. Supplement makers generally adjust the valepotriate content to some standardized value, and set the price according to the valepotriate content.

Vermifuge: A substance that kills intestinal parasites.

Vesicant: A substance, such as mustard, used to cause blistering, in the mistaken belief that the formation of blisters would help rid the body of toxins.

Vulnerary: Any herb used to promote wound healing. Examples include chamomile, comfrey, marigold, or sage.

White ginseng: The name given to air-dried ginseng root.

Yamogenin: A saponin contained in fenugreek and wild yams that prevents cholesterol from being absorbed from the gastrointestinal tract.

Appendix I: Commission E Approved Combinations

Combinations of herbs designed to relieve specific symptoms are sold under a variety of names. Even though federal law prevents manufacturers from making medicinal claims for specific products, combinations of herbs can be given names that clearly indicate the intended purposes. Thus, the proliferation of products with names like "Menstrual-eze," "ColdAway," or SleepEtime."

As a general rule, practicing physicians try to avoid fixed combinations of prescription drugs and would probably feel the same way about herbal products if they prescribed them. There is no guarantee that the dose of each drug/herb in the product is the amount necessary to achieve optimal benefit. And, in fact, fixed combinations are useful only if the ratio of the fixed doses contained in the product corresponds to the needs of the individual patient.

The Food and Drug Administration considers fixed-dose combination of prescription drugs as "new drugs." Clinical trials to prove safety and effectiveness are required before the product can be sold EVEN if all of the drugs contained in the combination product have already been approved for sale. Specifically, drugmakers must show that use of the combination they want to sell produces a better therapeutic response than any of the drugs in the combination when taken by themselves (as is true for some drugs used to treat high blood pressure), or that taking one drug makes side effects from the other drug less likely (one drug must act to reduce the incidence of adverse effects caused by the other).

No such rules apply to food supplements. Any manufacturer can market any combination with any name (provided someone else hasn't already trade marked it). A product labelled "ColdAway" might or might not contain herbs that will help cure a cold. One thing is for certain though: the combination of ingredients will almost certainly not have been tested for either safety or effectiveness. There may be evidence that the individual components contained in the product help relieve cold symptoms. But without clinical trials, there is no way to know whether combining the ingredients makes them more or less effective.

There are, however, very big differences between herbal combinations and prescription drug combinations. The most important of these differences is that, compared to combinations of prescription pain relievers or antibiotics, most of the herbs being combined are relatively non-toxic. Since the herbs are generally safe, combining several different ones, in much the same way as combining vitamins, may be a reasonable thing to do, and it may save money. Combinations of antioxidants and phytoestrogens not only make sense, but they sell at a discount to the price of the individual ingredients.

But not all combinations make sense. It is important not to lose sight of the fact that there is very little science to support such decisions. The combination may seem rational, but without doing clinical trials, there is simply no way to know whether a particular blend of herbs is good or bad. Unforeseen reactions may occur that render the combination less, rather than more, effective. For example, components of two different, nontoxic, herbs might compete for the same enzyme system in the liver and thereby increase the toxicity of both.

Experience is, however, a good guide. Years of experience in Europe have proven that the combinations listed below are unquestionably safe, and they may very well be effective. Commission E has reviewed the safety and effectiveness of a long list of fixed drug combinations. For the sake of convenience, the products are listed by the medical conditions they are used to treat. Only those combinations that Commission E knows to be safe and effective are listed.

Anxiety, Difficulty Sleeping
>Passionflower herb, Valerian root, and Lemon Balm
>Valerian root and Hops
>Valerian root, Hops, and Lemon Balm
>Valerian root, Hops, and Passionflower herb

Appetite Stimulation and Improved Digestion
>Angelica root, Gentian root, and Fennel
>Angelica root, Gentian root, and Orange Peel
>Angelica root, Gentian root, and Wormwood
>Angelica root, Gentian root, and Peppermint oil
>Ginger root, Gentian root, and Wormwood
>Peppermint leaf, Caraway seed, Chamomile flower and Bitter Orange Peel

Arthritis Symptoms, Muscle and Joint pain
>Camphor, Eucalyptus oil, and purified Turpentine oil (external use only)

Cold Symptoms
>Eucalyptus oil and Pine Needle oil (for inhalation only)
>Primrose root and Thyme
>Star Anise seed and Thyme
>Thyme and White Soapwort root

Constipation
>Senna leaf and Blonde Psyllium seed husk
>Senna leaf, Peppermint oil, and Caraway oil

Cough Suppressant (for use with dry coughs)
>Anise oil and Iceland moss
>Anise oil, Marshmallow root, Eucalyptus oil, and Licorice Root
>Anise oil, Marshmallow root, Iceland Moss and Licorice Root
>Anise oil, Marshmallow root, Primrose root, and Sundew
>Anise seed, Linden flower, and Thyme
>Camphor, Eucalyptus oil, and purified Turpentine oil (for inhalation)
>Licorice root, Primrose root, Marshmallow root, and Anise seed
>Marshmallow root, Fennel seed, Iceland moss, and Thyme
>Marshmallow root, Primrose root, Licorice root, and Thyme oil
>Primrose root, Marshmallow root, and Anise seed
>Primrose root, Sundew, and Thyme
>Sundew and Thyme

Expectorant (for use with productive coughs) (catarrh)
>Anise oil, Fennel oil, Licorice root, and Thyme
>Anise oil, Primrose root, and Thyme
>Anise oil, Ivy leaf, Fennel seed, and Licorice root
>Eucalyptus oil, Primrose root, and Thyme
>Gumweed herb, Primrose root, and Thyme
>Ivy leaf, Licorice root, and Thyme

Gallstones or Gallbladder Disease

Dandelion root with Dandelion herb, Celandine herb, and Artichoke Leaf

Dandelion root with Dandelion herb, Celandine herb, and Wormwood

Dandelion root with Dandelion herb, Peppermint leaf and Artichoke Leaf

Javanese Turmeric, Celandine herb, and Wormwood

Javanese Turmeric, Peppermint leaf, and Wormwood

Milk Thistle fruit, Peppermint leaf, and Wormwood

Tumeric root and Celandine herb

Gas and Flatulence (herbs to control are called carminatives) (dyspepsia)

Angelica root, Gentian root, and Caraway seed

Angelica root, Gentian root, and Peppermint oil

Anise seed, Fennel seed, and Caraway seed

Caraway oil and Fennel oil

Caraway oil and Fennel oil, and Chamomile flower

Caraway seed and Fennel seed

Caraway seed and Fennel seed and Chamomile flower

Ginger root, Gentian root, and Wormwood

Peppermint leaf and Caraway seed

Peppermint leaf, Caraway seed, Fennel seed

Peppermint leaf, Caraway seed, and Chamomile flower

Peppermint leaf, Caraway seed, Chamomile flower and Bitter Orange Peel

Peppermint leaf, Caraway seed, Fennel seed, and Chamomile flower

Peppermint leaf and Fennel seed

Peppermint leaf, Fennel seed, and Chamomile flower

Peppermint leaf, German Chamomile flower, and Caraway seed

Peppermint oil and Caraway oil

Peppermint oil, Caraway oil, and Chamomile flower

Peppermint oil, Caraway oil, and Fennel oil

Peppermint oil, Caraway oil, Fennel oil, and Chamomile flower

Peppermint oil and Fennel oil

Peppermint oil, Fennel oil, and Chamomile flower

Heart Failure

Lily-of-the-valley powdered extract, Squill powdered extract, and Oleander leaf powdered extract (NB: Commission approved this formulation, but it contains a very dangerous group of compounds called cardiac glycosides and should never, under any circumstance, be used without first consulting your physician)

Kidney Stone Prevention

Birch leaf, Goldenrod, and Java tea

Stomach Ulcers and Inflammation

Anise oil, Fennel oil, and Caraway oil

Licorice root and German Chamomile flower

Licorice root, Peppermint leaf, and German Chamomile flower

Urinary Tract Inflammation

Uva Ursi Leaf, Goldenrod, and Java tea

Appendix II: Unapproved, Potentially Dangerous Herbs

Herbs reviewed by Commission E were divided into three groups: (1) approved, (2) unapproved because there was insufficient evidence to decide, or (3) unapproved because the herb was found to be dangerous. Herbs falling into the last category are listed below. Mostly because of the way the German regulatory system works, the list is by no means inclusive. Very dangerous herbs, such as foxglove, the source of digitalis, cannot be sold in health food stores and, accordingly, do not make the list. Herbs listed below exert a variety of different effects, but they do have one thing in common: the members of Commission E felt the risks of using them far outweighed any potential benefits.

Many of the herbs on this list are discussed in detail in Chapter 6. The Commission's reasoning is not always easy to understand. In the case of coltsfoot, which contains dangerous pyrrozolidine alkaloids, the decision would seem to be clear cut. However, evidence against Roman chamomile is best described as slim. It was placed on the unapproved list because of the possibility of "rare allergic reactions." Readers will note that basil is also on the list. It was placed there because of concerns that it might be mutagenic. Does that mean that pesto sauce is also mutagenic? It is, after all, made from ground basil leaves. Readers will have to make their own decisions.

Angelica (seed and herb)
Basil
Bilberry leaf
Bishop's Weed fruit
Bladderwrack
Borage
Bryonia
Celery
Chamomile, Roman
Cinnamon flower
Coca
Colocynth
Coltsfoot
Delphinium flower
Elecampane
Ergot
Goat's Rue
Hound's Tongue
Kelp
Lemongrass, Citronella oil
Liverwort herb

Madder root
Male Fern
Monkshood
Mugwort
Nutmeg
Nux Vomica
Oleander leaf
Papain
Parsley seed
Pasque flower
Periwinkle
Petasites leaf
Rue
Saffron
Sarsaparilla root
Scotch Broom flower
Senecio herb
Soapwort herb, Red
Tansy flower and herb
Walnut hull
Yohimbine bark

Appendix III: How to do a Free Medline Search

The National Library of Medicine (NLM) made access to MEDLINE free in 1997. Since that time, public interest in MEDLINE has skyrocketed. According to a recent publicity release from NLM, the number of searches on MEDLINE has increased tenfold in just the last year. About 7 million searches took place annually before the first free MEDLINE search. There are now about 120 million searches annually, and one-third of them are being done by consumers. If you have access to the Internet, you can do your own MEDLINE searching. Just follow the easy steps outlined below. The process is illustrated here by doing a search for information about arnica.

First go to the National Library of Medicine's Web Site (http://www.nlm.nih.gov). There will be five large buttons on the top of the page (Figure #1). Click on the far left button which says "Search MEDLINE." The next screen will offer you a choice of two search engines - *PubMed* and *Internet Greatful Med*. Either will work equally well, but for beginners, *PubMed* may be simpler (Figure #2).

Once you click on *Pubmed* you will see a screen that says, *PubMed*. (Figure #3). To do a sample search, type "arnica" in the search box located just under the "search" button, and then click on "search." The search screen will be replaced by another with the results of the search. The top box will say "PubMed Query," and indicate how many references were found. In this case, 101 papers were found, and the individual papers are listed below (Figure #4). The references are listed by date with the most recent publications at the top of the list.

If you click on any of the individual papers, you can call up the reference. The first paper listed by is by two researchers, one named Ernst and the other named Pittler. The title of the paper is "Efficacy of homeopathic arnica: a systematic review of placebo-controlled clinical trials." This paper was printed in the journal named the *Archives of Surgery*, and it was published in 1998. To see what the paper was about, just click on the author's (Ernst) name. More details about the paper, and an abstract of the paper, will appear on your screen (Figure #5)

The abstract contains information about how the study was carried out and what the results were. In this case, a review of previous placebo-controlled clinical trials found that using arnica did not provide any apparent benefit. To find more articles about arnica, you can either go back to your original search list or you can click on the box in the top left corner (just above where it says "order this document") that says "related articles." Another new page will appear (Figure #6).

The top of the page shows the results. A total of 63 articles, apparently dealing with material similar to that described in the paper by Ernst, were found. The first paper on the list is, in fact, the paper by Ernst. It is followed by a list of other papers that the search engine believes are related. When you search for related articles, some of the results you get may be relevant while others are not. In this case, the second reference by Vickers, entitled" *Homeopathic Arnica 30x is ineffective for muscle soreness after long-distance running: a randomized, double-blind, placebo-controlled trial,*" is clearly about the same topic. If you would like to read the findings, just click on the author's name. The 7th paper on the list is by Pittler. It is about the effectiveness of peppermint oil in treating irritable bowel syndrome. The search engine probably assumed that it was related because (a) it is about an herbal medicine, and (b) it was written by one of the authors of the first paper (Ernst and Pittler).

One way to save time is to narrow your search. Using arnica as the single search word produced 63 possible references, only some of which may be relevant. A runner with sore legs might want to know whether taking arnica could help the aches and pains of overexertion. Instead of just typing in "arnica" as the search word, the runner could instead type in "arnica and pain." Instead of getting 63 hits, only 4 references are returned (figure #7), and all three are relevant. With a little practice, designing very complex searches becomes a relatively simple matter.

In some cases the reference will even contain an Internet link that will allow the complete paper to be downloaded, not just the abstract. Often too, the e-mail address of the author of the paper is given, making it a simple matter to contact the author. There is often a charge for the download, but it is usually modest. Alternatively, if you follow instructions on the first web page (Figure #1) you can contact a commercial service that, for a modest fee, will mail you a hard copy of the document in question.

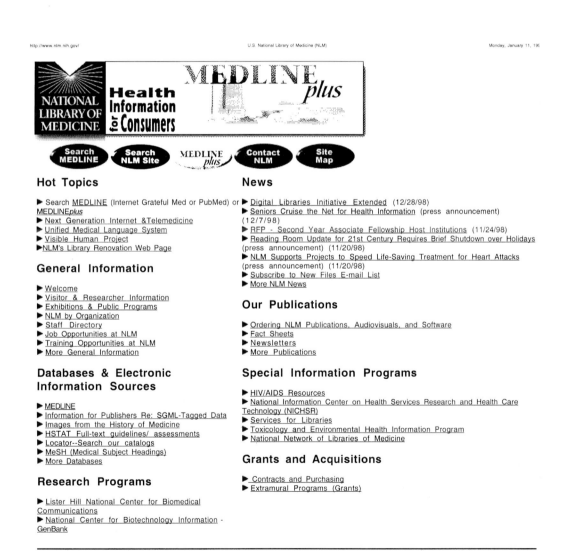

Figure 1

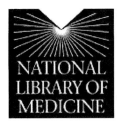

Search MEDLINE: PubMed and Internet Grateful Med

On October 22, 1998, NLM introduced MEDLINE*plus*, an easy-to-understand resource on various diseases and "Health Topics" for the public. MEDLINE*plus* includes information from MEDLINE, links to self-help groups, access to National Institute of Health consumer-related organizations, clearinghouses, health-related organizations, and clinical trials. MEDLINE can be searched directly using NLM's two Web-based products, PubMed and Internet Grateful Med. Below is a brief description of each system. Health consumers are encouraged to discuss search results with their health care professional.

PubMed

- Provides free access to MEDLINE.
- Sets of related articles pre-computed for each article cited in MEDLINE
- Can use Loansome Doc Document Delivery service (local charges and delivery methods may vary).
- Medical Subject Heading (MeSH) Browser.
- Citation Matcher
- Choice of Web search interfaces from simple keywords to advanced Boolean expressions. Field restrictions and MeSH index terms (main topics and subheadings) supported.
- Linkages to publishers' sites for full-text journals. Approximately 250 journals available, some by subscription only.
- Clinical query form with built-in search filters for diagnosis, etiology, therapy, and prognosis.
- Links to molecular biology databases of DNA/protein sequences and 3-D structure data.

Internet Grateful Med

- Provides free access to MEDLINE, AIDSLINE, AIDSDRUGS, AIDSTRIALS, BIOETHICSLINE, ChemID, DIRLINE, HealthSTAR, HISTLINE, HSRPROJ, OLDMEDLINE, POPLINE, SDILINE, SPACELINE, and TOXLINE.
- Effective September 1998 searches MEDLINE via PubMed's retrieval system.
  - Sets of related articles pre-computed for each article cited in MEDLINE
  - Linkages to publishers' sites for full-text journals. Approximately 250 journals available, some by subscription only.
- Can use Loansome Doc Document Delivery service (local charges and delivery methods may vary).
- Offers full range of Medical Subject Heading (MeSH) search features via UMLS Metathesaurus.
- Ability to limit searches by language, publication type, age groups, etc., using pull-down menus.

U.S. National Library of Medicine (NLM)
http://www.nlm.nih.gov/
Last updated: 21 October 1998

Page: 1

Figure 2

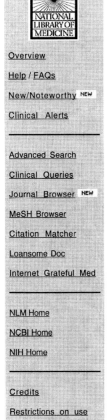

Overview

Help / FAQs

New/Noteworthy NEW

Clinical Alerts

Advanced Search

Clinical Queries

Journal Browser NEW

MeSH Browser

Citation Matcher

Loansome Doc

Internet Grateful Med

NLM Home

NCBI Home

NIH Home

Credits

Restrictions on use

PubMed

NLM's search service to access the 9 million citations in **MEDLINE** and Pre-MEDLINE (with links to participating on-line journals), and other related databases.

| MEDLINE | for: |

| |

Number of documents to display per page: | 20 |

Entrez Date limit: | No Limit |

- Enter one or more search terms.
- Author names should be entered in the form Smith JB, but initials are optional.
- Journal titles may be entered in full, as valid MEDLINE abbreviations, or as ISSN numbers (see Journal Browser for more information).

Questions or comments? Write to the Help Desk.

NOTICE: The PubMed data are for personal use only. Users are responsible for complying with all copyright and licensing restrictions associated with data.

Figure 3

NCBI *PubMed*   **PubMed QUERY**   PubMed | ?

arnica

Docs Per Page: | 20 | Entrez Date limit: | No Limit |

citations 1-20 displayed (out of 65 found), page 1 of 4

| Abstract report | for the articles selected (default all).

documents on this page through Loansome Doc

[No authors listed]   [See Related Articles]
[No title available].
Ukr Biokhim Zh. 1998 Mar-Apr;70(2):78-82. Russian.
[MEDLINE record in process]
PMID: 9848164; UI: 99064630.

Delmonte S, et al.   [See Related Articles]
Leukemia-related Sweet's syndrome elicited by pathergy to Arnica.
Dermatology. 1998;197(2):195-6. No abstract available.
PMID: 9840982; UI: 99026994.

Ernst E, et al.   [See Related Articles]
Efficacy of homeopathic arnica: a systematic review of placebo-controlled clinical trials.
Arch Surg. 1998 Nov;133(11):1187-90. Review.
PMID: 9820349; UI: 99036235.

Vickers AJ, et al.   [See Related Articles]
Homeopathic Arnica 30x is ineffective for muscle soreness after long-distance running: a randomized, double-blind,
placebo-controlled trial.
Clin J Pain. 1998 Sep;14(3):227-31.
PMID: 9758072; UI: 98429039.

Kostyshin SS, et al.   [See Related Articles]
[Selenium as a modifier of antioxidant protection and lipid peroxidation in microclones of Arnica montana L. as affected by
C-range ultraviolet rays].
Ukr Biokhim Zh. 1997 Sep-Dec;69(5-6):148-52. Russian.
PMID: 9606837; UI: 98269682.

Spettoli E, et al.   [See Related Articles]
Contact dermatitis caused by sesquiterpene lactones.
Am J Contact Dermat. 1998 Mar;9(1):49-50.
PMID: 9471988; UI: 98137826.

Lyss G, et al.   [See Related Articles]
Helenalin, an anti-inflammatory sesquiterpene lactone from Arnica, selectively inhibits transcription factor NF-kappaB.
Biol Chem. 1997 Sep;378(9):951-61.
PMID: 9348104; UI: 98006327.

Schaffner W.   [See Related Articles]
Granny's remedy explained at the molecular level: helenalin inhibits NF-kappaB.
Biol Chem. 1997 Sep;378(9):935. No abstract available.
PMID: 9348102; UI: 98006325.

Haraguchi H, et al.   [See Related Articles]
Antioxidative constituents in Heterotheca inuloides.
Bioorg Med Chem. 1997 May;5(5):865-71.
PMID: 9208098; UI: 97351816.

Youngson RM.   [See Related Articles]
Randomized trial of homeopathic arnica.
J R Soc Med. 1997 Apr;90(4):239-40. No abstract available.
PMID: 9155774; UI: 97300754.

Hart O, et al.   [See Related Articles]
Double-blind, placebo-controlled, randomized clinical trial of homoeopathic arnica C30 for pain and infection after total
abdominal hysterectomy.
J R Soc Med. 1997 Feb;90(2):73-8.
PMID: 9068434; UI: 97221388.

Hausen BM.   [See Related Articles]

Page: 1

Figure 4

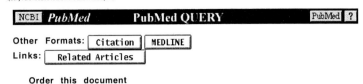

Arch Surg 1998 Nov;133(11):1187-90

Efficacy of homeopathic arnica: a systematic review of placebo-controlled clinical trials.

Ernst E, Pittler MH

Department of Complementary Medicine, School of Postgraduate Medicine and Health Sciences, University of Exeter, England, United Kingdom. E.Ernst@exeter.ac.uk

BACKGROUND: The efficacy of homeopathic remedies has remained controversial. The homeopathic remedy most frequently studied in placebo-controlled clinical trials is Arnica montana. OBJECTIVE: To systematically review the clinical efficacy of homeopathic arnica. MATERIALS AND METHODS: Computerized literature searches were performed to retrieve all placebo-controlled studies on the subject. The following databases were searched: MEDLINE, EMBASE, CISCOM, and the Cochrane Library. Data were extracted in a predefined, standardized fashion independently by both authors. There were no restrictions on the language of publications. RESULTS: Eight trials fulfilled all inclusion criteria. Most related to conditions associated with tissue trauma. Most of these studies were burdened with severe methodological flaws. On balance, they do not suggest that homeopathic arnica is more efficacious than placebo. CONCLUSION: The claim that homeopathic arnica is efficacious beyond a placebo effect is not supported by rigorous clinical trials.

Publication Types:

- Review
- Review, tutorial

PMID: 9820349, UI: 99036235

the above report in ⬜ Macintosh ⬜ Text format

documents on this page through Loansome Doc

Figure 5

NCBI *PubMed*   **PubMed QUERY**   PubMed ?

Docs Per Page: 20   Entrez Date limit: No Limit

citations 1-20 displayed (out of 103 found), page 1 of 6

    Abstract report   for the articles selected (default all).

    documents on this page through Loansome Doc

Ernst E, et al.   [See Related Articles]
    Efficacy of homeopathic arnica: a systematic review of placebo-controlled clinical trials.
    Arch Surg. 1998 Nov;133(11):1187-90. Review.
    PMID: 9820349; UI: 99036235.

Youngson RM.   [See Related Articles]
    Randomized trial of homeopathic arnica.
    J R Soc Med. 1997 Apr;90(4):239-40. No abstract available.
    PMID: 9155774; UI: 97300754.

Linde K, et al.   [See Related Articles]
    Are the clinical effects of homeopathy placebo effects? A meta-analysis of placebo-controlled trials.
    Lancet. 1997 Sep 20;350(9081):834-43.
    PMID: 9310601; UI: 97456644.

Plasek J, et al.   [See Related Articles]
    [Is homeopathic therapy more effective that placebos]?
    Cas Lek Cesk. 1996 Sep 18;135(18):575-9. Czech.
    PMID: 8998796; UI: 97103865.

Reilly DT, et al.   [See Related Articles]
    Is homeopathy a placebo response?
    Lancet. 1986 Nov 29;2(8518):1272. No abstract available.
    PMID: 2878144; UI: 87062977.

Vickers AJ, et al.   [See Related Articles]
    Homeopathic Arnica 30x is ineffective for muscle soreness after long-distance running: a randomized, double-blind, placebo-controlled trial.
    Clin J Pain. 1998 Sep;14(3):227-31.
    PMID: 9758072; UI: 98429039.

[No authors listed]   [See Related Articles]
    Trials of homeopathy.
    BMJ. 1991 Mar 2;302(6775):529. No abstract available.
    PMID: 2012859; UI: 91191183.

Kleijnen J, et al.   [See Related Articles]
    Trials of homeopathy.
    BMJ. 1991 Apr 20;302(6782):960. No abstract available.
    PMID: 1827743; UI: 91234914.

Bruseth S, et al.   [See Related Articles]
    [Homeopathy--the past or a part of future medicine]?
    Tidsskr Nor Laegeforen. 1991 Dec 10;111(30):3692-4. Review. Norwegian.
    PMID: 1780831; UI: 92141980.

Popova TD, et al.   [See Related Articles]
    [Homeopathy as a therapeutic system].
    Vestn Akad Med Nauk SSSR. 1991;(5):52-5. Russian.
    PMID: 1867003; UI: 91327721.

Borota R.   [See Related Articles]
    [Homeopathy].
    Med Pregl. 1998 Mar-Apr;51(3-4):197-8. Serbo-Croatian (Roman). No abstract available.
    PMID: 9611967; UI: 98274914.

Geller L.   [See Related Articles]
    [What is homeopathy]?
    Krankenpflege (Frankf). 1982 Nov;36(11):377. German. No abstract available.
    PMID: 6819398; UI: 83139790.

Figure 6

NCBI *PubMed*	**PubMed QUERY**	PubMed ?

arnica and pain

Docs Per Page: 20   Entrez Date limit: No Limit

4 citations found

Abstract report   for the articles selected (default all).

documents on this page through Loansome Doc

Vickers AJ, et al.   [See Related Articles]
Homeopathic Arnica 30x is ineffective for muscle soreness after long-distance running: a randomized, double-blind, placebo-controlled trial.
Clin J Pain. 1998 Sep;14(3):227-31.
PMID: 9758072; UI: 98429039.

Hart O, et al.   [See Related Articles]
Double-blind, placebo-controlled, randomized clinical trial of homoeopathic arnica C30 for pain and infection after total abdominal hysterectomy.
J R Soc Med. 1997 Feb;90(2):73-8.
PMID: 9068434; UI: 97221388.

Tveiten D, et al.   [See Related Articles]
[Effect of Arnica D 30 during hard physical exertion. A double-blind randomized trial during the Oslo Marathon 1990].
Tidsskr Nor Laegeforen. 1991 Dec 10;111(30):3630-1. Norwegian.
PMID: 1780819; UI: 92141966.

Kaziro GS.   [See Related Articles]
Metronidazole (Flagyl) and Arnica Montana in the prevention of post-surgical complications, a comparative placebo controlled clinical trial.
Br J Oral Maxillofac Surg. 1984 Feb;22(1):42-9.
PMID: 6365158; UI: 84128526.

Figure 7

Appendix V: Body Mass Index

One reason people take herbs is to lose weight. Any rational weight loss program, whether or not it includes the use of herbal supplements, must be based on realistic goals. It may be surprising to some, but valid assessments of the amount that needs to be lost cannot be made solely on the way you look in the mirror! Body Mass Index (BMI), defined as the weight in kilograms divided by the height in meters squared, provides a much better standard.

There are conflicting opinions on just what constitutes a normal BMI. According to the World Health Organization, the normal range for both men and women is 18.5 to 24.9 kg/m^2. Individuals with values of 25-29.9 kg/m^2 are considered "overweight," and those with values over 30 kg/m^2 are considered diagnostic for obesity.

The American Heart Association has adopted a somewhat more liberal set of criteria. Based on an extensive body of research, the AHA has set the normal range, for both men and women, at 21 to 25 kg/square meter. According to the AHA, a BMI of 25 corresponds to 110 percent of desirable body weight. Recently, the United States government tried to raise the normal range even higher, effectively legislating fat people into skinny ones. The increased values proposed by the government are not widely accepted, but those of the World Health Organization are disputed by very few.

BMI is a risk factor, similar to high blood pressure or high cholesterol. The higher the value, the more likely it is that something bad will happen. People with high blood pressure, high cholesterol, or high BMI are all much more likely to develop heart failure, renal failure, stroke, coronary artery disease, gallbladder disease, and even some cancers.

In case you do not have a calculator, or if you are unsure about converting inches to meters, use the formula below.

BODY MASS INDEX CALCULATION

1. Take your weight in pounds and divide by 2.2 to get kilograms
   (170 lbs / 2.2 = 77.272 kilograms)

2. Take your height in inches and divide by 39.37 to get meters
   (75" / 39.37 = 1.905 meters)

3. Take your height in meters and multiply the number by itself or in other words square the number (1.905 x 1.905 = 3.629)

4. Take your weight in kilograms and divide by your squared total to determine your Body Mass Index (77.272 / 3.629 = 21.292)

Appendix V: Useful Reference Books

A-Z of Traditional Herbal Remedies, by Michael Howard. First published in 1987 and reissued in 1997 by Senate Press, a division of Random House UK Ltd, Random House, 20 Vauxhall Bridge Road, London, SW1V 2SA. Only European herbs are discussed, and little or no modern medical information is provided. However, the descriptions of the plants and discussion of the folklore surrounding them is interesting and well described.

British Herbal Compendium, Volume 1: A handbook of scientific information on widely used plant drugs. A companion to the British Herbal Pharmacopoeia. Edited by Peter Bradley for the British Herbal Medicine Association, and first published in 1992. The chemical constituents of the most commonly used herbs are briefly described and the clinical applications are discussed. The official recommendations of the French, German and British governments for use of the herbs are also provided. Copies can be obtained through the American Botanical Council, PO Box 201660, Austin, Texas 78720-1660. Most physicians would find this a very useful reference.

British Herbal Pharmacopoeia, produced by the Scientific Committee of the British Herbal Medicine Association, and published in 1996.Copies can be obtained through the American Botanical Council, PO Box 201660, Austin, Texas 78720-1660. This provides descriptions of the microscopic appearances of the most common herbs and their chemical analysis, along with recommended assays for measuring individual components and determining purity. It will be of interest mainly to pharmacists and toxicologists.

Complete German Commission E Monographs, Therapeutic Guide to Herbal Medicines. Edited by Mark Blumenthal and published by the American Botanical Council in 1998. It is available from the Council (address and phone above). This important book contains translations of all of the Commission E monographs (reports) for the individual herbs, plus a well-written overview of the herbal drug industries in Europe and the United States. This is an indispensable reference but it is not perfect. The biggest problem is that the Commission stopped doing reviews in 1995. That means all of the monographs are at least five years old, and in some cases 10 years out of date. There have been major developments in the field in the last decade that consumers need to know about. Another very big problem is that none of the monographs contain any references. The Commission claims that at least 200 references were reviewed for each herb considered, but none are listed, so there is no way for the reader to either find out more or verify the conclusions reached by the Commission.

Guide to Medicinal Plants, by Paul Schauenberg and Ferdinand Paris. First published by The Lutterworth Press in 1977 (P.O. Box 60, Cambridge, CB1 2NT, United Kingdom). This is an excellent guide to over 400 medicinal plants. Sections on the botany and history are particularly strong. Only minimal medical information is provided.

Herbal Renaissance, by Steven Foster, published in 1997. This book is written for individuals who actually plan on growing their own herbs. The book contains excellent descriptions of the herbs and how to grow them, along with very good accounts of the history and past medical uses. More attention is devoted to the plants than to their medical uses.

Medicinal Natural Products, A Biosynthetic Approach, by Paul M. Dewick, published by John Wiley & Sons in 1997. Dewick, a Professor of Pharmacology at University of Nottingham, has written what is probably the single best book on the pharmacology of herbal medicines. Unfortunately, the book is written for toxicologists and pharmacologists and would be impenetrable to anyone without training in organic chemistry. Physicians will find this book incredibly useful.

The Honest Herbal, A Sensible Guide to the Use of Herbs and Related Remedies, Third edition, by Varro E. Tyler, Ph.D., published in 1993, by the Pharmaceutical Products Press, an imprint of Haworth Press, 10 Alice Street, Binghamton, NY 13904-1580. The book contains a wealth of sensible information and advice, but is now more than seven years out of date, and therefore contains no information about many exciting new developments in the field.

Rational Phytotherapy, a Physicians's Guide to Herbal Medicine, Third Edition, by Volker Schulz, Rudolf Hänsel, and Varro E. Tyler. Published by Springer-Verlag, Berlin, in 1998. As the title indicates, this is a reference work written mainly for physicians. It was recently translated from the German. It provides a very good overview of the issues. It is, however, already slightly out of date. The most recent references contained in the third edition are from 1995. Important new developments have occurred since that time.

Medicinal Plants of the World, Chemical constituents, traditional and modern medical uses, by Ivan A. Ross. Published by Humana Press, 1988. The book contains a compilation of scientific plant-use data from a variety of sources, with an extensive analysis of pharmacological effects and clinical tests. The book is highly technical, but should be of use to anyone with an interest in medicinal chemistry and herbal medicine.

Index